Praise for
BALANCE YOUR HORMONES, BALANCE YOUR LIFE

"Dr. Claudia Welch amalgamates Eastern medicine and Western science into a tidy and practical framework from whose clear perspective we can easily make sense of the complicated particulars of hormones and women's health."

—Dr. Robert Svoboda, BAMS, author of
Ayurveda for Women: A Guide to Vitality and Health

"A loving, compassionate healer and wonderful teacher, Dr. Claudia Welch has studied Ayurveda and Acupuncture extensively. She provides a new avenue and dimension of perception, integrating these two healing traditions to bring about holistic health."

—Vasant Lad, BAMS, MASc, Ayurvedic Physician,
author of *The Complete Book of Ayurvedic Home Remedies*

BALANCE YOUR HORMONES, BALANCE YOUR LIFE

BALANCE YOUR HORMONES, BALANCE YOUR LIFE

Achieving Optimal Health and Wellness Through Ayurveda, Chinese Medicine, and Western Science

Claudia Welch

DOCTOR OF ORIENTAL MEDICINE

Da Capo

LIFE LONG

A MEMBER OF THE PERSEUS BOOKS GROUP

Copyright © 2011 by Claudia Welch

Designed by Pauline Brown
Set in 10.5 point Berkeley Book by the Perseus Books Group

Library of Congress Cataloging-in-Publication Data

Welch, Claudia.
  Balance your hormones, balance your life : achieving optimal health and wellness through ayurveda, Chinese medicine, and western science / Claudia Welch.—1st ed.
      p. cm.
  Includes bibliographical references and index.
  ISBN 978-0-7382-1482-5 (pbk. : alk. paper) ISBN 978-0-7382-1499-3 (e-book) 1. Women—Health and hygiene. 2. Integrative medicine. 3. Hormones. I. Title.
  RA778.W2294 2011
  613'.04244—dc22

                                                                    2010049239

First Da Capo Press edition 2011

Published by Da Capo Press
A Member of the Perseus Books Group
www.dacapopress.com

Note: The information in this book is true and complete to the best of our knowledge. This book is intended only as an informative guide for those wishing to know more about health issues. In no way is this book intended to replace, countermand, or conflict with the advice given to you by your own physician. The ultimate decision concerning care should be made between you and your doctor. We strongly recommend you follow his or her advice. Information in this book is general and is offered with no guarantees on the part of the authors or Da Capo Press. The authors and publisher disclaim all liability in connection with the use of this book. The names and identifying details of people associated with events described in this book have been changed. Any similarity to actual persons is coincidental.

Da Capo Press books are available at special discounts for bulk purchases in the U.S. by corporations, institutions, and other organizations. For more information, please contact the Special Markets Department at the Perseus Books Group, 2300 Chestnut Street, Suite 200, Philadelphia, PA, 19103, or call (800) 810-4145, ext. 5000, or e-mail special.markets@ perseusbooks.com.

10 9 8 7 6 5 4 3

❧❦❧

For all women, perhaps especially the younger ones—
Jan, Noelle, Kali, Rachel, Luna, Josie, Ariel, Sujata, Hannah, Jessa,
Meralyn, Gemma, Jane, Magdalena, Chloe, Ella, Olivia, Janiya,
Mirabai, Vernit, and Ava.

May your lives be fulfilling, balanced, and joyful.

And for dear Lucy and Lillian. May
they each rest in profound peace.

❦❧❦❧

CONTENTS

PREFACE

A COUPLE OF NOTES

For people looking for medical counsel: Although the information, ideas, and perspectives contained in this book are based on Ayurvedic, Traditional Chinese, or Western allopathic principles or studies, and even though—in the case of Ayurvedic or Traditional Chinese Medicine—such perspectives have been employed for thousands of years, no part of this book should be taken or construed as medical diagnosis or treatment. One significant component of Eastern medical philosophy is that each person has individual, unique needs, so no single recommendation, no matter how sound, is sound for every individual. For any medical condition or personal medical, herbal, dietary, or lifestyle advice, always consult with a qualified health-care practitioner.

I'm not just saying this for legal reasons. There is always more to medicine than any one practitioner can know, not to mention more to an individual's health than an author can address without ever having even met that person. It is up to each of us to do our own search, find what works for us, and implement it. This book was born out of my own attempts to understand the sea of information available on women's health. The conclusions I draw are not facts. They are educated opinions.

For numbers and statistic buffs and critics: The data in many of the studies in this book describe the increased risk for an entire population—not the increased risk for an individual woman. Taken as the latter, they would be scarier. Taken as the former, they are still compelling numbers.

For Western-trained physicians: In my travels in the world, I haven't found any group who loves the perspective that this book presents more than you do. While Western medicine describes each individual hormone, Eastern medicine provides a context for understanding how they interact. This is heady, exciting stuff.

For everyone else: You don't have to have any background in either Western or Eastern medicine to understand the concepts in this book. Simple concepts are powerful and simply lay the framework for understanding complicated material in an easy and even enjoyable way. Bon voyage.

The Stress Epidemic

A couple years ago I spotted a bizarre headline in the *New York Times*. THE NEW MODERN WOMAN, AMBITIOUS AND FEEBLE,[1] it read. The article criticized certain popular TV shows for creating heroines who were driven, neurotic, anxiety prone, and undernourished. The author of the article decried these shows, concerned that viewers would emulate the shows' "ambitious and feeble" role models.

Although the headline was obviously a generalization about American women, it was not without merit. I am a Western woman who is also a doctor of Eastern medicine. Over the years I have seen that the medical problems of most women who come to me are rooted in a hormonal imbalance brought on by doing too much while getting too little physical and emotional nourishment, not unlike the feeble heroines. What's more, their hormones have been out of whack for an extended period of time. I'm not just talking about menopausal women. I mean women of all ages, women whose medical problems range from painful periods, mood swings, fatigue, and insomnia to infertility, uterine fibroids, hot flashes, heart disease, and osteoporosis.

Whereas Western medicine emphasizes the separate domains and functions of various kinds of hormones in the body, Eastern medicine emphasizes the context within which they exist and how they relate to each other. Combining Eastern and Western perspectives, we see two major types of hormones that affect a woman's health: stress hormones and sex hormones. Having the right balance of these hormones gives us plenty of energy, deeper sleep, healthier menstrual cycles, happier dispositions, easier menopauses, healthier hearts, stronger bones, and much, much more. When we experience stress (self-induced or otherwise), our body releases extra stress hormones until the "danger" resolves itself, thus throwing off our hormonal balance. When our whole lives are stressful, this imbalance becomes chronic. Healing begins when we start to live the life we really want to be living. Then we have less stress and the levels of stress hormones in our bloodstream drop. When our stress hormones are not rampant, our sex hormones have a better chance to work the way they are supposed to, and we experience the well-being that comes from having balanced hormones.

How Did We Get into This Situation?

> Advertising has us chasing cars and clothes,
> working jobs we hate so we can buy shit we don't need.
> —*FIGHT CLUB*, BASED ON THE NOVEL BY CHUCK PALAHNIUK

Many modern women mistake the feeling of being under stress for having energy, and putting ballast in the stomach for getting real sustenance. We think a woman has a lot of energy, for example, if she is a soccer mom *and* a full-time career woman. She starts running at dawn and doesn't rest until late evening, if she rests at all. Perhaps she grabs some fast food, a doughnut, or even healthy food, but she bolts it down to ground her so she can continue running. She's the human equivalent of the Energizer Bunny. She is driven by the need (or "ambition," as the headline writer called it) to do it all. But from the perspective of Eastern medicine, her health is becoming fragile, maybe even "feeble."

The Eastern concept of energy is quite different from that of our Western Energizer Bunny. In the East, energy is called *qi* (also spelled *chi*) or *prana* and it is the life force. Have you ever seen someone practicing tai chi or qi gong? If so, you've seen how the practitioner expends her energy—her life force—economically and efficiently, as an extension of her peace of mind. She nourishes her life force with whole and freshly cooked food that agrees with her, by breathing clean air, and by keeping good company. She has balance in her life. This balance, in turn, *affects* her life: Her equanimity is reflected in her hormonal levels. They, too, are in balance. She is happy and her health is hearty. Her life force, or qi, is strong and its flow unimpeded.

We'll go deeper into the concept of qi or *prana* later. (You can also see Appendix B for more discussion of *prana*). For now, let's get back to our poor Energizer Bunny. She needs help. It is one thing to go through a crunch period of high stress for a day, a week, a month, even two months. This happens to all of us, and our bodies, minds, and spirits can recover from it. We might even be able to tolerate it for a year or two. When we go through stressful times, we survive them by living on "credit," borrowing from our reserves of good health. When the stressful time passes, we regroup and rebuild.

Trouble arises when stress is prolonged and our reserves become too depleted. We no longer have the resources to combat the effects of the excess stress hormones in our systems. An overabundance of stress hormones outweighs the nourishing effects of our sex hormones and leads to the breakdown of bones, skin, muscles, and brain tissue. This is when we start feeling seriously off-kilter and require serious repair. While there is always hope that we can regain our health, it will be an uphill climb. It is far easier to maintain our health than regain it.

Eastern medicine teaches us that humans are an aspect of nature and are governed by her laws. Our minds are individual mirrors of the cosmic consciousness and our bodies are microcosms that reflect the state of the world around us. What happens to the one is reflected in the other. For example, look at what happens in the macrocosm of the economic world. When we experience financial crisis, often borne of spending money we don't have year after year, it becomes a sticky prospect to fully regain economic health.

In the microcosm of the world that is a woman's body, it is not uncommon for her to outspend her energetic and nutritional resources. Between holding down a job, maintaining relationships, and caring for her family, a woman often blows through the energy she "earns" from sleep, good food, and good company. Her daily needs repeatedly outpace her daily intake of energy. The result? She has to dip into her reserves, which depletes her core nourishment. This is no more sustainable than spending money we don't have. Just as there comes a time when we can no longer ignore financial debt, there comes a time when energy deficit becomes unsustainable. When that happens, it is not only economies that need bailouts. Our bodies and minds do, too.

How does hormonal imbalance come into this picture? When a woman is stressed, her body releases stress hormones. These hormones make her hypervigilant and they key up her nervous system until it is hypersensitive. In this state, she begins to experience even benign events as critical situations. This, in turn, stimulates the release of even more stress hormones. A vicious cycle begins. There is no easy resolution to the stress, because it is caused by not only external factors but ongoing internal factors, such as the woman's desire to meet all of her family's needs, her boss's needs, her friends' needs, and her own expectations.

The long-term oversaturation of a woman's cells by stress hormones throws her hormonal balance out of whack and triggers a host of maladies. True, some stressors are beyond our control: the death of loved ones, natural disasters, or the loss of a job, for example. But others stressors are ours to relieve, such as the stress created by our worldviews and values, our choices about what we deem essential or desirable in our lives, and the efforts we make to achieve those things. Credit problems are initiated in part by the belief that we need more than we can afford. To acquire or achieve those things, we put ourselves under stress so routinely that it becomes habitual. And as with all habits, we stop noticing we are doing it. We become so chronically stressed, we may not even realize it's not our natural state.

Maybe we know intellectually that our lives are stressful and need changing. Maybe we know this physically, as our bodies send us distress signals like headaches, irritable bowels, sleeplessness, hot flashes, feelings of tightness in our throats or chests, or overwrought emotions. Maybe we hear these pleas from our bodies, but we don't know how to stop running, pushing, overreaching ourselves. We are afraid that if we stop, something terrible will happen. We'll lose our jobs. Our lovers will leave us. Our families will collapse. Our personal worlds will come crashing down around our ears. So we keep going, going, going. And our hormonal balance becomes the victim.

 ## Are We Talking About You?

Try this little quiz. Check the things that apply to you.

- ☐ Do you jump when the phone rings?
- ☐ Do you feel anxiety about checking your mailbox?
- ☐ Do you dwell on the many things that could go wrong later today, later this week, month, or year?
- ☐ Do you commonly feel anxiety, stress, or worry for no particular reason?
- ☐ Do you commonly feel anxiety, stress, or worry for *any* reason?
- ☐ Do you commonly have anxiety about family members?
- ☐ Do you have panic attacks?
- ☐ Do you have depression?
- ☐ Are you exposed to any environmental pollutants or toxins, like smelly paints, plastics, industrial plants, city pollution, new construction, or renovation projects?
- ☐ Do you experience any of the following symptoms associated with your menstrual cycle: headaches, mood swings, acne, bloating, constipation, heavy or scanty bleeding, painful cramping, irregular periods, pain at ovulation, or bleeding between cycles?
- ☐ Do you use synthetic hormone therapy of any kind, like birth control pills, fertility drugs, or hormone replacement therapy for menopausal symptoms?

☐ Do you have hot flashes, insomnia, heart palpitations, accelerated heartbeat, thyroid trouble of any kind, low immunity, infertility, heart disease, osteoporosis, cancer, diabetes, adrenal burnout, or endocrine disorders?

If you answered yes to even *one* of these questions, it is likely your hormonal balance is affected.

To persevere on our busy course doesn't usually require courage. It takes an overly developed sense of responsibility—or a tendency to hope that everything will get better even if we don't do anything differently. What really takes courage is to stop—stop running, stop pushing, stop trying to please *everyone*, stop outspending our reserves. Just stop. Stop and begin to live the life we really want to be living.

When we do, I have found that our worlds do not come crashing down. On the contrary, if we take little steps to slow our pace and have more time, we find life becomes more enjoyable, even easier; and we begin to gain the confidence to slow things down further. The downward cycle becomes an upward spiral that gains momentum and delivers us into a life saturated with more joy than stress, more meaning than emptiness, and more health than disorder.

How to Change Course

The first step in achieving hormonal balance is to understand it. Most people, including doctors, are confused about hormones. The available information is at once exhaustive and conflicting. Health professionals who want to understand how hormones affect nearly every aspect of our health almost have to make it an extra part-time job. However, there is a simple way to grasp what these important biochemicals do. Basically, hormones can be separated into two easy-to-understand categories, which in Traditional Chinese Medicine (TCM) are called *yin* and *yang*. We will look at these in Part I. My point here is, you won't have to learn anything complex or scientific.

This may sound like I am reducing a complicated reality to a simplistic conclusion. But consider this: The phenomenally complicated mechanisms of computer programming can be boiled down to a sequence of zeros and ones. Zeros and ones. Like yin and yang, zeros and ones are two opposites that together describe and create something incredibly complex. Anyone who insists that hormones are extremely complicated is wrong. Einstein once said, "If you can't explain a concept to a six-year-old, you don't fully understand it." I'd add, "Or you're trying to get someone to buy something"—like hormone-replacement therapy, or even herbs and other remedies that offer only Band-Aids, not cures.

What is the cure? The secret is, there's no big secret to it. It is a general tendency of a student new to Eastern medicine to suspect that the real secrets of health lie in complicated solutions—perhaps an ancient recipe requiring the ash of a rare gem mixed with powder of an expensive root. It sometimes takes years of training and a good deal of experience to learn that the secrets are in the basics. There are three pillars that support our health and happiness. These are our diet, our lifestyle (including exercise), and how we manage stress. When there is a crack in any of these pillars, disease can creep in and take root.

Of course, changing our habits, even to balance our hormones and regain our health, isn't a piece of cake. Literally (usually) or figuratively. But it's not complicated or hard to learn. And it's really, really worth it.

One of the benefits of improving our habits is, we can often then avoid drugs and surgery. There is no question that there are times when they are crucial. They save lives. But surgery can have complications and drugs often have harmful side effects. You can end up in more trouble than you started out with. For example, in 2002, the *Journal of the American Medical Association* reported that in U.S. hospitals alone, as many as 106,000 people were dying *every year* as a direct result of adverse reactions to properly prescribed drugs. This didn't include the astounding numbers of deaths caused as a result of properly performed surgery, poorly performed surgery, or poorly prescribed drugs.[2] The fact that correctly prescribed drugs and treatments can cause illness and death in disturbing numbers might seem to violate the "do no harm" part of the Hippocratic oath. They are routinely used as first-response strategies, rather than using lifestyle, diet, and other less invasive tools.

In the original Hippocratic oath, along with the doing-no-harm part, Hippocrates swears to "prescribe regimens for the good of my patients according to my ability and my judgment." Eastern medicine is all about healthy regimens.

While there are certainly appropriate times for surgical or pharmacological intervention and natural herbs or remedies, we lean on them too often when we could achieve the same or better results—and without negative side effects—by practicing Eastern medicine, which addresses physical and emotional maladies first with lifestyle and dietary changes.

When we look at the Western science on hormones and then consider them from an Eastern medical perspective, some insights become very clear:

- Hormonal balance is essential to just about every aspect of women's health.
- Sex hormones and stress hormones are often misunderstood in a sea of conflicting and narrowly defined descriptions.

- Hormones can be understood easily, using the Chinese principles of yin and yang (or the corresponding terms in Ayurveda)[3] to describe how they work and interact.
- If we understand the effects of excess stress and poor nourishment, we can make more informed choices, change the direction of our lives, and regain health and happiness.

The Theory Behind the Stress Epidemic and This Book

Ayurveda and Traditional Chinese Medicine each have a set of fundamental principles and theories upon which they rely for diagnosis and treatment, and to describe the human body. Just as French or Spanish are different languages used to describe the same reality, Ayurveda and TCM are different languages that describe a reality they fundamentally see the same way.

It is beyond the scope of this book to introduce all fundamental principles of Ayurveda and Traditional Chinese Medicine. To do them all justice would require more page real estate than is feasible for this book, and to do more than a cursory job of it would introduce questions and confusion that would detract from our focus. (However, if you'd like a brief overview of both systems, see Appendix B.)

The purpose of the various theories is to explain different possible conditions and phenomenon. One theory may best explain one malady, another may more elegantly describe a different malady or aspect of reality.

In this book, we will be exploring the roles of stress and rejuvenation in hor- mones and women's health. There is no theory more applicable to these subjects than the one that underlies the relationship of duality. This relationship is described beautifully in both TCM and Ayurveda, and the theory behind it serves as the foundation for the perspective presented in this book.

Fundamentally, the relationship of duality is one of substance to energy, of passivity versus activity, of archetypal feminine versus masculine qualities. Respectively, these forces are called *yin* and *yang* in TCM, and *santarpana* or *brmhana* and *apatarpana* or *langhana* in Ayurveda. The TCM and Ayurvedic terms are synonymous but I'll use *yin* and *yang* in this book, as these are more familiar to, and easier to pronounce (*yin* rhymes with "in" and *yang* with "long," *not* "hang") for Western audiences than are their Ayurvedic equivalents.

The theory of yin and yang is distinctly understandable framework from which to understand stress, hormones, and the condition of the body and mind. It configures the quagmire of hormonal information into a construction that is easily navigated and feels surprisingly like common sense. It offers a thoroughly practical way to address imbalances, one you will be able to start using even before finishing this book.

As practical as they are, you don't have to believe in the concepts of yin and yang to benefit from this book. You can look at them as shorthand to describe two different types of complex biochemical activities at work in your body and mind. These activities have been researched and meticulously documented in Western medicine. What I am offering is a way of understanding them that is easy to grasp. As we get into the story of how hormones control health, it will be much simpler to understand hormones as either yin hormones or yang hormones than to memorize the names of the hundreds of hormones that flood our bodies, the glands that secret them, and the role each hormone plays.

How This Book Works

This book is in three parts. In Part I, we'll talk about yin and yang, how hormones work and, specifically, about what the sex and stress hormones do. This allows us to understand the root causes of our problems and why we crash.

In Part II, we'll look at the medical problems women suffer as a result of hormonal imbalance. I'll present the general Western medical approach, discuss its value, and explain how Eastern medicine would resolve these issues. (When I use the term "Eastern medicine," I am referring to both Traditional Chinese Medicine and Ayurveda.) When possible I'll also suggest some general things you can choose to do yourself for these specific ailments.

In Part III, we'll look at the basic tools to balance hormones through nutrition and lifestyle changes, including specific steps you can take. Obviously, it is beyond the scope of this book to prescribe for you individually, but Part III offers some nearly universal information and practices that are good for almost anybody. Sometimes universal steps are all that are needed, but if further tailoring of your diet or lifestyle is required for your particular situation, you can learn through self-study, by having a consultation with a practitioner of TCM or Ayurveda, or by taking a course. Whether you are already in a medical profession or are new to the study of medicine, you can find books, online courses, and other educational opportunities for learning these systems in Appendix A. This book will give you a foundation and framework to maximize the benefit of those resources so you can get started rebalancing your hormones and reclaiming your life.

Take-Home Messages from This Chapter

- Understanding how hormones work is quite straightforward when you look at them in terms of Eastern medicine.
- Balancing your hormones isn't rocket science.
- Expecting your health-care practitioner to give you the best advice on hormones is risky business. I have never met one who didn't admit to being confused about hormones.
- Anytime you take a pill to cure one thing, you cause something else to shift and risk getting side effects, sometimes pretty nasty ones.
- As a culture, we often ignore the fundamental causes of health and illness, and focus instead on how to fund drugs and surgery. Our health-care system really pays more attention to disease than to health. Of the $2.1 trillion spent in 2008 on medical care, ninety-five cents of every dollar was used to treat disease, not prevent it.[4]
- It is far easier to maintain our health than have to regain it. It's joyful and healthy to live the lives we want to be living—and it's attainable when we adjust our lifestyles and diets.

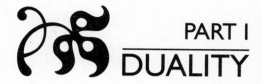

PART I
DUALITY

YIN, YANG, AND HORMONES

Foolish the doctor who despises the knowledge acquired by the ancients.
—HIPPOCRATES, THE FATHER OF WESTERN MEDICINE

ALTHOUGH EASTERN MEDICINE DOESN'T NAME AND EXPLAIN INDIVIDUAL HORMONES, IT GIVES US A COMPREHENSIVE CONTEXT IN WHICH TO UNDERSTAND HOW THEY WORK. IT IS AN EMINENTLY PRACTICAL AND USEFUL PERSPECTIVE THAT EXPLAINS THE FUNDAMENTAL CAUSES OF HORMONAL IMBALANCE AND THE REMEDIES FOR RESTORING IT. RATHER THAN LEARNING HOW TO MANIPULATE EACH AND EVERY HORMONE, WE WILL SIMPLY OPTIMIZE THEIR ENVIRONMENT THROUGH CHANGES IN NUTRITION AND LIFESTYLE, AND OUR HOR-MONES WILL SHIFT IN RESPONSE.

Hormones
AMBASSADORS OF
YIN AND YANG

Balancing our hormones is crucial to regaining full health. If we were in India, we might say it's the cheap and best way to stop feeling crummy. In this part of the book, we'll see how hormones work in a way that's simple to understand, remember, and put to use, day in and day out. We'll see what balancing hormones means and how to do it without taking drugs such as hormone-replacement therapy. In later sections of this book, we'll look at many specific medical problems women face and how to use the wisdom of Eastern medicine to heal them.

So what *are* hormones exactly and why does it seem like you need a medical degree to understand them? The problem is that there's a sea of information about hormones, and, worse, the waves in this sea are choppy and chaotic. You could easily drown in it. Much of this information—and many of the conclusions drawn from it—can be conflicting or confusing, even to physicians and serious students of various medical systems. I'm not going to swamp you with a comprehensive explanation of hormones as they are understood (or not) today. Instead, I'm going to sketch out some basic information about hormones from the perspective of Western medicine, then use the perspective of Eastern medicine to make it easy to understand.

Hormones are the ever-present servants of our mental and physical balance. Each is secreted in one part of the body, travels to another part, and influences it to do whatever the body needs to achieve (or regain) its equilibrium in the moment. That could be a signal to grow new tissue, metabolize nutrients in food, or increase the heart rate. Hormones are all-pervasive. They enter the cells of *every* tissue in our bodies and brains, and affect both our physical and mental well-being. Whereas some hormones (like the stress hormones) kick our bodies and minds into high gear, others (such as the dominant sex hormones, estrogen and progesterone) lead us to calm our minds and slow down so our bodies can replace depleted energy. Stress hormones stimulate our hearts to beat faster and increase blood pressure so we can leap into action. Sex hormones stimulate the monthly re-creation of the uterine lining and the production of breast milk after giving birth. Stress and sex hormones exert opposing influences, yet their ever-changing relationship serves to maintain equilibrium in the body and balance in the mind.

Stress hormones and sex hormones have a relationship with each other that reflects the duality present in physiology. Although they represent opposing forces, each supports the other. This is not a concept we often embrace in the West, but it is well understood in the East. Duality is found everywhere in nature. For example, although sunlight and water have opposing properties (one heats and the other cools), together they provide the essential elements for plant growth. They are in a relationship of duality. The sun provides the plant with warmth and the energy needed for photosynthesis, the process by which the plant receives nourishment. Water cools the plant and is one of the essential building blocks for photosynthesis. The plant needs both these opposing elements to thrive.

Eastern medicine has explored the concept of duality for millennia, and is adept at understanding the relationship and patterns of opposing forces that serve to benefit each other. We, as Westerners and as women, need to understand duality so we can grasp how stress and sex hormones, despite representing opposing energies, support and interact with each other to keep us healthy and whole.

Yin and Yang

Ayurveda and Traditional Chinese Medicine both hold that there are two fundamental (and opposing) principles that invigorate and nourish life. Yang is the energizing, activating, and motivating principle of life. Yin is the nourishing and building principle.

The easiest way to learn yin and yang is to consider some examples. In daily life, driving the car, making deals, playing sports, multitasking, drinking coffee, and eating spicy food are all predominantly yang activities. Sleeping, meditating, getting massage, and eating oatmeal all support yin. Yang is considered male energy, yin is considered female. Yang energy is hot, bright, fast, mobile, dry, energetic, and aggressive. Yin is cool, dark, slow, soft, substantial, stable, moist, and tranquil. Yang is daytime, yin is night. Yang is the movement of the wave crashing on the shore, and the undertow that draws back the water into the sea. Yin is the water that comprises the wave.

Yang is energetic. It's responsible for motivation, metabolism, transformation, and other active functions in the body and mind. It is considered a "reducing" principle in Ayurveda because being active reduces, or uses up, bodily reserves. Yang motivates our bodies and stimulates our minds. Yin is the nourishing principle that manifests as the substance of the body and calms the mind. All qualities of yin and yang manifest both physically and emotionally. Yin and yang are opposites that depend on each other for the whole to function. They continuously interact in a dance that creates and sustains life.

If we can understand yin and yang, we have a simple framework for understanding the function of any hormone in the body, and specifically the complex stress hormones (yang) and sex hormones (yin), whose relationship is at the root of women's health, good or ill. Whether we are talking about a liver cell, heart cell, fingernail cell, brain cell, or carbon molecule, each has form and substance. This is yin. Each also has an energy that organizes, transforms, and directs the substance. This is yang. Yin is mostly about mass, yang is mostly about energy. Yin is the thing operated on, yang is the operating force.

Consider how they function in a human being. As I mentioned earlier, every human being has a life force or vital energy. It remains in the body as long as there is life and leaves at the time of death. This life force is called qi in Traditional Chinese Medicine and *prana* in Ayurveda, and is a manifestation of yang. Yin is manifested through all the nourishing fluids that circulate in our bodies. If our yin and yang are balanced, our qi is robust. It flows smoothly, and we have sufficient nourishing fluids to irrigate our tissues and deliver nutrition to them. If yin and yang are out of balance, qi and nourishing fluids cease to flow smoothly and disease arises.

Throughout our lives, we need both yin and yang qualities to infuse and irrigate our bodies, minds, and emotions. We receive yin in the form of food, drink, and emotional comfort, all of which provide building blocks for our growth processes and give stability to our minds and contentment to our emotions. Once we have received yin, yang digests it. Yang transforms and organizes yin into biologically useful substances such as blood or bones. It also moves whatever we don't need out of our bodies in the form of waste. Yang qualities not only provide energy for metabolic processes, but for clarity of mind and happiness, too. Yang energy can even transform information into knowledge and knowledge into wisdom. It can determine whether an emotionally charged event will serve to create good judgment in future situations (that is, whether we "digest" the experience into something useful) or whether we become resentful, bitter, or depressed, unable to mentally digest what we experienced.

In Eastern medicine, yin and yang are opposing forces that act concurrently and constantly to maintain physical equilibrium. Consider the temperature of the human body. Ideally, it is 98.6 degrees Fahrenheit. The opposite forces of cooling (yin) and warming (yang) work together to maintain this temperature. One kicks in and the other recedes, or vice versa, as needed to keep our body temperature stable. When the yin and yang of our temperature system are out of balance and cannot rebalance themselves, crisis ensues. The same happens when our yin hormones and yang hormones are out of balance.

Whether we are talking about warming and cooling, sex hormones and stress hormones, or other examples of physiological opposites that coexist for mutual benefit, we can see that there is a tremendous intelligence at work. Every cell in our body—as well as in the greater universe—has to have a balance of yin and yang to function well. If these energies are out of balance, the cell, as well as the organism, must regain that balance to thrive. When we have a good balance of yin and yang, we feel healthy. If we have too much or too little of one or the other, we begin to see or feel signs of imbalance.

When we have the optimal amount and quality of yang, we have sufficient qi to feel energized, confident, focused, and engaged. What we eat and drink are efficiently transformed into blood, tissue, and energy to live our lives. If we have insufficient yang, our qi becomes depleted and we may feel fatigued, scattered, off track, chilly, out of sync, out of sorts, or out of step with the world around us. Without enough yang, our body's garbage-disposal system may go askew, ceasing to clean out what the body doesn't need, leading to problems like masses. We may encounter any number of other uncomfortable symptoms that accompany insufficient yang. We can also have too much yang, which leads to excessively fast, hard, hot, or aggressive energy. When that happens, we might get migraines or ulcers, or feel manic, restless, or angry. When such expressions possess our bodies and minds, our qi becomes stagnant, increasing irritability, restlessness, or pain.

We can also experience yin in healthy or unhealthy ways. If we have the optimal amount of yin, for example, we feel fulfilled, nourished, and content physically, emotionally, and spiritually. Menstrual flow is appropriate and sleep is sound and replenishing. If we have an excess of yin, we feel bloated, heavy, overweight, lethargic, stuffed up, and stuffed (as in overnourished). If we don't have enough of yin's cool, soft, moist, and tranquil properties, we may get hot flashes, feel emotionally isolated or fearful, or experience physical dryness or insomnia. We may become anemic or weak, have scanty periods, or experience dizziness. If both yin and yang are off, we may feel hot one minute and cold the next, and have weight fluctuations, bone loss, or mood swings.

In our bodies and minds, yin and yang energies manifest on a deep physiological level as hormones. Women's dominant sex hormones, like estrogen and progesterone, have a predominantly yin influence in the body, whereas stress hormones, like adrenaline or cortisol, have a predominantly yang influence. I say "predominantly" because even within each type of hormone—yin or yang— some individual hormones are more or less yin (or yang) than others.

Yin and yang may sound like black-or-white, all-or-nothing concepts but they are actually relative terms. Nothing that exists is totally yin or totally yang. They are simply yin or yang *in relation to other things*. In nature, for example, we see certain elements as more yin or more yang. Water, for example, being cooling, nourishing, and heavy, has a strong yin nature, so we say it "is" yin. Fire, being hot, light, and actively transformative is extremely yang, so we say it "is" yang. While it is common for something to be mostly yin or mostly yang, it is not possible to have one without at least a little of the other. This is nature's way of ensuring that there are always opposing forces present and available to maintain or regain equilibrium.

Eastern medicine teaches that we are affected physically *and emotionally* by every quality with which we come into contact. The general rule is: Like increases like. Western medicine recognizes this as well. For example, a study published in the journal *Science* in 2008 demonstrated that qualities like heat and cold affect both our emotional and physical well-being. In the study, people who held a warm beverage for ten to fifteen seconds or evaluated the warmth from a heating pad were more likely to "warm" to strangers and share with them than people who held a cold drink or evaluated the effect of a cold pack. And not only was the "warm" test group more open and generous with strangers, they perceived the strangers as warmer human beings as well. In another test, having subjects plot distant points on a graph actually led them to feel their relatives were distant.[1] This understanding of like increasing like will become important when we start learning how to balance our yin sex hormones and our yang stress hormones. For now, let us understand simply that engaging in motivating and activating activities will generally increase yang, whereas engaging in nourishing and nurturing activities will generally increase yin.

Sex Hormones
THE AMBASSADORS OF YIN

Women's dominant sex hormones serve to lubricate, nourish, and build us. They are yin. While there are many different sex hormones in the body, we'll be looking mainly at estrogen and progesterone. We can think of these two as Ginger Rogers and Fred Astaire, respectively. Remember what we discussed in the previous chapter about some yin hormones being more yin than others? Well, estrogen (Ginger) is more yin than progesterone (Fred), even though we say they are both yin. Estrogen is what we call in Traditional Chinese Medicine "the yin within yin." It provides nourishment, lubrication, and beauty. Progesterone (Fred) is the more yang of the two. It's called "the yang within yin," leading the dance and providing balance to Ginger's extreme yin.

Estrogen: Yin Within Yin

Yin is wet and nourishing. If there is one ultimately juicy hormone, it is estrogen, the Ginger Rogers of hormones. Estrogen is responsible for the development and maintenance of female sexual characteristics, like breasts, and stimulates the growth of the uterine lining. But the delights of estrogen are not confined to the reproductive organs and breasts. Every tissue in the body needs juice—lubrication and nourishment. Every single tissue in the body has been found to contain estrogen.

There are many kinds of estrogens in our female bodies. The three main ones are estradiol, estriol, and estrone. It is important to know a little about these, so we can understand that women don't stop producing estrogen after menopause and to understand which organs are doing all the work and what that may mean for us down the road. This information may be scintillating to some and, frankly, a tad tedious for others. You have full permission to skim, but better not to skip it altogether.

These are the three main estrogens and their glands of origin:

- Estradiol is produced in the ovaries and in the adrenal glands. It is considered the most potent of the three main estrogens. After about the age of fifty, or after surgery to remove the ovaries, it becomes the job of our adrenal glands to supply some of our estrogen, in the amounts we require (or to provide the biochemical precursors that our bodies can use to synthesize estrogen).
- Estrone is produced by the placenta during pregnancy, by fat tissue, and to a much lesser extent by muscle tissue. Estrone is the major estrogen for post-menopausal women, even though they will not be growing placentas, because the liver can transform estrone into estradiol and vice versa.
- Estriol is produced by the placenta and, to a lesser extent, by the liver. It is some-times called the "pregnancy estrogen" and is not a major player after menopause.

In general, one kind of estrogen or another is naturally synthesized in the body, either in the ovaries, the adrenal glands, or from other precursor hormones that can be made into estrogen. Progesterone, testosterone, and other hormones can serve as estrogen precursors. These precursor hormones are synthesized in the ovaries, adrenal glands, and throughout the entire body in fat, bones, muscle, skin, brain, and other tissue. Thus precursor hormones, body tissues, and even the ovaries[1] continue to provide estrogen after menopause. In fact, it is possible for an overweight woman to have more estrogen after menopause than a thin woman has before menopause, simply because of the amount of estrogen in her too-ample fat tissues.

To make estrogen, we also require aromatase and estrogen receptors. Aromatase is an enzyme that can instantaneously transform even precursor hormones, like testosterone, into estrogen.[2] Like estrogen, aromatase decreases after menopause; but happily, it also becomes more potent. Also like the estrogen precursors, aromatase is widely available in our bodies before and after menopause. It is found mostly in fat and muscle tissue, but also in bones, blood vessels, brain tissue, and breasts.

As for estrogen receptors, all we need to know for our purposes is that, although they decline after menopause, they are also found throughout the entire body.

Because every one of our cells needs yin, or nourishment, it is not surprising that we find estrogen (or its precursors) everywhere in the body, along with aromatase. With all the sources of estrogen production and the availability of aromatase and estrogen receptors, it is hard to imagine that we could ever have a shortage of estrogen. But we can. We'll see why in the next chapter, but here's a hint. The issue is not that we are not producing enough sex hormones, but that they are either insufficient to balance the effects of stress hormones on the body, or are even being sacrificed in our body's attempts to fuel our high levels of stress.

APPROPRIATE QUANTITY AND QUALITY OF YIN

If we have too little estrogen (yin), we may get vaginal dryness, dry skin, hot flashes, and night sweats. Although estrogen is vital to maintaining healthy yin in our bodies, too much of a good thing can also be problematic. If we have too much, we may gain weight, feel lethargic, get depressed, lose our libido, develop fibrocystic or tender breasts, retain water, get uterine fibroids, and have an increased chance of breast or endometrial cancer.

Just as we need the right quantity of yin, we also require the right *quality* of yin to ensure optimum nourishment and healthy hormones. Good-quality oils, foods, relationships, and sleep can nourish good-quality yin. As we will see in Part III, poor-quality yin, as we might expect from trans fats, for example, can create toxic sludge in the body that contributes to disease or disorder.

"GOOD" VS. "BAD" ESTROGEN

Highly toxic "bad" estrogen is related to the question of estrogen quality and quantity. Just as there is "good" cholesterol and "bad" cholesterol, there is "good" and "bad" estrogen. Whereas good cholesterol is said to prevent heart disease, bad cholesterol is widely expected to aggravate it. Similarly, good estrogen may help prevent cancer, but bad estrogen can greatly increase its risk.

We have seen that estradiol is the most potent estrogen produced in our bodies. It is created in the ovaries and adrenal glands. From there, the body converts it either to good estrogen (2-hydroxyestrone) or toxic estrogen (16 apha-hydroxyestrone). I have not encountered an explanation in Western medicine about why the body would choose to convert it to bad estrogen. According to Eastern medicine, whether the conversion is to good or bad estrogen depends on whether the liver, the body's metabolic processes, and the body's qi are functioning optimally. Bad estrogens are longer lived than good ones and stimulate breast cell proliferation, so they can be a factor in developing breast cancer, which is associated with an increased rate of cell production. There is also some indication that when estrogen is not metabolized in our bodies in a timely manner, it stagnates and then becomes problematic or "bad" estrogen.

Although poor-quality estrogen is a big problem, we can also have an inappropriate amount of good estrogen in the body. We can either have too much, or we can have an inequity of good estrogen in relation to progesterone, a situation often called "estrogen dominance."

Progesterone: Yang Within Yin

Let's turn our attention now to progesterone, the yin hormone that is more yang than estrogen. Progesterone prepares the uterus for the fertilized egg and maintains pregnancy, but perhaps its main function is to keep estrogen in check in a woman. It is produced in the ovaries until after menopause, in the adrenal glands of both men and women, and in the testes of men. Again, this is the Fred Astaire hormone, in contrast to the Ginger Rogers hormone, estrogen. Just as Ginger follows Fred's lead in the dance, estrogen follows progesterone's lead. For example, the body can make estrogen from progesterone, but it can't make progesterone from estrogen.

We can see that progesterone is more yang than estrogen in several ways. A woman's basal temperature (the temperature of her body first thing in the morning, upon waking) is warmer (a yang trait) during the progesterone-dominant phase of her cycle than in her more yin estrogen-dominant phase.[3] Yang represents the male counterpart to yin and, indeed, synthetic progesterone may actually have a masculinizing effect on female infants.[4] And, as yang represents energy and yin substance, progesterone prevents estrogen from creating too much mass in the body. You'll see what I mean shortly.

Like estrogen, progesterone has many effects on the body. First, it balances the effects of estrogen. Dr. John Lee, author of *What Your Doctor May Not Tell You About Menopause*, maintained a private practice for thirty years and dedicated about four decades to the study of hormones in women's health. In this book, he reports,

> Estrogen unopposed by progesterone was found to cause salt and water retention, increase blood clotting, promote fat synthesis, oppose thyroxin (a thyroid hormone), promote uterine fibroids, promote mastodynia (breast pain) and fibrocystic breasts, increase the risk of gallstones and liver dysfunction, and, more ominously, increase the risk of endometrial cancer, pituitary tumors (prolactinoma), and probably breast cancer.[5]

These signs all point to too much yin (substance) in the body relative to the balancing force of yang.

Progesterone would provide this balance. While estrogen stimulates the growth of the uterine lining, progesterone serves to hold the lining in place.

While estrogen promotes breast development and growth, progesterone helps protect against fibrocystic breasts (masses in the breasts). Excess estrogen increases body fat, fluid retention, blood clotting, and breast cancer, and creates other problems—each of which progesterone serves to counteract: It helps burn fat for energy, is a natural diuretic, normalizes blood clotting, and helps prevent breast and endometrial cancer.[6]

While progesterone and estrogen counteract each other in many instances, they also work together. As we saw earlier, estrogen can be made from progesterone. In addition, each serves to sensitize the receptors of the other.[7] The result is that progesterone primarily acts as a balancing force, supporting production of estrogen if there isn't enough, and opposing its effects if there is too much.

As progesterone is still one of the yin hormones, it also supports bone density. Dr. Lee found that it stimulates the building of bone tissue. Progesterone begins to decline at about age thirty-five in women. So we see it is not a coincidence that this is the same age when a woman's bone density begins to decline.

Just as estrogen can be made from progesterone, so, too, can stress hormones like cortisol. (The reverse is not true: You cannot make progesterone from estrogen or cortisol.) It follows that if we are deficient in either estrogen or cortisol, as long as we have enough progesterone, our body can use it to create the estrogen or cortisol it needs.

If progesterone levels are low, we may experience some symptoms similar to those of estrogen deficiency. This may be because there is not enough progesterone for the body to use as raw material to make estrogen. However, if we have ample estrogen but are deficient in progesterone, we may simply show signs of excess—unopposed—estrogen as I described earlier.

Too much progesterone relative to estrogen is not a common complaint. It is far more common—and troublesome—to have "estrogen dominance."

To recap, the major yin hormones in a woman's body are estrogen and progesterone. Estrogen can be made in any tissue in the body and serves to build and nourish us both before and after menopause. Progesterone serves to support estrogen and to act as the check in nature's check-and-balance system, so that estrogen's influence does not become dominant. Together, our Ginger and Fred interact in a constant yet ever-changing relationship as they engage in their graceful dance.

4

Stress Hormones
THE AMBASSADORS OF YANG

Sex hormones are the major yin hormones; stress hormones are the major yang hormones. Adrenaline and cortisol are the two major players for yang. They trigger the fight-or-flight response to real or perceived threats to our well-being and survival. This response causes us to be more alert and makes our hearts pump more blood to the big muscle groups that are responsible for helping us run, climb, or fight our way out of trouble. They are the survival hormones.

Just as we looked at two key sex hormones, estrogen and progesterone, we will focus here on cortisol and dehydroepiandrostenedione (DHEA)—a prohormone that balances cortisol in much the same way that progesterone balances estrogen. Using a metaphor from the entertainment world again, you can think of cortisol as Fred Flintstone (the yang within the yang) and DHEA as his wife, Wilma (the yin within the yang).

Adrenaline and cortisol are closely related. In fact, whenever adrenaline increases, cortisol levels rise.[1] Adrenaline provides a short-term stress response and decreases quickly. Cortisol increases when adrenaline does, but it stays active longer. When our cortisol levels are high, our recovery time after an adrenaline surge increases. Also, the more often we have adrenaline surges, the more cortisol is released with each surge. Although adrenaline and cortisol always function together, we are going to focus here on cortisol because of its long-term dominance in the body. (This will also avoid the repetition that would come from discussing both of them.)

So let's look at cortisol, the Fred Flintstone of yang stress hormones.

Whether a lion is chasing us or we are swerving to avoid a car accident, there are moments when we need to respond quickly or we will lose our lives. Say a big truck suddenly pulls out in front of you. Your heart starts to race, you break out in a sweat, and your blood pressure increases. You slam on the brakes, twist the wheel to the right, and avoid the accident. Your survival is due to the successful working of your cortisol. Thanks, Fred!

But if high stress becomes a way of life, cortisol becomes a permanent guest in your bloodstream. And cortisol, while essential, is problematic in excess. Happily, just as we saw progesterone balancing estrogen, there are substances that serve to counteract the effects of cortisol. One of these substances is DHEA, the Wilma Flintstone of stress hormones. DHEA is "the yin within yang" and balances the negative effects of cortisol. In this chapter, we'll see how the two work together, and we'll also look briefly at two other yang hormones, oxytocin and prolactin, the girlfriends that help Wilma (DHEA) balance the powerful, sometimes overbearing effect of Fred (cortisol).

Cortisol: Yang Within Yang

Cortisol is a yang stress hormone produced in the outer portion of the adrenal glands. It controls the metabolism of carbohydrates, fats, and protein, and plays an important role in infection-fighting, blood sugar balance, immune response, thinking, and other healthy functions. In excess, however, cortisol can cause problems. It is a risk factor for depression,[2] osteoporosis,[3] weight loss or gain, problems in the cardiovascular system, high blood pressure, and a host of other issues in women's health. There is a strong link between increased cortisol and depression, and solid evidence of lower bone mineral density in women with increased cortisol. This begins even before menopause and should be considered a serious risk factor.

Like other stress hormones, cortisol is released in response to any real or perceived stress, be it physical or emotional. Such stressors include overworking, fasting, infection, excess exercise, emotional upset, mental strain, and the presence of a threat to life.[4] Once cortisol has been released into the system, it is—like Fred Flintstone—loud, overexcitable, and hard to get rid of. It is released more slowly than adrenaline and lingers longer in the body. Once it has entered our systems, it remains active long after the real or perceived crisis has past.[5] Let's say you swerved and successfully avoiding hitting a big truck. The moment of danger passed. Afterward, you are driving along peacefully again, under no threat. But you are still drenched in stress hormones. Your heart is still racing; you are still sweating, charged up, and stressed out. There is no way to instantly turn off the yang stress reaction that had been instantly turned on.

Of course, we *need* to have our stress hormones released in quick spurts to help us get out of life-or-death trouble. But nowadays, they get triggered too often and in too-great quantities. We often have a version of fight-or-flight feelings in everyday circumstances like emotional or physical confrontations with a spouse, child, neighbor, parent, or boss. We may even have a stress response to the phone ringing, to checking our mail, or to hearing a loud or sudden noise. Sometimes the trigger for cortisol release has no external source but is within us. We feel stressed out, hyped up, pressured, and trapped in lives we don't want to be living.

In the modern world, many of us find ourselves in a near constant state of stress. When this happens, we have stress hormones like cortisol coursing through our bodies on a regular basis. The crunch comes when we don't have enough of these hormones available to satisfy the huge demand for them. Then our bodies will find a way—*any* way—to get us more. One way to get more is to sacrifice some of our sex hormones by transforming them into stress hormones. We have seen that progesterone can become cortisol. Good-bye, Fred Astaire; hello, Fred Flintstone.

Sadly, another source of stress hormones, if a woman is pregnant, is from her developing child. Studies have shown that an unborn baby's adrenal glands may enlarge substantially in utero to supply its mother with the stress hormones that her body is demanding. This can create problems for the mother and for the child. If a child is born with already overtaxed adrenal glands, Eastern medicine would suspect that she may have a naturally lower tolerance for stress and be especially prone to a hypersensitive nervous system and its related hormonal dysfunction from her day of birth onward.

Ironically, the more cortisol we have in the bloodstream, the more sensitive we become to stressful events. Even very small events such as being late for work or having a minor allergic reaction will trigger the release of even more stress hormones. We are caught in a downward spiral of stress provoking a hypersensitivity to stress. Pretty soon we begin to feel stressed out and battle ready (or battle fearful) most of the time. It becomes a way of life.

Too much cortisol circulating in the body leads to overall hormone resistance, including thyroid resistance. This means that the body becomes desensitized to these hormones and more may be required to do the same job. Eastern medicine would suggest that this winds up taxing the organs or glands that produce these hormones. Excess cortisol also hinders the optimal function of many other essential hormones, such as sex hormones.[6] Further, it promotes the breakdown of all yin in the body, including the bones, skin, muscles, and brain.[7] In excess, it can lead to protein breakdown, which in turn leads to muscle-wasting and osteoporosis, and blocks progesterone's ability to support bone density.[8] And it decreases libido. Many women mistakenly think that excess cortisol is directly responsible for their weight gain. This is not the case. Cortisol by itself actually breaks down tissue and can cause weight loss, but it can hinder the optimum function of insulin in a process that leads to the weight gain around the waist that many women find so hard to lose.

If cortisol is too high for too long, it causes accelerated aging,[9] even when normal amounts of estrogen and progesterone are circulating in the body. When cortisol is high, it relegates the body's resources to the extremities and keeps them on standby, so that the body can be ready to run or fight. This starves the body's vital organs of energy, and compromises the immune system. This process contributes to increased blood sugar, high cholesterol, heart disease, memory loss, and osteoporosis. A weakened immune system can also play a role in the development of cancer and recurring infections, especially of the respiratory system.

After a time, or after a particularly traumatic experience, this process exhausts the adrenal glands. Rather than responding to stressors by secreting stress hormones, they collapse and can no longer produce enough cortisol. Now our cortisol is too low, rendering us lethargic, numb, achy and vulnerable to infections, viruses, and other malignant influences. We may also develop allergies and diabetes. Put colloquially, we may feel crummy when our cortisol is either too low or too high and our hormonal balance is subsequently disturbed.

It can take years to reverse the pattern of low cortisol caused by spiraling stress. In addition from an Eastern perspective, stress seriously interferes with our qi, or life force. Qi works best when it is circulating smoothly. When we are stressed out, we tend to clench parts or all of our bodies, constricting the natural flow of qi until it stagnates, leading to tissue, organ, or system disorders.

In my experience, stress is at the root of most of women's health concerns. It sets off hormonal imbalance and causes qi to stagnate, conditions which can lead to everything from menstrual cramps and menopausal concerns to very serious illness.

APPROPRIATE QUALITY AND QUANTITY OF YANG

As with yin, it is important to have the right quality as well as quantity of yang. We have seen that too much or too little yang are both problematic. When we wish to support healthy-quality yang, we can breathe fresh air and engage in exercises that focus on the internal, smooth movement of qi or *prana*, which are manifestations of yang. Tai chi and qi gong are soft forms of martial arts that emphasize and support the free and easy movement of qi around the body. Some forms of yoga do this as well, focusing on our relationship with *prana* and encouraging its free movement. Other forms of exercise emphasize breaking a good sweat, fulfilling many modern women's goal of "getting a good workout." If exercise doesn't include fast movements or profuse sweating, many of us feel as if we're cheating. But this kind of exertion may actually increase stress and deplete our bodies. We will explore this more in Part III. For the moment, we can say that driven or competitive exercise, drinking coffee, pushing ourselves with blind ambition, exposing ourselves to toxic or irritant pollutants, and stressing out are all examples of actions that support poor-quality yang.

DHEA: Yin Within Yang

Just as estrogen is balanced by progesterone, cortisol's main balancing partner is DHEA. DHEA is a hormone precursor that can exert a weak hormonal effect. It's the Wilma Flintstone of stress hormones. While DHEA is more yang than estrogen or progesterone, it is more yin than cortisol. As Wilma does damage control for Fred, DHEA serves to buffer, balance, or antidote increased cortisol in the body. Like cortisol, it is also made primarily in the adrenals. It can act as a weak estrogen and can be used to make estrogen or testosterone. It is said to reduce "bad" cholesterol, increase muscle mass and energy, and build and repair protein. These are all qualities that are yin in nature and balance the negative effects of increased cortisol in the body, which we can consider the main job of DHEA.

Oxytocin and Prolactin: Bonus Buffers

Wilma has a couple of girlfriends that aid in damage control by counteracting the effects of excess cortisol. Oxytocin and prolactin are two very yin hormones that provide this function. Truly speaking, they are ambassadors of yin and might be more accurately placed in Chapter 3, but they have such a buffering effect on the body's stress response that it's more fitting to talk about them here, after we discussed about stress hormones.

Oxytocin and prolactin are naturally occurring hormones in both men and women, but are found in higher levels in women, which allow us to have different options for stress response than men. Although both men and women experience a fight-or-flight response to stress (which is created by the sudden release of stress hormones), women have these bonus hormones that offer an alternative plan of action.

Drs. Laura Cousin Klein and Shelley Taylor are authors of a study at UCLA on the role of oxytocin—sometimes called "the cuddle hormone"—in women's response to stress.[10] Their study showed a difference in the way men and women responded to stress. Whereas men tended to isolate themselves in response to stress, women found comfort in tending children and befriending other women. Klein and Taylor termed this the "tend and befriend" response and related it to the presence of oxytocin. The more oxytocin a woman has, the more this response will kick in. In addition, the more she "tends and befriends" others, the more her oxytocin levels increase. Thus, oxytocin serves to counter the effects of stress and produces a calming effect. Low levels of oxytocin (like high levels of cortisol) are associated with major depression.[11]

There is also evidence that the acute release of prolactin, the predominantly female hormone responsible for lactation, may reduce fear and anxiety and induce calmness.[12] It buffers the effects of stress.

Take-home message: We have the stress hormone cortisol, which serves a very yang (Fred Flintstone) purpose in the body. It activates and motivates. It's responsible for our survival in times of danger. But in excess, cortisol causes trouble in the body and mind. We also have more yin substances (DHEA, oxytocin, and prolactin) that act like Wilma Flintstone and serve to balance the effects of cortisol.

Our bodies require the motivation and activation of yang energy, but left unchecked, it is like having a world of men without women. The world needs both men and women the way each of us needs a balance between our drive to achieve and our nourishing resources. We need a balance of yin and yang.

Understanding How
Yin and Yang Hormones Interact

Travel, education, and the greater accessibility they provide afford us an invaluable opportunity to learn from the strengths and limitations of a variety of cultures. This is certainly the case in medicine and science, where the combined strengths of Eastern and Western perspectives give us a more complete understanding than either alone.

Consider a 2001 study, reported in *Psychological Review*, on cultural differences in systems of thought. Scientists showed Japanese and American people animated scenes of fish and surrounding underwater objects. One fish was distinguished in some way (bigger, faster, brighter, etc.). The participants were then asked to report what they had seen. The Americans referred to the focal fish within their first statement. If they were shown the focal fish in a different context, they were equally able to recognize it. In contrast, while the Japanese were equally likely to recall details about the focal fish, they referred to the background objects and environment about 70 percent more than the Americans did, mentioned the relation of the focal fish to inanimate objects about twice as often, and their recognition of the focal fish was negatively affected if it was shown within a different background. It was determined that, for the Japanese, the focal subject was "bound" to its context.[1]

If we apply this to the subject of hormones, we see that Western science has excelled at describing the focal fishes—each hormone, and its associated tasks and functions—in great detail, but considers less the context in which these hormones act and how they affect one another. If we apply an Eastern perspective to this picture, not only do we consider the function of the separate hormones, but how to define each in relation to the others, the context within which they are acting, and how they affect each other. We see that there needs to be a balance of yin and yang hormones, relative to each other, and when that balance is affected by unhealthy lifestyle and diet choices, our hormones reflect that imbalance: a terrain is established that favors disorder.

In the previous chapters we looked at each separate hormone—a rather Western approach. We also contextualized them a little, simply by comparing one with the other. We saw that:

- Stress hormones are yang, compared to our yin sex hormones.
- Of the stress hormones, cortisol is more yang than DHEA. Oxytocin and prolactin are more yin than either of them, and serve to antidote the effects of excess stress hormones.
- Of the sex hormones, estrogen is more yin than progesterone.

If we look at the relationships between estrogen and progesterone, and between cortisol and DHEA (along with oxytocin and prolactin), we see a pattern where at least one hormone checks the excess of another. Progesterone is brought into play to prevent estrogen from becoming too high. DHEA, oxytocin, and prolactin work together to prevent the pronounced negative effects that come from unchecked cortisol.

Applying the principles of Eastern medicine to these relationships, we see that they consist of a series of checks and balances that mirror the checks and balances between our yin sex hormones and our yang stress hormones. Our sex hormones serve to balance, buffer, mediate, and act as antidotes to our excess stress hormones, simply by providing more yin to the body. This relationship can work in the other direction, too, where yang balances excess yin, but modern culture tends to stimulate excess stress hormones, so it is more often the case that yin is required to provide checks and balances for excess yang (stress hormones).

The body will always want to buffer the effects of excess stress, because it is constantly striving for balance and health. It will try to scrounge material from wherever it can to create more of what is needed. For example, if there is too much cortisol in our bloodstream, our body will release more DHEA or sex hormones to counteract it. But the body can't always supply enough of everything to go around. When this happens, it needs to set some priorities.

Survival Always Comes First

Basically, the body works the way a hospital does. Emergencies get priority. Comfort is nice, but it's secondary to survival. This means that although the body enjoys the nourishing influence of yin sex hormones, it grants priority to yang stress hormones that will help us survive a crisis—get out of the way of a Mack truck, a hungry lion, a fifteen-foot wave, or an argument where we fear someone might hit us. We must first survive in order to reproduce. The bottom line is: *Sex hormones are nice but stress hormones are essential*. As you can imagine, immediate survival is a far greater priority than having supple skin, plump breasts, or even a healthy, nonirritable bowel. This is how our body's natural intelligence views things. If we run low on sex hormones or stress hormones or both, and there's not enough raw material available to make both, a choice must be made. And the body makes it: It prioritizes stress hormones.

We have seen that progesterone can be used to make estrogen when needed, but it can also be used to make cortisol. This is not a reciprocal relationship. Stress hormones cannot return progesterone's favor by shape-shifting into progesterone when the body requires more sex hormones. This reflects the body's priorities. When we are under chronic or extreme stress, any available resources are allocated to supporting the body's stress response instead of its reproductive function.[2]

This strategy of putting the needs of our survival systems first might work as a short-term arrangement, but for many of us, it becomes a way of life. Herein lies the problem. The adrenal glands have already had to work overtime to produce all the stress hormones getting triggered by our modern lives.[3] Then they have to pump out sex hormones or DHEA to reestablish the balance between yin and yang, which was thrown out of whack by all the stress hormones in the first place.

Little by little, we deplete both our sex hormones and our stress hormones. And because all these hormones—estrogen, progesterone, DHEA, and cortisol—are produced directly or indirectly in the adrenal glands or ovaries, it is not surprising that these organs burn out. They are not bottomless reservoirs that can subsidize a stressful lifestyle indefinitely without consequence. They have limitations, as do the rest of the endocrine organs, like the thyroid gland and the pancreas, for example. All endocrine glands secrete hormones, and when stress hormones are too high for too long, all the endocrine glands are at risk. When they burn out, the result is that our bodies cannot produce enough sex or stress hormones. The stage is then set for difficulties and discomfort. This is true at any age, but is especially pronounced during and after menopause.

Nature's Good Intentions for Us

Women experience a natural ebb and flow of hormones each month and across the span of their lives. We have more yin sex hormones during certain times of our monthly cycles than at others. Over the course of a lifetime, we have more sex hormones in youth (at puberty, our sex hormones increase wildly). At age thirty-five, progesterone naturally begins to decline. At around fifty, sex hormones decrease significantly. A postmenopausal woman produces 40 to 60 percent of the sex hormones that she did before menopause. In addition, by the time she is eighty, a woman has only 10 to 25 percent of the stress-tempering DHEA that a twenty-year-old does.

None of this is a problem. It's actually a perfect design. In youth we have plenty of yin sex hormones to balance the yang stresses of the world as we attempt to figure out our worldviews, ethical perspectives, careers, relationships, and how to manage emotional conflict. Youthful exuberance sometimes means bulldozing our way headfirst through life, a yang tactic that can easily create extra stress and consumes loads of yin. During this period, we need all the antidote for stress that we can get. Our ample yin sex hormones provide it.

But a postmenopausal woman doesn't require the high levels of yin sex hormones that she did during her teenage and child-bearing years. She no longer needs to make and sustain babies. Ideally, she has learned how to cooperate with life a bit more gracefully, stirring up as little extra stress as possible and moving through life with more ease, so she manages stress better and needs less of a buffer against its negative effects. Now she just needs enough yin sex hormones to provide whatever nourishment and lubrication her body still requires for daily balance.

So, while the amount of our sex hormones and DHEA levels decline with age, it is not aging (and our naturally diminishing hormones) that are at the root of our declining health. What disrupts our natural hormonal balance and eventually compromises our core health is the cumulative effect of excess stress hormones.[4] Our bodies "know" how much and which hormones we need to be healthy and comfortable at each stage of life—provided we do not have excess stress hormones circulating in the bloodstream—and they are hardwired to deliver accordingly.

Our life patterns, however, do not always reflect our wiring blueprints.

Too often we become more active and more stressed as we age, rather than less. Very few of us have figured out how to cope with stress, learn why we're on this planet and what we're supposed to be doing here, manage our daily stressors, and be fully engaged in our lives. This causes our life force, or qi, to stagnate, which leads to everything from migraines and irritability to organ failure, and it paves the way for adrenal burnout by the time we hit menopause. This, in turn, leads to osteoporosis, heart disease, and other often-avoidable maladies, because our adrenal glands are too burned out to provide for our postmenopausal sex hormone requirements and our chronically high stress-hormone levels have wrought their damage for decades. And let's not forget, it also means we are living lives we don't like. It's not that we are suffering now so we can enjoy life later. We are suffering now and we'll suffer for it later, too.

Simply put, our hormonal activity reflects the level of satisfaction we have with the choices we've made and the lives we are living. They are inextricably linked.

Imagine if, as girls and young women, we were educated in how to protect, appreciate, and nourish our yin. What if we were taught how to manage stress to avoid overusing and depleting yang though excess demand on our stress hormones? By the time we reach thirty-five—about halfway into the second stage of life—we could be well established in lives that reflected our values, lives that were full but peaceful. We would have some foresight and begin to slow down as we moved forward. We would stop and smell the roses. We would enjoy our lives. How many thirty-five-year-old women do you know who live like that?

Preparing for a healthy second half of life could not only pave the way for a more pleasant menopause and retirement, it could enhance the quality of the first half of our lives. It could keep our bones and hearts strong, our breasts healthy, our choices true. It could help us find our destinies and love our lives.

༜ 6 ༜

Why Not Just Take HRT/Synthetic or Bioidentical Hormones?

Over the past half century, while our natural hormones have been work-ing overtime, governing our cycles, fertility, and patterns, and attempting to find balance amid modern stressors, synthetic hormones have stepped in to become almost as ubiquitous as their natural cousins. As we have become accustomed to take synthetic hormones to prevent pregnancy, enhance its chances, or ease menstrual or menopausal discomfort, they have encroached on almost every stage of a woman's life. In a culture that loves a quick fix and instant gratification in its medicine as well as its food, entertainment, and exercise, syn-thetic hormones have become the solution to whatever hormonal mess we've found ourselves in. Unfortunately, they may cause more problems than they cure. Bioidentical hormones may be less malignant, and growing in popularity, but I still recommend them only when changing lifestyle and diet and taking herbal supplements aren't sufficient to address the hormonal imbalance.

Synthetic Hormones

One common form of synthetic hormones is hormone replacement therapy (HRT). Many menopausal women are now familiar with weighing the risks and benefits of taking HRT. Between the 1960s and 2002, it had become standard practice to prescribe them to menopausal women. Women loved what they did for their hot flashes and their skin. Prescribing physicians loved having something to give them. As it was standard protocol to prescribe them for *every* woman over a certain age, pharmaceutical companies, presumably, loved the profits.

It is easy to be wise in retrospect. By the time the bubble burst on Western medicine's love affair with HRT and its dangers were known, it had been given to menopausal women for thirty-six years. This changed abruptly in 2002, when the National Institutes of Health (NIH) reported that they were stopping a large-scale study of the effects of animal-derived estrogen plus progestin (a synthetic progesterone-like hormone) because of the alarming increase in risk of invasive breast cancer among study participants, as well as other unacceptable risks. The report from the NIH also showed a significant rise in the risk of heart attacks (a 29 percent increase) and stroke (a 41 percent increase) among women taking the synthetic hormones. (A year later, another NIH study would show that women taking synthetic estrogen and progestin had *twice* the risk of dementia, including Alzheimer's disease.) At the time the 2002 study was halted, its acting director, Jacques Rossouw, said the adverse effects of HRT applied to all women taking HRT for menopausal symptoms, irrespective of their age.

Whether to take synthetic hormones is not only a question relevant to menopausal women. It is a question for every woman. HRT is composed of the same hormones present in birth control pills and fertility drugs. During the time when perspective was changing radically on synthetic hormone replacement for menopausal women, almost nothing was said about the possibility that these results could apply to synthetic hormonal contraceptive methods. One exception was a couple of months after the Women's Health Initiative (WHI) study was halted, when *New York Times* journalist Gina Kolata reported that scientists said there was no reason to believe that the findings applied only to Prempro, the brand of synthetic hormones most widely prescribed for menopausal women. Until proven otherwise, they said, "Women and their doctors should assume that all hormone therapy that involved estrogen and progestin bears the same risks."[1] If the dangers of HRT are clear for menopausal women, why weren't younger women suddenly being cautioned about taking the Pill or using fertility drugs to increase their chances of pregnancy? The largest study we know of on the risks of synthetic hormones may have studied menopausal women, but the risks associated with synthetic hormone use may not be confined to menopausal women. Indeed, many of the same risks associated with HRT use are known to accompany the Pill.

In 2005, just three years after the NIH study was halted, the World Health Organization would reclassify the Pill from "possibly carcinogenic to humans" to "carcinogenic to humans." It became a Class 1 carcinogen, the same as tobacco and asbestos.[2] In their book, *The Pill: Are You Sure It's for You?* authors Jane Bennett and Alexandra Pope explore effects of synthetic hormonal contraception, especially the birth control pill, and address the popular misconceptions that it is both harmless and the most effective form of contraception.[3] We'll look at all these issues and some more of their history in detail later on, in the chapters on menstrual difficulties, birth control, fertility and conception, and menopause. It would be nice if simply taking a pill could restore balance to our hormones, but in my opinion the health risks of synthetic hormones have proven too great to take the chance.

Bioidentical Hormones

The idea of bioidentical hormones isn't new, even if it seems like it from recent publicity. Some physicians have been championing them for at least a few decades, and probably for good reason. Bioidentical hormones are pretty much what they sound like. The more often prescribed and used premarin and progestins—which I will call synthetic hormones in this book—vary slightly from the naturally occurring hormones in our own bodies. Bioidentical ones are exactly the same.

Because they are the same as our own, our bodies can recognize with confidence what bioidentical hormones are, why they are there, and what to do with them. This may be the reason women seem to tolerate them better than the "synthetic" ones. I am using quotations around "synthetic" here because, in a way, bioidentical hormones are synthetic, too. They start out in plant form, like a yam, and then undergo a refining process in a lab to isolate their active ingredients. Binders, additives, and further processing transform them into pills or creams.

Some physicians have extensively prescribed bioidentical hormones and reported overwhelmingly positive results with their patients and observations. Most of the data we have on bioidentical hormone use are anecdotal, from physicians prescribing them, because extensive studies, such as the NIH study on synthetic hormones, are prohibitively expensive to run.

Why wouldn't drug companies foot the bill to study them, the way they do for the drugs they produce? It turns out you can't patent naturally occurring substances—which bioidentical hormones are, as they are identical to the hormones a woman's body produces. No patent means anybody can make them. Without a monopoly, the marginal profits don't financially justify the major expense of comprehensive studies. Drug companies have motivation to foot the bill for such studies only if they will hold the patent on the drug being tested.

Perhaps due to lack of long experience or extensive studies (though this doesn't always stop us from using something, as we will see in the course of this book), bioidentical hormones are not used, or at least widely used, to address issues of birth control or fertility, but they do have a more significant history of addressing menopausal concerns, with positive results reported. We will consider their use for menopause more in Chapter 14.

While I respect the positive reports on bioidentical hormones, and have found my own patients respond very well to their use, I still rely on them as a last resort, usually only after addressing lifestyle and dietary habits and using herbal remedies to restore hormonal balance.

My caution with bioidentical hormone use is due to three factors:

1. *New-onset breast tenderness.* The first is that I have seen new-onset breast tenderness as a symptom women often begin to experience after starting on bioidentical hormones. Most physicians I've read about who are proponents of bioidentical hormones seem unconcerned with this side effect. But I'm not so sure it's safe. I suspect that, usually, when the body exhibits some signs of discomfort, it is generally a sign that the therapy carries with it some untoward side effects. Consider the 2009 Women's Health Initiative follow-up study reported in *Archives of Internal Medicine.* It followed seventeen thousand WHI participants and found that postmenopausal women who experienced sudden onset breast tenderness when they went on combination hormone therapy (synthetic hormone therapy, that is) faced an increased risk of breast cancer. After twelve months on HRT, women who experienced this sudden-onset symptom were about 50 percent more likely than were women without breast tenderness to be diagnosed with breast cancer over the next 5.6 years. This association was not seen with women in the placebo group.[4] Since this is the case with HRT, why assume that new-onset breast tenderness after beginning bioidentical hormones is benign? We're simply not sure bioidentical hormones are exempt from the short- or long-term health risks seen with HRT. Extensive long-term studies have not been conducted on bioidentical hormones as there have been on the synthetic ones.

2. *Lack of extensive studies.* Although that may sound overly critical, because I don't insist that such extensive studies be conducted with herbal remedies, there is a difference. Most herbal remedies do not involve isolating their active ingredients and so do not have such a concentrated effect on their consumers. Which leads to my last concern:

3. *The disruption of a natural balance.* When we divorce the active ingredients from the rest of the plant's compounds, we disrupt the natural balance of the plant's qualities—a balance arrived at after thousands, if not hundreds of thousands, of years of evolution. In Eastern medicine, the plant is used without disrupting that balance. Eastern medicine does not isolate active ingredients. We would rather retain the natural balance of the plant. This is generally a safer approach that aims to deliver the qualities the body and mind crave, through the raw plant, and let the body build what it needs from them.

For example, if a woman is stressed out and exhibiting too many yang qualities such as heat, anxiety, increased heart rate, panic, or insomnia, rather than giving her synthetic or bioidentical hormones, we would aim to balance her lifestyle and diet and then give herbal remedies if necessary. We might decrease the yang qualities, or increase the yin qualities in her lifestyle and, if needed, further nourish her yin qualities with more heavy, sweet, oily, dense food; herbs; or good-quality oils. The body is then free to refine these substances further, ultimately transforming them into hormones, proteins, fats, or tissue that it requires.

Thanks to a growing awareness of the ramifications of food engineering, we are learning that, the more processed the food, the less our bodies know what to do with it, and the more side effects are possible—both for us and for the world around us. This is true whenever we alter the natural properties of a substance. The human body has evolved over millennia to metabolize and make use of certain substances. Over the last century, technology has become adept at changing these substances down to the genetic level, but our bodies have not evolved at the same pace. Eastern medicine operates under a basic assumption: Nature is smart. We are wary of adulterating her products.

Take-Home Messages from Part I

Because of all the science we got into, this may not have been an easy section to get through. Whether you made the whole trip or just caught the drift, here are the take-home messages.

- Eastern medicine considers that there are two fundamental operating principles of nature around us and within us: (1) a nourishing and calming principle called *yin*, and (2) an energizing, mobilizing, and activating principle called *yang*.

- Within our bodies, sex hormones are predominantly yin and stress hormones are predominantly yang.

- Both yin and yang hormones are essential to the maintenance and preservation of our bodies as well as our species.

- Living a life that has a good balance between yin and yang—that is, between nourishment and activity—leads to balanced hormone levels before, during, and after menopause.

- Too much yin or too much yang throws off the balance in our minds, bodies, and hormones.

- When we live too stressful a life, we put great demand on our yang stress hormones and the main organs or glands that generate or secrete them. This creates a relative increase of yang, in relation to yin.

- When our stress hormones are in danger of running low, our sex hormones can shape-shift into stress hormones to meet the demand. This drains our sex hormones and results in hormone imbalance.

- Chronic hormone imbalance of this sort is at the root of most of the health problems women have, both pre- and postmenopause.

- Synthetic hormones, whether in the form of hormone replacement therapy or birth control pills, increase the risk of breast cancer, heart attack, stroke, and all forms of dementia. They are simply not worth the risk.

- Bioidentical hormones may not carry the same risks but are still best used as a stopgap measure while improving one's diet, lifestyle, and stress management.

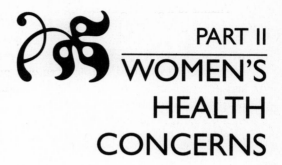

PART II

WOMEN'S
HEALTH
CONCERNS

Women's Health Concerns
AN OVERVIEW

My sister Samantha recently announced to me, "I hate when authors tell you that you have to understand the whole first half of their book in order to understand the second half." I nodded gravely—and didn't tell her that was exactly what I'd planned to say. Instead, upon reflection, I will say that browsing this part is encouraged and may yield some good insights. If you have opened this book directly to this part to troubleshoot—to see, for example, what to do about menstrual cramps or hot flashes—you'll probably learn something useful. However, it is equally true that much of the information in Part II builds on information addressed in Part I. A chief underlying cause for any of the conditions we will address here is hormone imbalance. Therefore, understanding hormonal balance is a prerequisite to understanding these issues more deeply.

Each chapter in Part II includes a section called "What Does Eastern Medicine Do About _____" followed by "What Should I Do?" These sections present an interesting challenge. As Westerners, we tend to look for a special medicine for each malady we encounter. However, just as optimal rainfall creates an environment ripe for all kinds of plants to thrive, optimal diet and lifestyle create an environment ripe for good health to overcome all kinds of health issues.

Although special herbs, dietary restrictions or lifestyle considerations may be uniquely applicable to each condition, there are certain principles that almost everybody can begin with. These principles are common to many health-care regimens that have proven successful. For example, Dr. Dean Ornish has demonstrated the benefits of many of these principles for heart health, and Dr. David Servan-Schreiber wrote about their anticancer value. Somebody else may demonstrate the effectiveness of these principles in combating depression. These principles create a physiological and psychological terrain that favors health and deters imbalance of all kinds.

Part III will address the principles of diet, lifestyle, and stress management, which are the main treatment strategies for *every* health concern we will discuss here in Part II. That being said, we will address some matters that are specific to each of these health considerations, some of which I will discuss here, and many of which would be best addressed in person with a Traditional Chinese Medicine practitioner or Ayurvedic consultant.

In the absence of compelling reasons for a different approach, I generally suggest a three-tier treatment strategy for regaining one's health:

1. Make appropriate diet, lifestyle, and stress-reduction changes first.
2. Use natural herbs and remedies when extra support is needed.
3. Use surgery, pharmaceutical, or bioidentical drugs in an emergency; as a stopgap measure when physical, mental, or emotional symptoms are unbearable; or to manage such symptoms when first-tier and second-tier strategies are insufficient.

At the end of Part III, after we've covered the elements of the first-tier strategy in depth, we'll revisit this philosophy and look at how to work with it.

• • •

Eastern medical perspectives can offer great clarity, but it is also sometimes useful to familiarize ourselves with Western science that supports these perspectives. When we can see where the two approaches agree, those more familiar with Western medicine become more comfortable with the Eastern approach. In the best of Eastern medicine, we usually do not offer a single remedy for a symptom. We recommend changes in lifestyle and diet, and perhaps the addition of herbal remedies. Then we watch and consider what happens to the person's whole system over time. It is not possible to study the effect of an herb someone is taking, for example, separately from the effects of the lifestyle and dietary changes she is making. If we want to evaluate the efficacy of this holistic kind of approach, it would be best to use an outcome-based method of evaluation.

Just as it takes a combination of a stressful life, poor diet, and inappropriate exercise to arrive at a state of imbalance, it requires changes to all of these to treat the root causes of imbalance.

While we may not be able to rely on scientific studies to prove everything we are doing to heal ourselves, we can certainly apply common sense to the issues that affect us and arrive at our own conclusions. We can acquire a basic understanding of hormones and women's health, and how they are affected by the manner in which we live our lives. Armed with this education, we can begin to make choices that restore, support, and maintain balanced hormones, healthy bodies, and deeply contented spirits.

Feeling Crummy
OUR BEST EARLY-
WARNING SYSTEM

During our first consultation, Elaine told me that she'd felt stressed out for about a year. Her thinking was foggy, she wasn't sleeping well, she had little energy, and she suffered frequent heartburn. Her period had become a little lighter than it had been a year ago, and she felt little twinges of ache in her right ovary around ovulation. Nothing, she said, was bad enough to take painkillers or to affect her work, but she just didn't feel right. She had gone to her Western medical doctor, seeking some explanation, but all her blood work and other tests came back normal. Although Elaine was glad nothing serious was going on, she was disturbed, too. She had never sought acupuncture or Ayurvedic counseling before, but she came to me because she was unwilling to accept that her recent emotional and physical changes might be here to stay. She was seeking a way to return to the level of health she had experienced before.

Long before a disease has progressed far enough for Western medicine to diagnose it, there are signs that something is wrong. Like Elaine, we may just feel crummy. Nothing big. Just little things that don't significantly alter our lives or lifestyles or even show up on a Western medical chart, blood test, X-ray, urine test, ultrasound, MRI, or thermometer. But they hover in the background, affecting our quality of life and giving us the nagging feeling that all is not right with our world. This may be the wisdom of intuition, because all may not, in fact, be right with our world.

We live in a world that has a love affair with yang qualities, to the exclusion of yin. Spiritual goals, emotional equanimity, and physical nourishment are sacrificed for professional or social ambition. Success is measured by our ability to set and meet professional or peer-related goals, to climb the ladder as fast as we can. Many of us, oblivious to other means of measuring success, have adopted these ubiquitous values as the settings for our personal autopilots. We are so committed to this default course that we don't even notice when we start feeling crummy. Or we notice it, but ignore it in favor of pushing on. Or maybe we aren't even aware of the difference between feeling whole and healthy, and feeling crummy.

Here are the symptoms of "feeling crummy." Even if they are mild or intermittent, they tell us that something is out of balance with our yin, yang, or both. We experience:

- Confused or foggy thinking
- Little aches and pains
- Stress, irritability, or depression
- Poorer short-term memory than normal
- Heavier or lighter periods than usual
- Fatigue or lethargy
- Hot flashes
- Insomnia
- Mild headaches
- Minor digestive complaints, such as gas, bloating, heartburn, constipation, or loose stools
- Lack of appetite

To balance our hormones, we need good-quality yang and good-quality yin daily. There is no herb, supplement, or drug that can entirely take the place of having an appropriate daily diet, lifestyle, and stress-management routine. I suspect this is why Hippocrates swore to "prescribe regimens for the good of my patients." There is no way pills and potions can counteract the effects of all the stressful things we expose our bodies and minds to, throughout our days and our lives.

We can support good-quality yang by doing appropriate exercise, taking time to inspire ourselves daily, and engaging in mentally stimulating activities. Indulging in a stressful, overly ambitious, frantically busy life fosters poor-quality yang.

We can nourish good-quality yin by ensuring that our diets consists of healthy food, taking time every day to enjoy solitude and quiet contemplative time, and engaging in loving relationships. We promote poor-quality yin if we indulge in lethargy or inactivity and eat poor-quality food such as junk food, fast food, or highly processed or refined food.

What Does Eastern Medicine Do About "Feeling Crummy"?

Feeling crummy is about so much more than feeling crummy. It belies imbalance in your body, mind, and, more than likely, your hormones. Eastern medicine addresses all medical problems first and foremost by establishing a healthy diet, the first pillar of health.

Eastern medicine recommends eating mostly whole, freshly cooked food that is mostly vegetarian. Our bodies have evolved to know how to digest and assimilate these foods. Cooking them helps us digest them easier. Whole foods include vegetables, fruits, whole grains (like brown rice, millet, quinoa, and oats), beans, honey, maple syrup, dairy, and meats. It is best to eat organic, when possible, especially dairy and meat. The fresher these foods are, the better. It is best to avoid canned, frozen, or leftover foods.

The second and third pillars of health are, respectively, lifestyle and stress management. These are like the red and white stripes of a candy cane. They are intertwined aspects of the same structure. They support each other and cannot exist separately. If we have an appropriate lifestyle, this goes a long way to manage our stress; likewise, the things we do that especially serve to manage stress become incorporated into our lifestyles. Having a daily routine is a crucial part of health. When the body adjusts to a daily routine, and learns to count on it, the nervous system can relax. Ayurveda prescribes a routine where we do the same things at the same times, daily if possible. In Ayurveda, a healthy, low-stress lifestyle means having a daily routine that includes such elements as getting appropriate regular exercise and sufficient sleep, meditating or having some other nourishing spiritual practice, and doing self-massage and special breathing exercises.

What Should I Do?

> We cannot do everything at once, but we can do something at once.
> —CALVIN COOLIDGE

Making dietary and lifestyle changes like those just described may seem difficult. The most common reason I hear for not being able to make these changes is time. There's not enough of it. And if we cut out some of the things we currently do to make the time, we're afraid our lives will fall apart. But there is more than one way to live a life. What I have found over and over again is, if we cut out something to make room for crucial dietary and lifestyle elements, our lives don't fall apart.

When we start with a couple of changes that feel doable, our lives begin to improve. As we begin to feel better and become more motivated to make more changes, they begin to improve exponentially. In fact, not only does life not fall apart, we find it gets better than we ever dared hope. If we start by taking baby steps toward these goals (as I describe), strength and stamina can improve, and our nervous systems can find relief and begin to heal. We can begin to remember what health feels like.

HOW TO JUMP-START IMPROVING YOUR DIET

Without stressing yourself out, see if you can take one (or more) of the following steps. When you are ready, take another one. You don't have to reinvent your entire diet in one day or one week or one month. Do what you can, and when you can, add something else or take something away. A longer, more detailed discussion of optimal diet, lifestyle, and stress-management techniques can be found in Part III, and you'll find even more suggestions for relevant books and Web sites in Appendix A. Here are some basic guidelines to begin with.

1. Start by making a list of whole foods you like. Are you partial to fresh fruits? Grains like millet or quinoa? (Don't confuse whole grains with products made of whole wheat flour. Flour is ground-up grain and does not have all the benefits of whole grain.) See if you can find recipes that use whole foods you already like. (You'll find some on my Web site, www.drclaudiawelch.com, via a link from my Articles and Publications page.) In Appendix A, I've also listed some cookbooks that rely on whole foods—with recipes that are satisfying and delicious.

2. Once you've found recipes that you like, try to begin by eating freshly cooked, whole foods one day a week. Oatmeal, cracked wheat, and creamed buckwheat (one of my favorites) are all examples of whole-grain breakfasts. One breakfast I learned to make in Colombia is quinoa cooked with fresh ginger and whole milk. Add some maple syrup and it's a real treat. One of my husband's and my favorite dinners is organic brown or basmati rice; steamed broccoli with olive oil, sea salt, and fresh lemon juice drizzled over it; and fried tofu. To get you started, here are some suggestions of simple whole foods and how to prepare them.

Whole Grains

Here's a simple starter stir-fry that's easy to prepare and is delicious in its simplicity:

Quinoa with Simple Veggies
Serves 3 to 4

INGREDIENTS
1 CUP QUINOA
2 TABLESPOONS EXTRA-VIRGIN OLIVE OIL
  (ORGANIC, IF POSSIBLE)
1 CUP DICED ONION (ANY KIND)
1 CUP DICED CARROT
1 CUP DICED CELERY
2 CUPS WATER
FRESHLY GROUND BLACK PEPPER
SEA SALT OR ROCK SALT

First, prepare the quinoa. In a fine-mesh strainer, rinse the quinoa well under cool water (make sure you rinse it, to remove the natural bitterness). Set aside.

Pour the olive oil into a heavy-bottomed, medium-size saucepan over medium heat. Add the onions, carrots, and celery, and sauté until the onions are translucent. Add the rinsed quinoa, along with the water. Bring to a boil, then lower the heat to simmer. Cover and cook until the water is absorbed, about 15 minutes. Add salt and pepper to taste.

Rice and Stir-Fried Veggies

INGREDIENTS
1 CUP RAW ORGANIC WHITE OR BROWN OR WILD, UNPOLISHED, UNBLEACHED RICE
2 CUPS WATER
2 TABLESPOONS EXTRA-VIRGIN OLIVE OIL (ORGANIC, IF POSSIBLE)
1 MEDIUM-SIZE ONION
2 TO 3 CUPS CHOPPED VEGGIES (SEE NOTE)
1 TABLESPOON GRATED FRESH GINGER
SOY SAUCE OR TAMARI
FRESHLY GROUND BLACK PEPPER

Wash the rice in a strainer. Let drain. Place in a heavy-bottomed saucepan with the water. Bring to a boil over medium-high heat, then lower the heat to a simmer. Cover and cook until the water is absorbed and the rice is tender. The time varies according to the kind of rice, although it will generally be about 20 minutes for white rice and about an hour for brown rice.

In another pan, sauté the onion in the olive oil, over medium heat, until translucent. Mix the veggies and ginger into the onion, lower the heat a little, and cover the pan. Check and stir every few minutes to be sure the veggies are not sticking on the bottom. If they begin to stick, add about 1/4 cup of water and cover again. Cook until the veggies are tender. The time will vary according to what vegetables you are using, but it is likely to be about 15 minutes. Add soy sauce and black pepper to taste. Serve either over or next to the rice.

NOTE: YOU CAN USE ANY VEGGIES THAT APPEAL TO YOU, SUCH AS CARROTS, BROCCOLI, KALE, BELL PEPPERS, ZUCCHINI, SUMMER SQUASH, MUSHROOMS, AND SO ON. CHOP VEGGIES THAT TAKE LONGER TO COOK SMALLER THAN VEGGIES THAT COOK MORE QUICKLY. FOR EXAMPLE, CHOP CARROTS SMALLER THAN BROCCOLI.

Replacing rice with other whole grains or pastas:

- Try experimenting with kasha or millet by cooking them the same way as the rice (a one-to-two ratio). Note that you usually don't need to wash these grains.
- Organic soba noodles (buckwheat pasta) are a delicious, healthy change from regular pasta. Cook according to the directions on the package and serve with vegetables or sauce.

Beans

- Soak a cup of aduki or black beans overnight (at least 8 hours) in cool water. The next day, sauté some diced onions in extra-virgin olive oil along with about 2 tablespoons of grated fresh ginger. Place the mixture in a large stockpot. Add the beans and enough water to cover them by 2 to 3 inches. Add a couple of strips of kombu and bring to a boil. Lower the heat to a simmer and cook until the beans are soft. Then remove the kombu and add some tamari and freshly ground black pepper to taste. Serve with rice and steamed kale, chard, or spinach.

- Eat tacos made with whole or refried pinto beans. You can cook the pinto beans like the aduki or black beans, as above, but without the ginger. Substitute salt for the tamari.

- Buy or make some hummus. It's a blend of cooked, mashed chickpeas, tahini (ground sesame seeds), olive oil, lemon juice, salt, plus garlic, if it agrees with you. Eat it with whole-grain flatbread, or as a dip for raw veggies in the summer or steamed veggies in the winter.

Hummus

INGREDIENTS
2 CUPS DRIED CHICKPEAS, SOAKED OVERNIGHT (SEE NOTE)
5 TO 6 CUPS WATER
½ CUP TAHINI
3 TABLESPOONS SOY SAUCE OR TAMARI
JUICE OF 1 MEDIUM-SIZE LEMON
1 CLOVE GARLIC, CRUSHED, IF IT AGREES WITH YOU
FRESHLY GROUND BLACK PEPPER

Drain the soaked chickpeas and place them in a heavy-bottomed saucepan (or pressure cooker if you have one and know how to use it). Add the water and bring to a boil. Lower heat the heat to a simmer and cook until they are very soft. It may take a few hours. When they are soft, turn off the heat and allow to cool. Then drain the chickpeas, saving the water in a dish. In a medium-size bowl, mash the chickpeas into a paste, adding some of the water you saved, if you want a thinner consistency. Mix in the rest of the ingredients well. Eat immediately or save in a sealed container in the refrigerator, where the hummus will keep well for a few days. Use as a sandwich spread, with lettuce, sprouts, cucumbers, or tomatoes, or as a dip for crackers or raw veggies.

NOTE: PUT THE CHICKPEAS IN A BOWL AND COVER WITH ABOUT 4 INCHES OF WATER. THEY WILL SOAK IT UP BY MORNING.

Whole Vegetables

- Steamed veggies with a drizzle of olive oil and fresh lemon or lime juice.
- Vegetable soups (It is ideal to make your own, but if you purchase boxed or canned, make sure to look at the ingredients, as most packaged soups rely on salt and highly processed, hard-to-pronounce-or-digest chemicals for flavor.)
- Sautéed vegetables (most veggies do well sautéed in 2 tablespoons of olive oil).
- Baked yams.
- Roasted potatoes, onions, carrots, peppers, and cauliflower. Dice, coat with olive oil, and add a bit of thyme, oregano, salt, and pepper. Bake in a single layer on a cookie sheet at 400°F until done, about 35 minutes. Turn them every 7 to 10 minutes.
- Salad, if in the summer or in the middle of the day when the heat in the environment supports our digestive capacities. Make sure to mix dark, leafy greens (forgoing iceberg lettuce, for the most part) with other fresh veggies, such as grated carrots, cucumbers, or sliced radishes or red bell peppers. Try making your own salad dressings, rather than relying on store-bought varieties that often contain high-fructose corn syrup, monosodium glutamate (MSG), and other additives and preservatives.

Dairy

- Add some mild, white farmer cheese to a salad or to steamed veggies for extra grounding influence.
- Warm rice pudding made with milk
- A couple of hours before bed, have a cup of hot, whole milk with a pinch of saffron, nutmeg, and cinnamon, sweetened with a tablespoon of pure maple syrup. If you are lactose intolerant, try soy, rice, almond, or hemp milk. (Hemp milk is made from the seeds of the hemp plant, but contains none of the mind-altering THC that is found in the more famous, less legal, use of hemp.)

Additional Considerations

- Avoid eating too many flour products, especially ones made from refined white flour. Many of us begin our day with toast and cold cereal made from flour, have a sandwich for lunch, eat cookies or a pastry for a snack, and for dinner have pasta and a flour-based dessert, such as cake. Although flour is a convenient, quick way to satisfy cravings and appetite, having a lot of it tends to clog the digestive system and smother the digestive ability. It's like putting waterlogged wood on a fire. Bread and pasta made from whole wheat, whole brown rice, or buckwheat are less clogging and often tasty. Including some flour in our diets on a regular basis is fine, but it's still better to avoid having it at every meal and to instead eat whole grains. Enjoying the occasional bagel, cookie, slice of pie, or grilled cheese on white bread is not the end of the world, but doing so more than a few times a week starts to tax the digestive system. If the digestive system is unhealthy, doing so even a couple times a week may be too much.

- In addition to lowering your intake of white flour, avoid alcohol, refined sugar, and more than one caffeinated beverage (8 to 12 ounces) daily. These items often hinder the digestive process or aggravate the nervous system and end up acting like poison in the body.

- If you drink coffee, buy organic coffee. More about this in Chapter 13.

- Make a list of the processed foods you now eat. See which can be most easily eliminated or can be replaced by a whole-grain substitute. If you do buy processed foods like cookies and breads, at least read the ingredients list. The fewer ingredients, the better. The more mystery ingredients—the ones that sound like chemicals instead of food—the less the chance that you are purchasing anything that could be called "whole."

- Switch to buying organic meat and dairy products. Buy organic produce, grains, and beans whenever possible.

- Top ten foods to buy organic: any meat, any dairy, celery, peaches, strawberries, apples, blueberries, spinach, kale, and potatoes. (The Environmental Working Group [EWG] regularly updates their "dirty dozen" list of fruits and veggies with the most pesticide residue, at www.foodnews.org/sneak/EWG-shoppers -guide.pdf.)

- Avoid hydrogenated fats (lard, shortening, margarine) and never eat trans fats.

- Artificial sweeteners are okay—for killing ants. My husband and I put a little of one brand on our counters to kill ants. It doesn't work quite as well as boric acid, maybe because the ants don't seem to like it that much—an example of the natural intelligence of ants, perhaps, because artificial sweeteners are crummy for us. Don't use them.

- Avoid iced drinks, especially with meals. Cold liquid hinders the digestive process.

The Wisdom of Michael Pollan

Most of these points, though based on ancient Eastern medicine and my own experience, sound a little like a CliffsNotes version of Michael Pollan's excellent and entertaining book *In Defense of Food*. If you haven't read it, you're missing one of the best modern books I know on diet and whole food. It's listed in Appendix A. I love it when current insight and perspective, based on solid, sophisticated modern research, resoundingly agrees with ancient Eastern medical philosophy. Pollan's book is a prime example.

HOW TO JUMP-START IMPROVING YOUR LIFESTYLE

As with the jump-start information about diet, when you read the following suggestions, choose one you can start with, and start as small as you need to. Make it your daily routine. When you are comfortable doing this, add another of the elements to your routine. Detailed explanations of each of these elements are in Chapters 25 (on lifestyle) and 26 (on stress management).

1. Wake as early as you can (predawn is ideal) and meditate, e templation, or read inspirational material. Do this for five t longer, depending on the nature of your spiritual practice. I meditation practice, this could be a time of prayer, or for gent cises that you can learn from a yoga practitioner. In any case, should quiet the mind. This is useful for calming the spirit and ...e pace for a less stressful day. Again, feel free to start in increments as brief as five minutes. Do whatever you can do.

2. Apply warm oil to your body. This can take as little as 2 to 3 minutes or as much as twenty (see Chapter 26). This has an incredibly calming effect on the nervous system. Having a less trigger-happy nervous system means less stress hormones are circulating, and this leads to more balanced hormones.

3. Bathe, dress, then exercise for 20 to 30 minutes. This can be a combination of brisk walking, gentle stretching or yoga, tai chi, qi gong, hiking, or biking, depending on your energy and stamina.

4. If you won't have time to cook later in the day, cook in the morning for the rest of the day. Try to avoid keeping hot foods or liquids in plastic containers. If you keep food in plastic containers, just make sure it is cool before you put it in them.

5. Have breakfast, lunch, and dinner at the same times every day.

6. Remember to breathe deeply throughout the day.

7. Slow down, in general. Stop multitasking. It dissipates energy. Studies have also shown that multitasking has a detrimental effect on mental processes, even when you are not engaged in it. Do one thing at a time. This will encourage focused, calmer energy. We'll look at this more closely in Part III.

8. As one of my teachers told me when I was eight years old, "Keep good company. Good company makes a man great." Spending time with loving people who have healthy habits supports our own healthy habits.

9. Watch less than ten hours of TV a week. I'll talk more about this in Chapter 25.

10. Spend the evening quieting the mind and body, in preparation for bed. If you have insomnia or don't sleep enough, see the suggestions in Chapter 25 in Part III. However, you may find your sleep difficulties will resolve by themselves after a few weeks of following these basic lifestyle and diet guidelines.

11. Retire at the same time each evening.

This routine is one that usually works for just about anybody, health permitting, but can be modified for individuals according to their special needs or considerations. And, if daily doesn't work for you, doing this three times a week will still begin to create a great foundation. You'll notice that most of the to-do list happens even before breakfast. This sets the tone for the day (much the same way early childhood sets the stage for life), and ensures that some of the most important things we can do to maintain or restore our health will not get lost over the course of the day. It's sometimes more effective to work the really important things into morning routines, before the demands of the day crowd them out. Although simple, these might be the hardest changes. They also might be the most important and rewarding.

If we opt not to make the lifestyle and dietary changes necessary to improve our lives, we may run into problems. The nature of these problems will be determined by constitution, stage of life, environment, and genetic disposition. In the following chapters we will look at how our life stages and health conditions are affected by the way we think, eat, and live.

Menstruation

Why We Have Cycles

Menstruation is evidence of a woman's fertility. It reflects the condition of yin and yang in her body. When the quality and quantity of yin is healthy, she has a healthy, moderate flow. As long as her yang is balanced, she will enjoy regularly timed cycles. When yin and yang are out of balance in quantity or quality, she may suffer from painful, heavy, scanty, or irregular periods, headaches, skin breakouts, or extreme emotions accompanying her cycle. A woman's menstrual cycle is a great indicator of her hormonal balance, and when it is accompanied by unpleasant symptoms, she can change her lifestyle or diet to help restore balance and end her symptoms.

Although the obvious reason for a woman's cycle is fertility, menstruation has other beneficial effects. Scientist Margie Profet of the University of California at Berkeley received the MacArthur Genius Award in 1993 for thinking outside the box about menstruation. Profet suggested that a woman's menstrual cycle may have evolved in part to protect the health of her reproductive organs. If so, taking hormones that block or stop a woman's periods would place her at higher risk for disease in these organs. Let's look closer at Profet's theory.

Menstrual blood is rich in immune cells and is the only blood in the body that doesn't clot. This means that when menstrual blood flows, it freely bathes and cleanses the uterus, cervix, and vagina with its antibacterial, antiviral properties. Profet suggested that the evolutionary purpose of our monthly discharge of menstrual blood is to protect a woman's reproductive organs from invasive disease. This is especially important when a woman is sexually active, as sperm cells invariably have bacteria that hitch rides with them. Although cervical mucus usually inhibits the passage of these bacteria into the upper reproductive tract, this mucus is much more permeable during ovulation to allow the sperm's passage to the waiting egg.[1] Once allowed passage, the sperm finds the endometrial lining, which remains until it is clear that this month's egg has not been fertilized. If the woman does not become pregnant, her endometrial lining sloughs off, creating her menstrual flow, depriving any invasive bacteria of a permanent home and exerting its antibacterial, antiviral effects.

Aside from being particularly important for a woman to have her period when she is sexually active, there are other causes of inflammation or bacterial infection in the reproductive system, and a woman's cycle may help suppress these invaders as well. For example, women who use intrauterine devices (IUDs) often experience a flow that is heavier than their pre-IUD cycles. IUDs can cause chronic inflammation. The cycle of a woman who uses an IUD may become heavier to cleanse this area and decrease the potential for disease to get the upper hand in an organ crucial to our species' survival.

This raises the question as to how a woman's reproductive health is protected during times when she naturally doesn't menstruate; namely, during pregnancy and after menopause. The answer is that postmenopausal women have thicker cervical mucus, which creates more of a barrier. This is also true for the first seven months of pregnancy. So during these times, it is less necessary for a woman to have a period to guard against pathogenic factors—infectious agents or germs that may cause trouble in her reproductive organs. During the last two months of pregnancy, a woman's cervical mucus becomes more permeable, which is why doctors often advise women to have their partners use condoms during this time, to prevent the introduction of sperm-borne pathogens.[2]

If Profet is right, it is unhealthy to suppress menstruation, especially when women are sexually active.[3] This is an especially timely concern with the increased availability and popularity of chemical birth control that seeks to all but eliminate a woman's cycle.

A woman's healthy cycle is indicative of her fertility, which in turn is evidence of her baseline good health. Evolution has invested many millennia and showed remarkable success in the design of a woman's reproductive patterns and organs. Over the last couple decades, however, menstruation seems to have fallen out of favor. There are now methods of birth control designed to liberate women from what is seen as an unnecessary burden. What evolution took ages and pains—no pun intended—to create, we are trying, in record time, to bypass with the assistance of synthetic hormones.

Eliminating Cycles

There is a modern trend to think that periods create trouble in more ways than one. Not only can they cause pain and inconvenience, they also increase a woman's lifetime exposure to estrogen, because estrogen spikes monthly with her cycle. The concern is that a modern woman has more periods over the course of her life than did women in earlier times. Women of those bygone eras are presumed to have menstruated fewer times due to later onset of menarche, more pregnancies, and shorter life spans. They also had a lower incidence of breast cancer. Therefore, some believe that the modern prevalence of breast cancer is associated with women having more menstrual cycles and thus more lifetime exposure to estrogen. The argument goes that doing away with a woman's period, or at least a number of them, will reduce her chances of breast cancer.

It's true that increased exposure to estrogen is linked to an increased risk of breast cancer.[4] The more cycles a woman has in her life, the greater her overall exposure to monthly surges in estradiol. This means that the later a woman gets her period, the earlier her onset of menopause, the more pregnancies she has, and the longer she nurses, the less she is exposed to these surges. As we might expect, then, less breast cancer is seen in these women than those with more periods over the course of their lives, whether because of early menarche, late menopause, fewer babies, or shorter duration of nursing.[5]

There has been a movement over the past decade or so that follows this line of thinking to a pharmaceutical conclusion. If women take birth control pills—that is, synthetic hormone therapy—for each day of their cycle, then they would not have a period at all. John Rock, the original promoter of birth control pills, gave women placebo pills for one week of every month, not so that they would have an actual period—which is eliminated for women on the Pill, but so they would have enough "breakthrough bleeding" that the pattern would resemble a natural cycle, and thereby be less likely to draw opposition from the Church. One current theory is that women would benefit from being on hormone therapy so consistently that even the breakthrough bleeding that accompanies the Pill is eliminated. Stopping or severely limiting the frequency of a woman's cycle, the argument goes, would decrease a woman's lifetime exposure to estrogen and thereby decrease her risk of breast cancer.[6]

This thinking, in part, has led to synthetic hormone prescriptions that result in fewer or no periods. Take Seasonale, for example. Women take Seasonale for eighty-four days in a row. Then they stop it for seven days and bleed. The result is only four weeks per year when they bleed.

This is thought provoking. Even aside from the possibility that Margie Profet is right about the disease-preventive role of monthly periods, attempting to reduce a woman's lifetime exposure to estrogen by giving her a daily dose of synthetic estrogen and progestin (a synthetic progesterone-like hormone) seems ironic. Yes, taking hormone replacement therapy like this will reduce the estrogen surges present in a natural menstrual cycle, and will thereby reduce a woman's overall lifetime exposure to estradiol, a potent natural estrogen. But it will also increase her lifetime exposure to synthetic hormones. Remember that birth control pills are synthetic hormones, as is HRT. We have seen how detrimental synthetic hormone replacement can be, and, ironically, how synthetic hormone therapy itself may increase the risk of breast cancer. It also carries a risk of blood clots, strokes, and other serious side effects.

It would be more useful to identify and eliminate the causes of a woman's hormone imbalance that in itself leads to increased risk of breast cancer and other disorders. Some causes are poor dietary and exercise habits, environmental stressors, pollutants, and psychological stress. We have seen that the most common type of breast cancer actually decreased when women went off HRT—the same hormones present in synthetic birth control prescriptions. Considering the side effects of synthetic hormones, one of which is increased breast cancer if the pill is taken before a woman reaches her early twenties, it seems a risky gamble to use them to reduce her chances of breast cancer—especially since there are so many other things a woman can safely and effectively do to reduce those risks. We'll look at this in depth in Chapter 13.

We have already discussed problems related to synthetic hormone use. It increases the risk of heart attacks, strokes, blood clots, Alzheimer's, and possibly hearing loss. Remember, too, that there is reason to suspect that synthetic hormones are problematic for all women, not only postmenopausal women. There are further considerations as well, not the least of which is that replacing the body's naturally occurring hormones is tricky business.

The body's hormonal demands and levels naturally change on an hourly basis.[7] Whereas the body's natural feedback mechanisms relay how much of which hormone is needed at any given time, synthetic hormones suppress and replace the body's natural hormonal response. Synthetic hormones are neither taken in the context of that sensitive feedback loop nor balanced by other naturally occurring substances. Thus, they cannot deliver the exact level of hormone needed in the bloodstream at any given time. This consistent over- or underdosing may cause problems that may eventually strain our organs or glands to the point where we begin to experience side effects that were not apparent earlier. It's just like eating a high-fat hamburger with fries. This may have some mild immediate effects, like heartburn, but it is only the cumulative effect of habitual use that will enable us to see the real effects. If we routinely eat hamburgers and fries for years, our organs or vessels will be strained enough to deliver more serious side effects, such as high blood pressure or thickening of plaque on the artery walls.

SIDE EFFECTS OF ELIMINATING CYCLES

When we turn to synthetic hormones to limit the frequency of the cycle, we can experience serious side effects.

Debbie was twenty-five years old when she came to see me. Although her periods had never been painful, irregular, or associated with mood swings, she felt they interfered with her sex life and were inconvenient. She went on Depo-Provera, an injection of synthetic progestin, so that she would not have periods for three months.

After gaining ten pounds and developing moody cycles of rage and depression, she decided that the inconvenience of having a monthly period was not as big an issue as the side effects from the Depo. When her first three months were up, she decided not to get another Depo injection. She did not expect what would follow. She bled for nine days and stopped for three. Then she bled for fifteen days and stopped for seven, bled again for twenty days and stopped for nine. This irregular heavy bleeding continued for months. Debbie was soaking through four pads an hour on the days she bled. She became anemic and exhausted. It took five months for her cycle to return to normal. When I teach a class full of women and ask for a show of hands of those who have experienced firsthand, or know a friend who has experienced, a similar reaction to Depo, there are always hands raised. This is not surprising considering its impressive list of potential side effects, which includes irregular, heavy or loss of menses, headaches, nervousness, mood changes, breast tenderness, decreased sex drive, acne, hair loss, muscle pain, heart palpitations, jaundice, blood clots, severe allergic reactions, infertility, severe depression, heavy or prolonged vaginal bleeding, five- to ten-pound weight gain that occurs in more than 70 percent of its users, and irreversible loss of bone density with prolonged use. Synthetic progesterone in the form of Depo-Provera has been seen to cause rapid proliferation of breast cells, a condition that predisposes to breast cancer, and there is conflicting evidence that it increases the risk of cervical cancers. It also causes bones to leak calcium, possibly predisposing a woman to osteoporosis after menopause, so it is recommended not to take Depo-Provera for more than two years.

A small number of women may be motivated to take synthetic hormones to limit their lifetime estrogen exposure, but this isn't the main reason young women are taking them and physicians are prescribing them. The main reason is for birth control, and the second is for menstrual difficulties, both of which we'll discuss shortly.

What Does Eastern Medicine Do About Menstruation?

A fundamental difference between Western and Eastern medicine is the issue of control. Western medicine believes it can control a woman's cycles and health better than nature can. From an Eastern perspective, intentionally stopping a woman's period will lead to stagnation in her reproductive organs and to adulteration of the natural intelligence of the body—both conditions that lead to health concerns ranging from irregular heavy bleeding like Debbie's, to endometriosis, tumors, endocrine disorders, and other serious conditions.

In Eastern medicine, menstruation is considered a natural physiological process that reflects the condition of a woman's overall health and the balance of her yin (sex) and yang (stress) hormones. If a woman's yang hormones are balanced, her cyclic timing is regular. When her yin hormones are balanced, she has both good-quality and -quantity yin, and her cycle is neither scanty nor too heavy.

Traditional Chinese Medicine and Ayurveda agree that a woman's cycle should naturally be about twenty-eight days from the first day of her period to the first day of her next period. Her cycle should be three to five days and have healthy, moderately bright red blood in a moderate amount. She should have no cramps or discomfort and no emotional upset before, during, or after her cycle.

If her cycle follows this natural rhythm, it is a good indication that her hormonal balance and general health are in good shape. If she is on birth control pills or other forms of synthetic hormones, they will mask the true condition of her health by covering up hormonal imbalance. If a woman is having difficulty with her cycle, Traditional Chinese Medicine and Ayurveda will address issues in her lifestyle and diet and then may treat her with herbs and or acupuncture to restore a balanced rhythm to her cycle and health.

In the following chapter, we will see what happens to a woman's cycle if she has insufficient yin, too much poor-quality yin, or conditions reflecting a state of stagnation in her reproductive organs, and how to address those issues. In general, if a woman is consuming a diet that offers good quality nourishment, or yin, and an exercise and meditation routine that supports healthy yang, her cycle should be painless and regular.

What Should I Do?

1. Follow the three pillars of health described in Part III: appropriate diet, lifestyle, and stress management. (Suggestions for how to get started in these areas were listed on pages 46–52.)

2. Avoid contraception or medication that eliminates or reduces the frequency of your menstrual cycle, especially if you are sexually active.

3. If you are currently taking synthetic hormones, be sure to consult with a qualified health-care practitioner to learn how best to eliminate them from your system, but still practice some form of effective birth control if you are not ready to have babies. (See Chapter 11.)

4. If you have irregular or painful cycles, read the following chapter, on menstrual difficulties, and consult with a qualified practitioner of Traditional Chinese Medicine or Ayurveda.

5. Read *Taking Charge of Your Fertility: The Definitive Guide to Natural Birth Control, Pregnancy Achievement, and Reproductive Health* by Toni Weschler, MPH. This book is a wonderful guide to learning about your healthy cycle and to troubleshooting irregularities.

ఌ 10 ఌ

Menstrual Difficulties

Many Western physicians prescribe birth control pills to help manage the pain and heavy bleeding that some women experience with their cycles. This, birth control pills undoubtedly do, but we have already seen that there is a price to be paid for choosing this solution to the problem. Eastern medicine takes a less risky approach.

Like other medical systems, Traditional Chinese Medicine and Ayurveda excel at treating certain disorders but can take longer to resolve other complaints. In my experience, menstrual difficulties usually respond beautifully to treatment with TCM or Ayurveda. Let's look at the three most common problems: scanty or absent periods, heavy or painful periods, and irregular periods. We'll particularly consider how they can be addressed without resorting to synthetic hormones.

Scanty or Absent Periods

The quantity of flow of a woman's cycle, like everything else, reflects her balance of yin and yang. As yin relates to substance, a scanty cycle usually indicates a lack of good-quality yin—or good-quality nutrition, most commonly due to not eating enough or to exercising too much.

It is well known and documented that a woman's period may become scanty or irregular, or even disappear if she engages in strenuous athletic activities, or if she has insufficient nutrition. Intense physical training consumes a lot of yin. It is important for a woman to replace that yin, otherwise her nourishment in general and her sex hormones in particular will diminish.

According to a study published in the *Journal of Clinical Endocrinology and Metabolism*, eating more can reverse cases of exercise-induced absence of periods.[1] When estrogen is reduced due to excessive exercise over a prolonged period, it not only affects the menstrual cycle but may also contribute to increased risk of heart disease and dangerously low bone density.[2] Appropriate exercise and diet supports good bone density; excessive exercise and insufficient nutrition can decrease it.

Jennifer was a runner. She was twenty-seven. She was very slender and ran three to five miles a day, about five times a week. After running for a year, her periods had become very light. She bled only a little and only for two days. After another two years of running, she started missing a period every couple of months. When she came to see me, she had not had a period for a year. She and her new husband knew they wanted children and she was concerned about her fertility.

I told Jennifer that, according to Eastern medicine, she really needed to restore her yin and that it would be ideal if she could trade running for a gentler form of exercise. She was resistant to this idea, as running kept her emotionally stable. If she missed her training, she said, she would slide into depression and frustration. We came to a compromise. She would substitute half of her running days with yoga days. On her yoga days, she would do an hour of a slow, stretchy form that focused more on circulation of *prana* than on straining muscles, and fifteen minutes of slow alternate-nostril breathing—a form of *pranayama* (breathing exercise). Jennifer didn't need to change her diet, which was already healthy and nourishing. She was simply expending way more energy than she was taking in. She couldn't eat enough to sustain the demands of her excessive exercise routine. Within three months of beginning her revised exercise routine, Jennifer's periods returned, albeit lightly. They were regular, and she was more confident that, when the time came, she could become pregnant. She developed her own yoga and *pranayama* routine that she became as attached to as she had been to her running, and she began to consider joining a yoga teacher's training program. After about two years, her cycle had normalized and she became pregnant.

Jennifer's story is not uncommon. When women become addicted to the endorphin high that accompanies serious training, this can outweigh the reality of their diminishing yin and disappearing cycles. Asking a devoted runner to stop running can be about as fruitful as asking a heroin addict to switch to mint tea. Although it might be crucial for her hormone balance that she stop running and switch to a gentler, more yin form of exercise, it may be necessary to introduce this change gradually.

What Does Eastern Medicine Do About Scanty or Absent Periods?

A scanty menstrual flow is usually an indication of blood deficiency. In Traditional Chinese Medicine, we see blood as a subset of yin, so we say that there is insufficient yin to support a woman's menstrual flow. A woman will usually develop insufficient yin for one of two reasons. The first is that she is not consuming enough. The second is that she is burning through food, drink, and rest faster than she is replenishing it. In either case, the nourishment that would go to nourish the blood of her menses is diverted to support other life preserving organs or functions.

While evolution would like to support reproduction, it prioritizes the woman's own survival and health, and will sacrifice reproductive ability for it. If a woman's body is very low in yin, it will siphon off the yin that would normally go to maintain the blood necessary for a menstrual cycle and allocate it to the internal organs that are necessary for survival. Women who develop scanty or absent periods due to insufficient yin are usually underweight.

Our society places a great emphasis on being thin and this has a strong effect on women, who often diet excessively to try to obtain that cultural ideal of thinness. If she finds her period is getting lighter or that she is missing one occasionally, it is a sign that she may not be getting the good-quality yin that her body needs to create a healthy period. Also, if a woman's exercise routine causes her to sweat a lot, this is another indication that she is spending yin that is vitally important to replace.

A woman can nourish good-quality and quantity yin by eating a wholesome, nourishing diet appropriate to her current requirements (we will discuss this in Part III), including good-quality oils, and by engaging only in gentle to moderate exercise so she avoids depleting more yin. We would also suggest she be sure to get plenty of rest and good-quality sleep, avoid stress—which gnaws away at yin—and prescribe blood-building and nourishing herbs.

One less common reason for scanty or absent periods is a mechanical blockage, whereby a channel, vessel, gland, or natural function is blocked or affected by a mass or tumor. This would usually occur more in a woman who is overweight and would be considered either an insufficiency of yang or a presence of too much poor-quality yin. Eastern medicine would usually treat this by ensuring that the woman engage in sufficient exercise, that her diet has good-quality yin and not too much of it, and would consider herbs and natural remedies that would serve to dissolve any blockages.

What Should I Do?

1. Take careful notes about your cycle's duration and other details (consistency, etc.). Consult with your primary care physician—bringing your detailed notes

with you—to determine the cause. Whatever the cause, as well as seeing your gynecologist, consult with a qualified practitioner of Traditional Chinese Medicine or Ayurveda (see the Appendix A) to support you with appropriate lifestyle, diet, and herbs.

2. If the cause of your scanty or absent periods is a deficiency of yin, there are very nourishing herbs that can help, including:

   • In Ayurveda: *shatavari*, *vidari*, or *ashwagandha*, depending on your current condition. (If you have breast lumps or uterine fibroids, you should consult with your Ayurvedic diet and lifestyle consultant before using *shatavari*.)
   • In TCM: *Dang gui*, *shan yao*, *sheng di huang*, and *shu di huang* are just a few of the many herbs that could be appropriate.

3. Whether you have too much or too little yin, eat a nourishing diet of whole, unrefined, freshly cooked foods. Consult Part III of this book for guidance. (Suggestions for how to get started with a healthy diet are listed on page 46.) An Ayurvedic practitioner can help you adapt the general guidelines for your particular constitution.

4. If you have insufficient yin, your diet should include the following high-quality yin foods:

   • A glass of warm milk with a pinch of cinnamon, nutmeg, or saffron, an hour before bedtime. If you tolerate dairy, this can be cow's milk. Ideally this will be organic unhomogenized milk (the homogenization process renders it less digestible). If you don't tolerate dairy, you could use almond, soy, rice, or hemp milk.
   • Baked orange yams or squash, carrots, or stews of seitan or tofu cooked well with fresh ginger and onions.
   • Warm, cooked whole-grain breakfast cereals such as oatmeal, cream of wheat, and cream of rice.
   • Warm beverages that are naturally caffeine free.
   • High-quality, organic, cold-pressed olive oil or other high-quality oils.

5. If you have insufficient yin, include a very gentle exercise routine in your life. Gentle forms of exercise such as walking or stretchy forms of yoga, tai chi or qi gong, for example, do not eat up as much yin as do vigorous forms of yoga or other strenuous exercise (such as running).

6. If you have too much poor-quality yin in your body, follow the directions for diet and exercise in Part III, consult with your primary care practitioner and a practitioner of TCM or Ayurveda to develop a more vigorous exercise routine and consider other options for removing masses or tumors if they are causing blockages in natural channels or functions.

Heavy or Painful Periods

When menstrual flow is too heavy or painful, conventional medicine may diagnose uterine fibroids, endometriosis, or dysfunctional uterine bleeding (DUB), or may be unable to find any cause that shows up on its various diagnostic tests.

UTERINE FIBROIDS

Uterine fibroids are hard or soft masses of muscle tissue that can appear in any layer of the uterus and are almost always benign. They may exist without any symptoms, or can cause abdominal, back, or menstrual pain; a feeling of weight or pressure in the lower abdomen or bladder; frequent urination; constipation; infertility; and, most commonly, heavy or irregular menstrual bleeding. Bleeding can be so heavy that a woman may have to change both a pad and tampon every half hour.

Uterine fibroids range from microscopic in size to three pounds or even larger, expanding the uterus as if there was a full-term pregnancy. If they are small, they may cause no problems. However, if they are large or in a crucial spot, they can block the fallopian tubes, prevent implantation of the embryo, or otherwise hinder conception. As many as 80 percent of women may get uterine fibroids, and the risk is increased by obesity—a sign of excess, poor-quality yin. Fibroids are estrogen dependent and hormone sensitive, and their growth can be stimulated by estrogens and even by progestins (synthetic progesterone-wannabe hormones) designed to counter some of the negative effects of estrogen. Natural progesterone alone may help the situation.[3]

Because uterine fibroids are hormone sensitive, they often enlarge during pregnancy, when hormone levels are higher, and shrink after menopause. There also may be a genetic component involved.[4] Certain oral contraceptives may help stabilize bleeding fibroids in a minority of women.[5] But because this approach is of questionable efficacy, more dramatic drugs are often prescribed. These drugs, called GnRH-agonists, serve to halt a woman's natural production of hormones, thereby starving the fibroid. They also put the woman into a chemically induced menopause and increase her risk of osteoporosis and other disorders associated with stopping a woman's natural production of hormones.

A hysterectomy, the surgical removal of the uterus, is sometimes necessary to treat uterine fibroids or endometriosis, although perhaps not as frequently as it is used. Uterine fibroids are the most frequent reason given to warrant a hysterectomy. At about 770,000 per year, hysterectomies outnumber almost all other types of surgery performed in the United States.[6] And this number is two to three times the number of hysterectomies performed in other countries. In March

2000, Dr. John Lee reported that representatives on a panel of doctors and researchers at UCLA concluded that 76 percent of the hysterectomies performed on a group of five hundred women in the United States did not meet criteria for appropriateness of recommending the procedure.[7]

Dr. Vicki Hufnagel, in her book *No More Hysterectomies*, argues against surgery to remove the uterus. In most cases she prefers what's called female reconstructive surgery (FRS), even if the woman is older and has a fast-growing fibroid.[8] Dr. Hufnagel encourages early use of FRS to remove the fibroid, rather than a wait-and-see approach, so that it doesn't grow and cause further damage within the uterus, fallopian tubes, and so on. Her book, which includes a section on how this procedure is performed, is worth a read for women considering their options for dealing with fibroids.

While FRS is one alternative to a hysterectomy, there are other surgical options as well. Myomectomies remove the fibroid but leave the uterus. There is also a procedure called uterine artery embolization (UAE) that works by starving the blood flow to the fibroids. Yet another procedure, myolisis, involves cauterizing the vessels that provide the blood supply to the fibroids, after shrinking them with GnRH-agonist drugs for a few months. However, this procedure also weakens the integrity of the uterine wall and so is not recommended for women who may wish to get pregnant.[9] The point is that there are options besides hysterectomies, and if your doctor is not familiar with alternatives, you may wish to find one that is.

One school of thought goes something like this: "Hey, if we're in there anyway, why not remove your ovaries, because they could become cancerous later on and cause you trouble." Although future trouble is possible, if there is no reason to think it is probable, it may be more prudent to suppose that nature has a good reason for endowing us with ovaries and it may cause more harm than good to remove them (unless they are clearly diseased). Aside from the problems associated with removal of a major endocrine organ and depriving the body of the hormones it would have provided, follow-up surveys on women who had elective surgery to remove their ovaries revealed that these women had a higher risk of dying over the course of the study's time frame, an increased vulnerability to lung cancer and heart disease, and double the risk of developing Parkinson's disease compared with women who kept their ovaries.[10]

ENDOMETRIOSIS

Another major cause of heavy bleeding is endometriosis, a condition whereby cells that belong to the uterus lining migrate outside the uterus, invading local tissues and organs and sometimes migrating as far as the lungs or even the nose. When a woman's uterine lining sloughs off each month, creating her cycle, endometrial cells that have migrated outside of the uterus do so too, but unlike the cells inside the uterus, they don't have an exit path. The resulting internal bleeding can cause inflammation, cramping, and sometimes incapacitating pain and scarring that may lead to infertility. Endometriosis is stubborn. It can even recur after a hysterectomy, so it is useful to try to resolve it without surgery. It is exacerbated by estrogen and exposure to estrogen-like pollutants, such as dioxin.

Physicians are now analyzing studies that link other estrogen-like pollutants to endometriosis. Eighty years ago there were only twenty-one reported cases in the world. In 1994 there were five million in the United States alone, and a German study showed that women with endometriosis were more likely to have higher levels of PCBs.[11] Endometriosis is itself linked to an increase in breast cancer, ovarian cancer, malignant melanoma, and some autoimmune disorders like fibromyalgia and lupus.[12] These associated conditions may also be the result of exposure to pollutants, so addressing one condition successfully may benefit all of them.

DYSFUNCTIONAL UTERINE BLEEDING

Yet another cause of heavy bleeding is dysfunctional uterine bleeding, which is usually due to excess unopposed (meaning, without the balancing effect of enough progesterone) estrogen's building a uterine lining that has insufficient support. Sometimes this is called "estrogen dominance." Again we see problems that occur when sex hormones are out of balance.

A woman's recourse to treatment in modern medicine seems fairly limited. She may be given the option to take synthetic hormones or be advised to consider a hysterectomy or other surgical solution. These options carry the risk of side effects.

PAINFUL PERIODS WITH NO OBVIOUS CAUSE

Painful periods are a very common complaint for women. Often there is no DUB or endometriosis, no fibroids, no discernable masses, or any other cause identifiable by Western diagnostic tests, and yet a woman will have painful periods. Women are often told to use Advil or some other similar medication for pain, and they assume this is normal and that they need to accept that they will have painful periods throughout their lives.

What Does Eastern Medicine Do About Heavy Bleeding or Painful Periods?

Eastern medicine teaches that no woman should have an uncomfortable menstrual cycle and recognizes various causes and treatment strategies for painful or heavy bleeding. Menstrual pain might be common, but it is not normal or necessary. There are many possible imbalances that can lead to painful or heavy cycles. We can look at the most common causes, all of which involve some kind of stagnation. Whenever there is stagnation, there is pain.

Ayurveda considers that the reproductive system is comprised of a group of channels and vessels through which the woman's qi, eggs and menstrual blood migrate. These channels or vessels can become constricted or blocked. Once constricted or blocked, the qi or *prana*, blood, yin, or material that would normally migrate smoothly through them will stagnate or begin to move in the wrong direction. For example, in endometriosis, the cells of the uterine lining proliferate and move outside the uterus.

Eastern medicine considers that constriction of the reproductive vessels can be a result of stress or coldness. The vessels can also become blocked by excess, poor-quality yin that tends to stagnate, becoming a mass, or by qi that stagnates long enough that it stops moving and transforming yin, which then becomes a mass. When qi stagnates, it causes a dull, moving pain. Pain becomes fixed and worse as masses and blockages develop.

The main reasons that qi will stagnate are insufficient physical movement, or vessels that constrict, restricting the natural movement of qi. There is an important concept in Eastern medicine: The structure of the body reflects the state of qi in the body, and the qi reflects the condition of the spirit. If our spirit is calm and harmonious, qi flows smoothly in our body. If qi is flowing smoothly, the bodily tissues and channels will be well formed, lubricated, and nourished. If the spirit is discontent, the body may constrict and disturb the normal movement of qi, and the structure of the body will likewise become disturbed.

Consider this: When we are stressed out, we often hold our breath and clench our bodies. Where we clench varies. Some women hold their stress in their shoulders, others in their abdomen, and others in their reproductive organs. Eastern medicine teaches us that bodily tissues will coalesce around what the body's energy is doing. If your life force is flowing smoothly, your blood and tissues will be healthy and supple. If it stagnates, blood will stagnate and you will get ischemic muscles (muscles with decreased blood flow). The longer qi and blood stagnate, the more stubborn the pain will be and the greater the chance that masses, fibroids, or endometriosis will develop. In the case of reproductive stagnation, a woman may have a pattern of holding stress in that area, or there may be something in her lifestyle that is encouraging stagnation there.

Eastern medicine usually treats stagnant qi or yin with dietary and lifestyle changes, acupuncture, and what Traditional Chinese Medicine calls "blood moving herbs," all prescribed according to the woman's specific condition, constitution, and current requirements. Often it is also helpful to add a regimen of castor oil packs. Castor oil has an astounding ability to penetrate through the tissue, dissolve obstructive masses, and relax and open vessels. (See Appendix E for directions on how to make and use castor oil packs). In this case, castor oil packs can break up the stagnation in and around the uterus, relax the tissues and blood vessels, and support free movement of qi. I have found it rare for a woman not to find relief within three months, if she adheres to an appropriate diet, lifestyle, and an herbal and castor pack regimen.

A study in the peer-reviewed magazine *Alternative Medicine* in 2002 demonstrated the efficacy of acupuncture and herbs for managing or curing uterine fibroids. There was evidence that either could be effective alone. In one case where acupuncture was used without herbs, a woman's fibroids shrank enough that she was able successfully to conceive. Treatments of fibroids with herbs alone showed an overall effective rate of 92.4 percent.[13] Because the risks and negative side effects of acupuncture and herbs are small, it seems prudent to explore these options before resorting to treatments that we know are fraught with risk, such as drugs or surgery.

Using these complementary therapies is very different from taking a wait-and-see approach. Lifestyle and diet changes can be very difficult to adhere to. After all, your diet and lifestyle pretty much make up your life. Then add some herbs and castor oil packs, and it can feel as if you're putting out an effort equal to at least a part-time job. Not to worry. What starts out feeling like an overwhelming change becomes simply routine after a while and may end up taking no more time than your previous lifestyle and diet.

Whether surgery is required or not, it is important to address the underlying imbalance or stagnation that leads to pain, fibroids, endometriosis, or dysfunctional uterine bleeding. A Traditional Chinese Medicine or Ayurvedic practitioner will look to identify the cause leading to the stagnation, unravel it, and support a woman in appropriate lifestyle, energetic, and dietary changes that will counteract the pattern of stagnation and will encourage free and easy movement of energy and blood through the reproductive area. These changes will, as a positive side effect, serve to balance her hormones. In fact, in one of those chicken-and-egg situations, it is not clear if balancing the hormones through Eastern practices solves the stagnation or solving the stagnation serves to balance the hormones. The truth is that the two are inseparable and it is impossible to address one without affecting the other.

What Should I Do?

1. Suggestions for how to get started with a healthy diet, lifestyle, and stress-management techniques were listed on pages 46–52, but this is covered in depth in Part III.

2. Be sure your diet is appropriate. A good diet encourages the right amount of good-quality yin in your body. Too much good yin or any poor yin will aggravate the condition. Having too much good yin is like overeating at Thanksgiving or some other feast. Even if the food is high quality and nourishing, too much of a good thing becomes problematic. You feel heavy, gain unnecessary weight, and get indigestion. Poor-quality food delivers poor-quality yin, regardless of the quantity, as we will see more in Part III. Educate yourself on Ayurvedic principles of constitution and diet or work with an Ayurvedic diet and lifestyle consultant.

3. Develop an appropriate exercise routine to support the movement of qi in your body. See Chapter 25.

4. Reduce stress. Stress creates constriction in the body, which interferes with the free flow of qi, creating stagnation that leads to heavy bleeding. See Chapter 26.

5. Check with your primary care practitioner to make sure nothing serious is going on. If you can safely avoid or postpone drugs or surgery, you might consult with a TCM or Ayurvedic diet and lifestyle consultant to see if stagnant qi in the uterus is causing your pain or heavy bleeding. Both the Chinese and Ayurvedic systems use herbs to address this; I have found the Chinese herbs especially effective in this case. *Tong jing wan* is a good common formula. I usually tailor a formula for my patients that includes the following raw, dried powdered Chinese herbs (your practitioner should be familiar with these): *tian san qi, chuan xiong, hong hua, shan yao,* and *dang gui.*

6. Try using castor oil packs, according to the directions in Appendix E. While this is time consuming, it can be an incredibly powerful therapy, well worth the time.

Irregular or Missed Cycles

There can be many reasons for irregular or missed cycles. It is important to see a Western medical doctor, because bleeding between periods can be a sign of a serious disorder or can at least help to narrow down the cause. Although it is good to rule out serious conditions, usually the causes of irregular periods are not so pernicious and are easily treated with Eastern medicine.

Sometimes the causes are healthy, such as pregnancy or nursing, both of which naturally cause missed periods. Otherwise, we see that hormonal irregularity underlies irregular periods. This can be caused by various factors, including weight gain or loss. Although excess weight can be a cause, it is more common for low body weight to cause missed or irregular periods, for the same reasons that it causes scanty periods. Because of this, disorders such as anorexia nervosa or bulimia nervosa or too much exercise, can be related, as they contribute to weight loss. Other factors, such as illness, stress, or travel, can throw off the hormonal rhythms and cause a missed or irregular cycle. If the travel, stress, or illness passes, the cycle should return to its normal rhythm.

Pharmaceutical and recreational drugs can also run havoc with our natural hormonal rhythms. Indeed, some pharmaceutical drugs are specifically designed for women to miss their cycles. We talked about this practice, and its associated risks, in Chapter 9 (see page 55). Finally, there can be problems with various organs—problems that can interfere with healthy hormonal cycles. For example, women can have cysts on her ovaries, or a condition called polycystic ovarian syndrome (PCOS), that, while often benign, can sometimes lead to irregular periods. There can be disorders of the liver, the bowels, and other organs that can lead to irregular periods.

There are many different causes of irregular cycles, but there are a couple of shared considerations. One is that we can be sure that the woman's hormonal rhythms are off and she will need to restore hormonal balance. Another related consideration is routine. If there is no routine in life, how can we expect our bodies to maintain certain routines or rhythms?

One endocrine organ that is not fully understood is the unassuming pineal gland. This pea-size, pine cone–shaped gland is found near the center of the brain, between the two hemispheres. It is known to be associated with our daily and seasonal biorhythms and is suspected of being susceptible to the influence of sunlight and moonlight. How this communicates with the hypothalamus to regulate hormones is not entirely known, but there is some evidence that it does.[14] This helps explain why women's cycle-related acne, PMS and irregular cycles can sometimes clear up just by taking a walk outdoors at the same time every day.

A woman's menstrual cycle is a clear indication of her state of hormonal balance—that is to say, her balance of yin and yang—nourishment and energy, or substance and stress. The combination of attention to lifestyle, diet, herbs, and natural remedies is generally impressively successful at addressing many menstrual disorders and regulating a woman's cycle, by restoring balance in the body and spirit.

What Does Eastern Medicine Do About Irregular or Missed Cycles?

This section will be brief, as irregular or missed cycles is so closely related to the sections on heavy and scanty bleeding. One of the first questions we ask is whether a woman's irregular period is also heavy or if it is scanty, and we would address the heavy or scanty bleeding as described earlier. Sometimes this is enough to solve the irregularity at the same time. If it isn't, we need to look further. We would consider the condition of her various organs and their related functions. This would be a good time to see a qualified practitioner.

Although there are many causes for irregular cycles, usually one or more of three main factors are involved: stagnation of qi, lack of sufficient yin, or hormonal imbalance. If qi stagnates in the reproductive organs, there will be an obstructive influence in the channels of blood or qi, and we would treat it similarly to how we treat heavy bleeding. If deficient yin is the problem, we would ensure that the woman's diet and lifestyle support proper nourishment, and we would treat it similarly to how we treat scanty periods. If the woman's hormone balance is off, we look at the role that stress plays in her life and try to balance this. If stress is high, stress hormones are likely to be high, which disturbs the balance of sex hormones, as we saw in Part I. The timing of a woman's cycle is governed by these hormones, so high stress is almost always involved in irregular cycles.

Traditional Chinese Medicine excels at regulating menstruation through acupuncture and herbs. Both Ayurveda and TCM consider and treat the associated scanty or heavy bleeding and Ayurveda encourages adherence to an appropriate daily routine that involves time outdoors, exercise, and diet.

What Should I Do?

1. Consult with your primary care practitioner and a qualified practitioner of TCM or Ayurveda to determine the cause of your irregular cycles and tailor a lifestyle, diet, and herbal plan.
2. Consider if your cycle is irregular and heavy or irregular and scanty, and address this as described in previous sections, along with the irregularity. Sometimes just addressing the causes of scanty or heavy bleeding will be enough to restore regularity.
3. Follow the three pillars of health described in Part III: diet, lifestyle, and stress management. This will help no matter what the cause of your irregular periods. (Suggestions for how to get started in these areas are listed on pages 46–52.)
4. Focus on your daily routine. If your daily rhythms are regular, this encourages regular physiological functions.
5. Walk outdoors for about a half hour, preferably at the same time every day. Your exposure to the natural light and nature's rhythms may support your pineal gland to support your own internal rhythms and natural cycles.

Birth Control

Historical and Current Practices

Birth control is not a modern quest. In the past, a woman might eat bees, spit into a frog's mouth, jump up and down and backward after sex, or wear weasel testicles, just to name a few ancient methods of contraception.[1] In a second-century display at the History of Contraception Museum in Toronto, there are vaginal plugs made from honey combined with crocodile and elephant dung.[2] Although most women today would probably not experiment with the contraceptive effectiveness of pachyderm excrement, many have freely (though often unknowingly) experimented with supplements derived from pregnant mares' urine. This is the basis for Premarin, the leading estrogen-replacement therapy (ERT) offered to menopausal women. Premarin is not prescribed as a contraceptive; however, birth control pills contain the very same sorts of synthetic hormones. We have seen significant enough problems with the side and aftereffects of synthetic hormones that some experts even suggest that postmenopausal women should not take them at all, not even in the short term.[3]

While the forms of contraception used today include female and male sterilization, condoms, and other methods, synthetic hormonal contraception is the most common practice.

In 2004, in the United States alone, 11.6 million women used birth control pills. And, in 2010, more than 100 million women worldwide[4] used the Pill for contraception, menstrual pain, or skin improvement. The total number of women exposed to synthetic hormonal contraception is even larger, as this figure doesn't include women using the "morning-after pill" or other forms of hormonal birth control available in the United States since 2000, such as the hormonal contraceptive patch, the levonorgestrel-releasing intrauterine system, the hormonal contraceptive ring, the hormonal implant, and the ninety-one-day regimen of oral contraceptives.[5]

RISKS ASSOCIATED WITH SYNTHETIC
HORMONAL CONTRACEPTIVE METHODS

As we saw earlier, one thing was not discussed much when the house of cards that supported the near-universal use of synthetic hormone replacement therapy (HRT) for menopause was collapsing: the fact that the very hormones prescribed for menopause were—and are—also prescribed in phenomenal numbers as birth control for younger women. The same synthetic hormones that are in HRT are in birth control pills, implants, injections, some IUDs and vaginal rings. As I mentioned in Chapter 6, a few lonely scientists were sufficiently bold to point out that there was no reason to believe that the findings applied only to Prempro, the brand of synthetic hormones most widely prescribed for menopausal women. They said, "Women and their doctors should assume that all hormone therapy that involves estrogen and progestin bears the same risks."[6] Prescriptions for HRT for menopausal women, and the Pill for women in childbearing years, are unique cases in the world of medicine, as they are both designed to be taken long term by healthy women rather than ill women. Whether or not the women remain healthy after taking them is another matter.

If older women increase their chances of breast cancer, heart attack, strokes, and dementia by consuming synthetic hormones for menopausal symptoms, why is it okay for younger women to take these drugs?

Aside from many of the same issues we saw with menopausal and post-menopausal women's use of synthetic hormones—such as increased risk of breast cancer, stroke, and heart disease—many women report difficulty finding a type of birth control pill with side effects they can tolerate. Uncomfortable side effects include bleeding between menstrual periods, skipped periods, nausea, change in weight, bloating, increase in vaginal infections, depression, and mood swings. More serious side effects can include gall bladder disease, changes in blood levels of fatty substances, increased blood pressure, worsening of migraine headaches, and an extremely rare liver tumor. Synthetic hormonal contraception impedes normal function of a woman's ovaries, thereby interfering with their beneficial effects, some of which are healthy bone production and maintenance.[7] Some, like Depo-Provera, may cause significant bone loss, among many other disorders.[8] Those at greatest risk of developing these problems are over thirty-five, smoke, or have other health problems like diabetes, high blood pressure, heart or vascular disease, or blood cholesterol and triglyceride abnormalities.

Usually, the lower the dose of synthetic hormones, the fewer side effects. That's helpful to know, but even if there are no obvious side effects now, synthetic hormones may be taking a silent toll that will show up many years later, or when a woman's constitution suffers some other strain, such as diabetes or other health problems.

BREAST CANCER

One study showed that after less than a year of use synthetic progestin-only pills, there was a 60 percent greater risk of breast cancer. If a woman develops breast cancer before age forty-four, the chances are good that she has used combined oral contraceptives, meaning synthetic estrogen combined with progestin.[9] If she uses the Pill before age twenty, her risk of breast cancer may double.[10] When we see this sort of correlation, it is no wonder that in 2005 the International Agency for Research on Cancer (the World Health Organization's cancer research group) reclassified the Pill from "possibly carcinogenic to humans" to "carcinogenic to humans."[11]

HIGHER LEVELS OF CRP

Higher levels of C-reactive protein (CRP) have also been linked to women's taking oral contraceptives. Higher levels of CRP are associated with an increased risk of heart disease.[12] When the liver detects inflammation in the system, it produces CRP, which is not found in the blood under normal circumstances.[13] This leads us to wonder if oral contraceptives directly or indirectly increase inflammation in the body.

If taken before a woman is twenty, there is evidence that birth control pills reduce levels of important vitamins such as B_6 and folic acid and increase the risk of breast cancer. They suppress ovulation, the normal functions of the ovaries, and the production and action of a woman's natural hormones. They replace her natural rhythms and hormones with synthetic hormones and imposed rhythms.[14] Suppressing natural ovarian hormones might be a questionable idea, as they are necessary to build and maintain bones.

DIMINISHED BONE DENSITY

One reputable study showed that, over the course of two years, young women who led sedentary lives lost 1 to 2 percent of their bone density.[15] Conversely, young women who engaged in regular aerobic exercise and resistance training, such as weight lifting, increased their bone density by 1 to 2 percent *unless they were taking oral contraceptives*. Women using oral contraceptives did not increase their bone density, *even* if they were exercising.

INCREASED PLAQUE

The University of Ghent measured plaque in the blood vessels of 2,500 healthy men and women and found that women who had used the contraceptive pill when younger had a 20 to 30 percent increase in plaque in their carotid and femoral arteries by the time they reached late middle age.[16]

The question arises: Is there any age at which it is safe to take synthetic hormones? Studies have shown that it is risky during and after menopause, it puts women in their thirties at more risk, and it is not safe for woman under age twenty. This seems to indicate that there are risks of synthetic hormone use at any stage of a woman's life.

It is unclear what the effects of hormonal manipulation will be on succeeding generations, but some consider it a definite cause of iatrogenic disorders (symptoms or illnesses brought about by a physician's treatment) in its present-generation users.[17]

CONTRACEPTIVES THAT ELIMINATE THE CYCLE

There are risks associated with every type of synthetic hormonal contraception, but perhaps especially forms that eliminate a woman's cycle. In Chapter 9, we looked at the side effects of Depo-Provera, one of the common contraceptives in this category. In that same chapter, we also looked at Margie Profet's theory that menstruation suppresses pathogenic activity in women's reproductive organs, especially when they are sexually active.[18] Yet health-care practitioners and educators often recommend synthetic hormonal contraceptives due to their perceived convenience. One of my niece's high school health education instructors actively pushed synthetic hormonal contraception as the superior form of birth control. When my niece voiced her concerns over the side effects, she felt her concerns were dismissed as being radical and uninformed.

My niece's concerns were not trivial and it is nice to see young women considering effects beyond what is skin deep. Indeed, cosmetics are a common reason for a woman going on birth control pills, as they are regularly prescribed and taken for skin problems. If a woman is taking birth control pills for this reason, however, she might consider that one possible (and permanent) side effect is a spotty darkening of skin on her face.

It is curious to note that, while many women seem tolerant of having their ovarian function disturbed by the use of synthetic hormones, men are apparently less tolerant of similar effects on their physiology, perhaps because they are visible. In one study, both men and women took synthetic hormones to prevent conception. The concoction stopped ovulation in women and sperm production in men. When one of the men experienced the side effect of shrunken testicles, all further male Pill trials were halted, with the agreement that any such Pill would have to be proven safe before experimentation should proceed.[19] If women's ovaries were on the outside of our bodies, and the negative side effects were actually cosmetically visible, would we be less tolerant?

EDUCATE YOURSELF

We are generally a culture that expects immediate or at least quick gratification of our desires without giving much forethought to the consequences. We expect to find a quick and easy solution to pregnancy prevention, one that does not involve having to learn about our own fertility cycles. The question of what is a truly safe and effective form of contraception is not an easy one, nor is it one we can necessarily trust that our health care educators are experts on. If we rule out synthetic hormonal contraception, the other commonly prescribed forms are diaphragms, cervical caps, intrauterine devices (IUDs), and condoms. But to trust diaphragms, condoms, and the spermicidal jellies and lubricants used with them or alone, we have to trust that the chemicals in those jellies and lubricants are harmless to the delicate reproductive tissues they bathe. There is not a great track record to assure us that the chemicals in these lubricants are not damaging to our delicate tissues. Consider that by 2004 the World Health Organization, the Joint United Nations Programme on HIV/AIDS, and the U.S. Centers for Disease Control had all raised concerns about Nonoxynol-9 (N-9), then a common ingredient in condom lubricants and in a vaginal cream. This cream had been in use for fifty years before N-9 was found to deteriorate or irritate the cell linings of the rectum and vagina.[20] Compromising this first line of defense in the reproductive system makes it easier for viruses or bacteria to invade.

Although IUDs do not rely on chemical jellies for their effectiveness, their use can lead to uterine discomfort, heavy cramping, and even ectopic pregnancy, all signs that Traditional Chinese Medicine interprets as indicators of stagnation of qi in the uterus. As we saw in Chapter 10 and will see in the next chapter as well, uterine stagnation is not desirable.

FERTILITY AWARENESS

To learn about the various forms of birth control and the natural alternatives in detail, I recommend reading two highly informed and accessible books. The first is *Taking Charge of Your Fertility: The Definitive Guide to Natural Birth Control, Pregnancy Achievement, and Reproductive Health* by Toni Weschler, MPH, the book I mentioned on page 59. The second, Jane Bennett and Alexandra Pope's

The Pill: Are You Sure It's for You? is the first book I've come across that outlines the drawbacks of synthetic hormonal contraception so clearly. Both books, especially the former, explore effective pregnancy prevention through learning about and cooperating with your own fertility cycle. Weschler provides detailed directions, explanations, and illustrations to guide a woman to learning the fertility awareness method (FAM). There is a prevalent misconception that FAM or natural family planning (NFP) are ineffective forms of contraception. This misconception stems partly from people—including experts—mistakenly associating FAM or NFP with the infamous, imprecise, and inaccurate "rhythm method." There is an old (and somewhat tired) joke: "What do you call a couple who practices the rhythm method?" The answer: "Parents." While this may be an accurate description of users of the rhythm method, it does not do justice to the nature and practice of FAM or NFP. This unfortunate association, coupled with the misconceptions that FAM or NFP are difficult, time-consuming techniques that most women will not willingly learn and practice, gives them undeserved negative reputations. If learned well and practiced diligently, they are effective forms of birth control, even if a woman's cycle is irregular. They are both based on a woman's learning her signs of fertility. The main difference between them is that NFP practitioners choose, often due to religious reasons, to abstain from sex during the woman's fertile days, whereas a FAM practitioner may choose to use barrier methods of contraception during her fertile days. Either way, once a woman learns about her own fertility, she can use her knowledge either to prevent or support conception for the remainder of her fertile life. And she can do so without the inconvenient to tragic side effects of most other forms of birth control.

Katie first came to my office when she was twenty-two. She was looking for alternative forms of birth control. She had become sexually active at seventeen years old, but quickly found that she was allergic to the latex in condoms. She tried a diaphragm, but its spermicidal jelly unduly moistened her vaginal tract and the consistent dampness led to yeast infections. When Katie turned to birth control pills, she had to try one kind after another to find one she could tolerate. The first made her gain weight. The next gave her mood swings. The third, headaches. Because none of these methods had worked well for her, she wanted a natural solution to birth control. I put her in touch with a woman who specializes in helping women take charge of their own fertility. (See Appendix A.) Katie is now thirty-one and has been married for five years. Since she learned about her own cycles and used this knowledge to help prevent pregnancy, she has not used birth control devices or prescriptions and has not become pregnant.

What to do to prevent unwanted pregnancies is a question every woman has to answer for herself. But given the downside we saw with the use of synthetic hormones, chemical lubricants, spermicides, and IUDs, the solutions that make the most sense to me are NFP or FAM, with a minimal use of barrier forms of birth control, such as condoms. This minimizes tissue exposure to possibly damaging influences and increases self-awareness. It can be very empowering for a woman to know her own cycle and take responsibility for her actions and choices. Just as we do well to consider the consequences of indulging in fast food, we benefit from increasing our self-awareness and responsibility around sexual interaction.

Having said this, I leave ample room for the possibility that other forms of birth control may be more appropriate for certain women at certain stages of life. For example, if a woman is having sex with multiple partners or she is unlikely to take the time to effectively learn FAM, it may be more appropriate for her to use condoms, as they both help prevent the spread of AIDS and sexually transmitted diseases, and they don't require her to take time to learn about her own physiology.

What Does Eastern Medicine Do About Birth Control?

There are two primary ways Eastern medicine addresses what we today call birth control. One is with herbs and the second is with special exercises to suspend a woman's fertility until she requires it. Neither is an option I would recommend for most women.

Currently, there is very little reliable information on herbal remedies for birth control. While there are reports of certain herbs used for contraception, not enough people are using them or documenting their efficacy for me to feel comfortable recommending them. I also have a concern that some of these herbs, if taken to prevent pregnancy on a regular basis, would be inappropriate medicine for some women to take long term. Eastern medicine considers that what works for one woman may damage another. The herbs that are used for contraception might be fine for a woman of one constitution to take, but might cause trouble in another.

Qi gong, tai chi, or yoga are all forms of exercise that, when optimally practiced, move energy smoothly throughout the body. Qi gong exercises that affect women's fertility are documented in ancient Taoist texts. These exercises were mostly practiced by Taoist nuns, to reverse the flow of a woman's downward-moving qi, which is essential for her period, and send it from her uterus and ovaries to nourish other internal organs. These practices also suspend her monthly cycles. Were she to desire children, she would stop her exercises, her period would return, along with her fertility.

These exercises might be effective for birth control purposes, but their main purpose is to stem the monthly loss of vitality that occurs with a woman's monthly bleeding and use it to irrigate her body. I do not doubt that these exercises can be effective, but they were taught, in times past, to unmarried women who spent much of their lives engaged in meditation practices and qi gong. For a woman to use these exercises today, she might do them enough to stop her period, but not enough to then circulate that qi smoothly throughout her body. Thus, instead of benefiting her, these practices could harm her, as she would run the risk of simply creating stagnation in her uterus and other local physiological systems.

Amber was a thin, pale woman reluctant to show emotion. She came to me when she was forty-three. In her midthirties, she had practiced a qi gong regimen designed to suspend her periods. She had an office job at the time, working forty-five hours a week, and had a boyfriend with whom she wanted to have sex without worrying about getting pregnant. She spent thirty minutes a day doing the qi gong and, as long as she continued the exercises, she didn't get her period. This worked, but her relationship eventually ended, and she felt she no longer needed to continue the exercises. She stopped them and her cycle returned. Amber came to me because of digestive complaints, including severe constipation, which had begun during the time she was doing the exercises.

Amber's digestive complaints are easily explained with Eastern medicine. Although she did enough qi gong to stop the natural downward flow of energy in her reproductive area, this also affected her digestive organs. Instead of stimulating the normal peristaltic movement of her intestines, her energy stagnated, affecting her natural digestive function.

When these Eastern systems of medicine were being developed, environmental and social factors were different than they are today. A woman may have been expected to be either monogamous or celibate her entire life, have as many babies as came along, and perhaps be more in touch with her own fertility cycles.

What Should I Do?

1. Consider alternatives to synthetic hormonal contraception.
2. Receive expert counsel (make sure it is expert) on the fertility awareness method (FAM) and consider using this in combination with barrier methods when necessary.
3. Read *Taking Charge of Your Fertility: The Definitive Guide to Natural Birth Control, Pregnancy Achievement, and Reproductive Health*, by Toni Weschler, MPH (see Appendix A). This book makes learning FAM a friendly, even exciting process. It is a method that will work even if your periods are irregular.
4. If you are using or considering the Pill, read *The Pill: Are You Sure It's for You?* by Jane Bennett and Alexandra Pope. This is also listed in Appendix A.

Fertility and Conception
THE FOUR CRUCIAL ELEMENTS

According to Eastern medicine, if a woman gains, maintains, or regains the health of her menstrual cycle, the more likely she will be fertile. So the first step in conceiving is to be sure her cycle is healthy.

We know that a woman's cycle, and therefore her fertility, are negatively affected by exposure to environmental toxins, low sperm counts, infection-related scarring in the reproductive organs, hormonal irregularities, diet, low body fat, smoking, drug and alcohol use, and other factors. A combination of these factors causes an estimated 6 million American couples to be confronted with infertility.

Ayurvedic medicine considers these factors and how they relate to the four crucial elements necessary for conception and childbearing: the egg, sperm, reproductive system, and timing of conception. If all these elements are healthy, the woman's pregnancy and her baby are likely to be healthy.

The Egg

A woman has up to 2 million oocytes—immature eggs—when she is born. This number is whittled down to roughly 250,000 by the time she is an adolescent. From this reservoir, about 400 oocytes will mature and be ovulated over the course of her lifetime. This impressive repository of egg cells remains inside the ovaries until a monthly surge in hormones beckons forth the Chosen Egg of the Month. From the time this Chosen Egg hears the call, it takes about 110 days for it to concurrently mature and travel from the depths of the ovary to the surface, to be released from the follicle in the process of ovulation.[1] Scientists think that a process called "polarity" affects this egg during this preovulatory time. *Polarization* is the term for the process whereby the various components of an egg are organized within it. They are beginning to see that the polarization process may have a direct bearing on whether the egg is viable or not, and that it may indicate the presence or absence of long-term health challenges for the human whose life starts with this egg. The phenomenon of polarity is causing scientists to look at environment, nutrition, and events that may affect the polarization process of an egg three to four months before conception occurs.[2]

If a woman is well nourished, well rested, engages in appropriate exercise, and has balanced emotions, chances are that her hormones are balanced and her egg's maturation process will progress unhindered, resulting in a healthy mature egg. And if the egg is healthy and well when it encounters the sperm, then the first of the four crucial elements is in place.

IN VITRO FERTILIZATION, DONOR EGGS, AND OTHER TECHNOLOGIES—AND UNEXPLORED RISKS

If, for some reason, a woman's eggs are not viable, she may turn to in vitro fertilization (IVF), to an egg donor, or to other assisted reproductive technologies (ART) to assist her in her quest for motherhood. Ironically, the customer base for fertility drugs—which are designed to manipulate a woman's endocrine system and her naturally occurring hormones—includes many women who turned to synthetic hormones for much of their lives to *prevent* pregnancy.[3] (Fabio Bertarelli, a Swiss billionaire, is the owner of Serono Laboratories, which manufacturers seven out of ten of the world's fertility drugs. Bertarelli told the *Wall Street Journal*, "Our usual customers are women over thirty who have been taking birth control pills since they were teenagers or in their early 20s."[4])

Although using assisted reproductive technologies may certainly help a woman realize her desire to conceive, this course has consequences, expenses, and risks for both the mother and the donor, if a donor is involved. From an Eastern medicine point of view, before deciding on IVF, donor eggs, or similar technologies, we would first want to understand the whole process, then consider its overall effect on the donor and the resulting embryo.

IVF

If a woman requires assistance conceiving, she may turn to IVF. In this procedure, she is given fertility drugs to stimulate her ovaries to release multiple eggs in her ovulatory cycle. (Normally she would release just one.) Then the eggs are collected and fertilized with her partner's sperm outside her body, and the resulting embryos are inserted into her uterus, where implantation may or may not occur. This is not always a comfortable process. One woman describes it as, "PMS times 1,000."[5] And it is not without risk.

IVF results in multiple births more often than is the case with natural pregnancies, and multiple births carry greater risks. In fact, the fertility drugs themselves carry risks. Although studies are not conclusive, many give cause for
caution. For example, research by Alice Whittemore, PhD, at Stanford University
School of Medicine found ovarian cancer was about three times greater in
women who had taken fertility drugs and had borne children as a result. The
risks were even greater for women who took the drugs but did not eventually
give birth.[6] There have not been many conclusive studies, and the drugs' connection to cancer had not been studied seriously, at least as of the year 2000.
The connection is serious enough, though, that the FDA required a warning of
the risk of increase in ovarian cancer with such fertility drugs as Pergonal, Clomid, and Gonal-F. Even though Whittemore found cause for concern, she also
found there was a feeling, at least with some physicians, that the risks were a
necessary sacrifice in the cause of learning about the process of conceiving and
birth control.[7] It is possible that in women's quest to become pregnant and their
physicians' quest to assist them, risks are being minimized and important information is being overlooked.

Because synthetic hormones (like those used in fertility drugs) affect ovarian
function, we must wonder at the effect they will have on the woman's eggs. We
might also question how the mechanical process of some IVF practices might affect the successful development of the egg or the developing embryo. If a needle
is injected into the egg, for example, the polarization process is altered, and we
do not know the long-term consequences of such interference. Some scientists
who are engaged in this study, while proponents of assisted reproductive medicine, are concerned that these technologies are being employed before they are
proven safe.[8] Their concerns are that some of the interference practices, like the
needle in IVF, may lead to health problems—possibly as the result of a disturbed
polarization process—in the person born, and that these problems may show up
perhaps as far as fifteen to twenty years down the road. There has been very minimal follow-up research on the health of people who were born with the help of
assisted reproductive technologies.[9]

Egg Donors

What about using an egg donor? Let's look at a sample plan for what the donor
goes through.[10] First, to shut her ovarian function down, the donor injects herself
in the abdomen with the drug Lupron for three weeks. This prevents her eggs
from maturing and her follicles from developing, mimicking menopause, no matter what her age. She can expect the mood swings and hot flashes one might get

with a sudden onset of menopause. Next, she switches to injections into her hip of drugs designed to kick-start follicle-stimulating hormones, which will stimulate her ovaries to send a crop of eggs (instead of the usual single egg) to the surface of her ovaries, each of which is now the size of an orange (instead of its usual size of a walnut). Then she gets a shot of human chorionic gonadotropin (hCG). Thirty-six hours later, under general sedation, ultrasound probes are inserted in the donor's vagina and threaded up to her ovaries, where a needle penetrates each of them, sucks out their eggs, and transfers them to a petri dish. There sperm are injected into the eggs. If the procedure is successful, the resulting embryos are transferred to the prospective mother's womb.[11]

In 1999, ads in Ivy League school newspapers offered up to $50,000 to the right donor ("right" often including traits like physical fitness, tallness, and high SAT scores). Perhaps the large sum was to offset the dangers of hormonal and ovarian hyper stimulation and the small risk of suffering a stroke. But what if the process jeopardizes the donor's chances of having her own children later in life? In 1999, Karen Synesiou, co-owner of the Center for Surrogate Parenting and Egg Donation, put it this way, "If you get an 18- or 19-year-old who has been stimulated four or five times and her ovaries stop functioning because of all the scarring, she is going to want to sue someone for being infertile."[12]

Health Risks

In 2004, the Associated Press reported a story of a couple who went through five years trying to have a baby, including trying IVF for three cycles, and finally had a successful pregnancy through a donor egg implantation. Sadly, their daughter was born without the cells needed to make her liver function, a condition that the doctor said was "not even described in medical literature."[13] Now, it is certainly possible that this sort of anomaly was not due to IVF procedures. But it is also possible that it was, as these procedures are relatively new, without a long or strong track record of safety. Our desire to have children should not stop us from scrutinizing the reality and the risks to the mothers, donors, and children who suffer the effects associated with assisted reproductive technologies.

In 2000, Stanford's Whittemore told Ms. magazine that in her years researching and writing on assisted reproductive technologies, she found there was little effort to analyze the health risks associated with them. Dr. Marsden Wagner, former director of Women and Children's Health for the World Health Organization, is quoted as saying there was "almost no effort to examine the reality behind the hype," and that dangerous health risks for babies resulting from such technologies are significant and "some of the best-kept secrets." He added, "Four times as many IVF babies die around the time of birth than babies conceived naturally . . . and there is also a higher risk that these babies will have some sort of handicap."[14]

Whittemore called for comprehensive research on the health risks of assisted reproductive technologies, for proper clinical research procedures to be applied to newly proposed methods, and for meaningful informed consent and full disclosure for all patients.[15] History has warned us of the trouble that can arise from ignoring such advice. Consider the 1971 finding that the drug diethylstilbestrol (commonly called DES), which was prescribed for decades to prevent miscarriages, caused a rare type of reproductive cancer in the *daughters* of women who took the drug.

WHAT EASTERN MEDICINE SAYS ABOUT THE EGG

In Eastern medicine we would question the prudence of manipulating a woman's eggs and fertility in this manner. Traditional Chinese Medicine and Ayurveda describe a substance called *jing* or *ojas*, respectively. It is something we are born with and it is a life-giving, immune-enhancing, age-inhibiting, and rather mysterious substance that is more substantial and concentrated than qi or *prana* and contributes to a person's overall vitality. A woman's eggs are a reflection of the health of her *jing*. In Traditional Chinese Medicine we consider that a woman is born with a certain amount of *jing*, which can be protected through proper rest and nourishment and which she uses throughout her life. Some is released each month through ovulation and its accompanying hormones. It is also used in the normal course of life. As a woman's *jing* dwindles, her physical stamina may decline. She may hasten this process if she squanders her *jing* on a life that is too stressful or if she has habits that are detrimental. She can also preserve and protect her *jing* by having an appropriate lifestyle and diet. A Taoist perspective suggests that as a woman ages, her *jing* transforms to wisdom and, as she learns to navigate life with less strain, she preserves her *jing*.

There are certain factors that consume *jing* at a quicker rate than would naturally occur. These factors include chemically forcing a larger crop of eggs than normal to be released from the ovaries in any given month and detrimental lifestyle or dietary habits that deplete *jing*. Western medicine supports the concept that lifestyle choices can affect reproductive vitality. We know, for example, that smoking can render a woman years older in reproductive terms and significantly reduce her chances of successful IVF treatment.[16]

WHAT IT ALL MEANS

Whatever effect this information and these questions have on the future of assisted reproductive technologies, one take-home message for us is that a woman's egg is quite possibly vulnerable to her dietary, environmental, and lifestyle choices for months *before* she actually conceives. We can see why this might be so by considering the developing fetus. As its organs and systems are forming, they can be damaged by disturbing influences. It has long been known and accepted that a fetus is more vulnerable to such influences than a child who, in turn, is more vulnerable than an adult. In general, we can say that the younger a human is, the more vulnerable it is to its environment.

It is possible that this trend extends to the egg development, months before conception. Thus a developing egg and its polarization process may be even more susceptible to environmental factors, including the mother's emotions and lifestyle, than is the developing fetus. We know that a fetus is extremely sensitive to environmental factors. It is especially vulnerable, for example, to even very minimal exposure to chemical pollutants. (It is difficult to avoid all such exposure because chemicals like phthalates are found in plastics, lubricants, solvents, cosmetics, personal care products, medical equipment, toys, paints, and packaging, but it is worth the effort to minimize exposure where possible.)

We will see, in Part III, how chemical pollutants affect us, but it is even more important to be aware of these factors when our babies (and our eggs) are developing. A team of scientists at the University of Rochester, New York, found that even minimal exposure to numerous chemicals was linked to a higher risk of genital abnormalities in baby boys. The team, which examined 134 boys, found that women with higher levels of phthalate-related chemicals in their blood were more likely to give birth to boys with undescended or small testicles, small penises, or a shorter distance than usual between the genitals and anus. Abnormalities were even found in women exposed to levels *below* those found in 25 percent of U.S. women. Professor Richard Sharpe, of the UK Medical Research Council's Human Reproductive Science Unit in Edinburgh, considered these findings significant because they offer important evidence that phthalates may cause adverse effects not only on reproductive and genital development, but on many bodily tissues, including the brain.[17]

A study at the University of Missouri has experts concerned that chemicals in oral contraceptives and some man-made chemicals, like ethinylestradiol and bisphenol A, may lead to fetuses having damaged prostates and urethras. Frederick vom Saal, professor of biological sciences at the university, said the results indicate that even small amounts of such estrogenic chemicals may permanently disrupt a fetus's cellular control systems and render the baby's prostate vulnerable to disease.[18] Meanwhile, in Great Britain, Professor Roger Kirby, urologist at St George's Hospital in London and spokesman for the nonprofit Prostate Research Campaign, agreed that environmental factors could be contributing to the rise they are seeing in prostate cancer and the fact that they are seeing it more often in younger people.[19] Cause and effect can have a very long tail, as economists call it: When these same young men grow up, they may contribute to fertility issues themselves.

The Sperm

Just as the quality of a woman's *jing* or *ojas* is reflected in the quality of her eggs, the quality of a man's is reflected in the quality of his sperm. Although women are often initially suspected if there is trouble conceiving, male problems account for 35 to 40 percent of fertility trouble. Perhaps this is not surprising considering the changing colors of the tapestry that is male fertility, virility, and overall reproductive health.

Between 1938 and 1991, men's sperm counts in twenty-one countries, including the United States, plunged an average of 50 percent, while testicular cancer tripled.[20] This was reported by Danish endocrinologist Niels Skakkebaek, who suspects this is due to the men having exposure in utero and as newborns to estrogen-like chemicals in their mothers' blood and milk.[21]

In May 2004, the *New York Times* reported results of a study on mice that determined that parents could incur *genetic* damage by breathing soot from factories or highways and that this damage can be passed on to their offspring.[22] A similar Canadian study in 2002 revealed that mice living in a polluted environment (in this case downwind from steel mills) passed on twice as many DNA mutations to their offspring as did mice that lived in cleaner environments.[23]

Besides affecting a man's children, pollutants damage his sperm. In 2004, BBC News reported that although successful conception may not be affected by whether the father smokes, that smoke may damage the chromosomes in his sperm.[24]

Along with the usual suspects of environment and diet, it is worth considering the effects of lifestyle on a man's reproductive health. For example, it has been found that bike riding for more than short periods on traditional bicycle seats (the ones with a narrow back and a pointed front) lowers the sex drive and causes impotence in men. It can even cause small calcified masses in the scrotum.[25]

A man's procreative ability and the health of his sperm (and that sperm's effect on the developing child) may be affected throughout his life by his lifestyle and dietary choices. It is even possible that he was more vulnerable while he, himself, was in utero, and perhaps especially vulnerable during the few months before he was conceived. Of the roughly 500 million sperm ejaculated during sex, about 4,000 reach the egg. Of these, only one sperm will penetrate and fertilize the egg. Just as a woman's egg is susceptible to influences for three to four months before conception, a man's sperm may be as well. Some years back, I attended a presentation at the University of New Mexico by Dr. Paul Magarelli, a board-certified reproductive endocrinologist and infertility specialist in southern Colorado and New Mexico. I learned that it takes about three months for sperm to get from the somniferous tubule (where sperm are produced) to ejaculation. As we saw above, this is roughly equivalent to the egg-maturation period. Modern science has only recently begun to consider the issue of polarity when it comes to women's eggs. It may be that sperm are equally vulnerable to their environment during their three months before ejaculation.

Ayurvedic medicine teaches that both men and women should prepare for conception at least three months before they will try to conceive. It is ideal for each of them to undergo a cleansing and rejuvenating routine, ending three months before conceiving, to ensure their bodies and emotions are healthy. This has a beneficial effect on the Chosen Sperm and the Chosen Egg that together will become a new human being, as well as on the nuclear family to whom the child is born, and ultimately, on the local and global community to which we all belong.

The Reproductive System

The health of the uterus and associated reproductive tissues, hormones, and organs, is reflected, at least in part, by the presence of a healthy cycle. Ideally, there should be an absence or resolution of ovarian cysts, uterine fibroids, dysfunctional uterine bleeding, pelvic inflammatory disorder, yeast infections, herpes, other sexually transmitted diseases such as chlamydia and gonorrhea, or other local imbalances. Also ideally, before trying to conceive, a woman would follow an appropriate lifestyle, and a dietary and herbal regimen that would help resolve or manage any of these conditions. Again, this leads us to consider the teachings of Ayurveda to prepare for conception.

What constitutes an appropriate diet will vary from woman to woman. (Eastern medicine is loath to offer a one-size-fits-all approach to diet; what is medicine for one woman may be poison for another.) Again, we can look to yin and yang. To conceive, we need sufficient good-quality yin in the form of adequate blood flow through the uterus, good-quality eggs, sufficient fluids, and balanced sex hormones. If a woman doesn't have enough stored energy in the form of good-quality yin, she may have difficulty ovulating, lose her period altogether, or be unable to sustain a pregnancy. If she has excess poor-quality yin, problems such as obesity or blocked passageways may hinder the conception process.

Our modern love affair with yang—with ambition, stress, and a life on the go—contributes to many of the obstacles to conception. If a woman has too much yang, high levels of stress hormones and depleted yin hormones, she may need to slow down, relax, and indulge in some high-quality yin to be able to conceive.

The Nurses' Health Study, begun by Harvard Medical School professor Frank Speizer in 1976, looked at 18,555 women and considered the effect of diet and other factors on ovulatory infertility. Ovulatory infertility is where there is a problem related to the maturation process or release of a mature egg.[26] This study was considering what we could call poor-quality yin versus good-quality yin. As you will see, the findings were exactly in line with what we would expect according to Eastern medicine.

First, some background. When it comes to diet, there is a choice between poor- and high-quality yin. Good-quality carbs such as brown rice, pasta, whole grains, beans, whole vegetables and fruits, fats, proteins, and dairy are considered high-quality yin, provided they are digested well. Poor-quality carbs, fats, proteins, dairy, and poorly digested food are considered poor-quality yin. Examples of poor-quality carbs are those that are quickly digested, such as white breads, sugary sodas, cold breakfast cereals, white rice, potatoes, and highly processed flour products. In the Nurses' Health Study, women who had the highest glycemic load—that is, those who were eating the most of these poor-quality carbs—had up to 92 percent more chance of ovulatory infertility than did women with the lowest glycemic load[27]—those who consumed slow-digesting carbs. The amount of carbs consumed was not anywhere near as important as the quality of carbs.

Like poor-quality carbs, poor-quality fats can have a disastrous effect on ovulatory fertility. In the Nurses' Health Study, trans fats were directly linked to ovulatory infertility, even at only four grams per day—that's roughly two tablespoons of margarine or one doughnut. Whereas unsaturated fats increase insulin sensitivity (that's a good thing) and calm inflammation in the body, trans fats do the opposite.

The quality and quantity of protein was also found to be important. Although it is common for women to be concerned about consuming enough protein, it was found that women who ate the most protein were 41 percent more likely to have problems with ovulatory infertility than were women who consumed the lowest amount.[28] This, it seems, was because of the effects of animal protein on the problem. Eating nuts and beans rich in protein had a beneficial effect, in addition to their containing fiber and many minerals. Women who received their protein from plant sources were considerably less likely to have problems with ovulatory infertility than did women who got their protein from meat. Adding animal protein increased the problem. Whether or not women consumed animal protein, adding plant protein such as beans, peas, tofu, soybeans, or nuts offered them modest protection.

One result of the Nurses' Health Study that may have been surprising outside Eastern medical circles, related to dairy. The study found that one to two daily servings of whole milk (or foods made from it) was beneficial, but nonfat and low-fat milk were harmful. In fact, the more nonfat and low-fat milk a woman consumes, the more likely she will have difficulty getting pregnant. Removing fat from dairy changes its composition of sex hormones. Eastern medicine is not a fan of adulterating foods to begin with, and to take some of the yin (fat) out of a food that is designed by nature to be a rich source of good-quality nourishment—good-quality yin—is altering its nature and defeating its natural purpose.

Of course, too much of a good thing is not good in just about any case. In the Nurses' Health Study, the beneficial effects of whole-milk ice cream, for example, were seen at two half-cup servings a week. A little rich good-quality yin can go a long way. (This isn't permission to eat a gallon of Breyer's ice cream every day.)

Diet isn't the only area where we can get yin. Good-quality sleep and relaxation promote a calm spirit and support nourishment essential to health and conception, but too much sleep or lounging may serve to increase yin beyond a healthy level, if there is already adequate yin.

As with yin, good quality and quantity of exercise, a yang activity, is important. Enough exercise will support a good flow of energy and substance in the body. Too much will drain the yin and may increase stress hormones, throwing sex hormones off balance, to the extent even of eliminating a woman's period. Sometimes doctors prescribe no exercise for women having difficulty conceiving, if it is clear they need more nourishment.

Physical and mental exercises are yang activities. If we have too little of these in our life, our qi or *prana* can become stagnant, leading to problems conceiving as well as other disorders. Too much of them can consume yin, increase stress hormones and throw off hormonal balances.

Establishing reproductive health consists of regulating the cycle and the hormones, having good quality and quantity of yin in the diet and lifestyle, and good quality and quantity of exercise and mental activity to support healthy yang.

Timing of Conception

Timing is the fourth and final crucial element, when looking at conception from an Ayurvedic perspective. This includes the optimal time of the month to become pregnant, the age of the parents when they are attempting to conceive, and other more obscure considerations. For example, Eastern medicine looks at the season, the phase, and position of the moon and planets; the day of the week; the environment; and the emotional state of the parents at the time they conceive. Ambitious parents may even consider which nostril they are breathing through, which way they are facing, and other minutia.

Although it is possible that each of these factors has an effect on the process of conception, most of us do not have sufficiently subtle awareness to accurately make use of them. In addition, we can take this idea too far and in our attempts to control all possible factors related to conception, risk having delusions that we can control the whole process. We may even develop rigid ideas of what is right and wrong. This may not only hinder conception but, if Nature has a sense of humor, it will turn our ideas of perfection into mincemeat. For most of us, it may be sufficient to calmly consider the environment into which we are considering inviting a soul. Is this an appropriate time of life to have a child? Does our home feel good? Is our relationship harmonious? Are our minds calm? These factors may have an effect on the process and chances of conception as well as on the resulting child.

Western medicine also has something to say about the less obscure considerations. It is interesting that perhaps the most useful information for preventing pregnancy can actually be used to *achieve* it. In Chapter 11, I talked about fertility awareness and the book *Taking Charge of Your Fertility: The Definitive Guide to Natural Birth Control, Pregnancy Achievement, and Reproductive Health* by Toni Weschler, MPH (see Appendix A). This book gives a comprehensive description of how to chart and interpret your signs of fertility, how to pinpoint if there is an impediment to conception, how to identify what the impediment is, and how to maximize the chances of conception. I cannot recommend this book highly enough. If every woman was familiar with the knowledge this book presents, there would be far fewer expensive, often unnecessary procedures that women would undergo to increase their chances of conception. Instead, a woman would be confident about when she has the best chance of conception and would be an educated and full participant in her efforts to conceive.

PARENTAL AGE

The age of the parents must also be taken into consideration. Generally, it is optimal for a woman to conceive between the ages of eighteen and thirty-five, when she is physically, mentally, and emotionally well equipped for motherhood. For men, it is preferable to father a child before a man is in his fifties. While it is common knowledge that the risks of carrying and delivering a child increase as a woman ages, the risks associated with aging fathers are not as widely known. Increased paternal age has been linked to schizophrenia and autism, and a large Swedish study recently found that the older the father, the more likely his child is to develop bipolar disorder as an adult. The oldest fathers in the study were 35 percent more likely than the youngest to have children who would go on to develop bipolar disorders as adults. Fathers aged fifty-five years and older were 1.37 times more likely to have affected children than were fathers twenty to twenty-four years old.[29] This study supports a previous hypothesis that advancing paternal age is a risk factor for neurodevelopmental disorders.[30]

Although the Swedish study showed that the mother's age had no statistically significant effect on whether her child developed bipolar disorder later in life, a woman's chances of miscarriage increases with age, the quality of her eggs declines, and her likelihood of conception decreases. In a study by the National Institute of Environmental Health Sciences, there was a 50 percent decrease in the likelihood of pregnancy between women in their early twenties and those in their late thirties. When having intercourse at the most fertile time of their menstrual cycle, women aged nineteen to twenty-six had a fifty-fifty chance of conceiving. From age twenty-seven to thirty-four, those chances decreased to 40 percent. From age thirty-five to thirty-nine, the conception rate dropped below 30 percent.[31] After age thirty-five, a woman's chances of miscarriage also increase. A twenty-five- to thirty-five-year-old who conceives has a 15 percent chance of miscarriage; however, a forty-year-old woman has a 40 percent chance.[32]

Despite this reality, there is a modern trend for couples to wait until their late thirties and forties—older for men—to have children. Modern medicine is responding to the challenges accompanying this trend by attempting to manipulate physiology, through assisted reproductive technologies or other treatment options. For example, scientists are experimenting with freezing slices of a young woman's ovarian tissues for later return to her so that her younger, more viable, healthy eggs can be used later in her life. They are also experimenting with sucking the nucleus out of an older woman's egg and transferring it into the cytoplasm of another woman's younger egg. Aside from this practice, which is not widely practiced, egg donors, IVF and other assisted reproductive technologies have become common practice.

One visible cross-section of women who are having babies later in life is Hollywood celebrities. When we see one of these women smiling, glowing, and pregnant on the cover of supermarket magazines, we may receive false or misleading impressions. "Not one of us can take fertility for granted," says Robin Roberts, president of the support group Resolve of Greater Los Angeles. "In hearing about the technology, people assume there will be an answer. Hollywood actresses and other successful women over 40—who are likely using donor eggs—give the illusion that our fertility can be extended, and it can't."[33]

Certain lifestyle choices can render a woman's reproductive age older than her actual years. Smoking, as I mentioned earlier, can add the equivalent of ten years to a woman's reproductive age. This not only decreases her chances of conception and increases her risk of miscarriage at any age, it reduces the chances of successful IVF treatment and decreases the chances of a live birth resulting from an IVF pregnancy.[34]

As we saw, Traditional Chinese Medicine considers that people have progressively less *jing* as they age, or as they injure it through inappropriate lifestyle or choices such as smoking. As a woman's *jing* decreases, her chance of miscarriage increases, as do the chances of problems with the developing fetus or resulting child. As a man's *jing* decreases, he risks passing on an increasing number of disorders to his offspring.

Even though there are risks, known and unknown, associated with assisted reproductive technologies, I don't mean to imply that their use is never appropriate. It may be ideal to avoid them, but such decisions are never made in a vacuum, using nothing but logic as the fuel to drive them.

If a couple were unable to conceive, Eastern medicine would counsel that they work first on regaining their own health before trying to bring another being into the world. If they regain their health sufficiently, they may be able to conceive without the aid of assisted reproductive technologies. However, if the woman is still unable to conceive and her desire to have a child is so consuming that she feels her life will not be complete without one, this desire will affect her spirit. If her spirit cannot be assuaged through adopting a child or finding another solution, its disturbance could affect first the qi or *prana* of the mother and then her own bodily tissues further. In cases like this, it may be that this suffering outweighs the suffering associated with taking advantage of assisted reproductive technologies to help her fulfill her desire.

What Does Eastern Medicine Do About Conception?

In general, if a couple wishes to conceive, Eastern medicine counsels the mother to consider her overall health, including the health of her eggs and reproductive organs; asks the father to consider his overall health as well as the health of his sperm; and suggests that both of them choose the appropriate timing for conception. If a woman's menstrual cycle is irregular or troubled, or her reproductive organs are in disorder, or if the man's sperm is scanty, Eastern medicine will address these imbalances first, through lifestyle, diet, and herbs, if possible.

Rather than target the specific troubled organ, egg, or sperm, we first address the overall physical and mental well being of both parents. Ayurveda recommends that the couple undergoes a cleansing process called *panchakarma*, well supervised by an experienced practitioner. This process should end three months before trying to conceive.

Panchakarma is a unique aspect of Ayurvedic medicine. It is a detoxification regimen designed to rid the body of toxic material. Using an individually prescribed combination of warm medicated oil massage, steam, and detoxifying herbs and therapies, toxins from the deeper tissues of the body are encouraged to move into the gastrointestinal tract, from where they can be eliminated. This practice has been utilized in India for thousands of years and is only beginning to gain acceptance in Western countries over the last decade or two. (See Appendix A for a brief description of *panchakarma* and where to receive it.)

The mental and emotional health of the parents is considered of paramount importance because we understand that a person's physical tissues and processes are only as healthy as the qi or *prana* flowing through them, and that qi, in turn, is only healthy and free flowing if the spirit is calm.

Whatever a woman's age, Eastern medicine suggests she spend some time gaining, regaining, or building her strength and health before getting pregnant, even if it is easy for her to conceive. Addressing and, if possible, resolving such issues as obesity or diabetes, for example, will have a good effect on a woman and may well increase her chances of conception and healthy pregnancy. Eastern medicine suggests resolving even minor imbalances before conceiving. If a woman's body and mind are healthy, her reproductive health is more likely to be optimized. Instead of focusing on just the reproductive organs, sometimes it is beneficial for a couple to temporarily forget about trying to conceive and, instead, spend some time trying to get healthy and enjoy healthy living.

Jane's story is a clear illustration of this. She came to me wanting to get pregnant. She regularly smoked pot, enjoyed wine every evening, and was very overworked in her life. Her plan was to quit the pot and wine and to reduce her workload once she got pregnant. But she had had a lot of trouble conceiving. We discussed a new strategy, based on the possibility that her child did not have a suitable place to land. It was as if she were inviting a guest to enter when her door was nailed shut. We developed a new plan in which Jane immediately cut back to part-time work, quit pot and alcohol, began to eat nourishing food, and started a simple yoga practice. In this way she would create a life that was an invitation for her child. Within months of following her new plan, Jane got pregnant.

GET QI TO MOVE SMOOTHLY

A key maxim of Eastern medicine is that the nourishing fluids of the body (blood, lymph, menstrual blood, etc.) follow and imitate whatever the qi or *prana* is doing. If the qi is stagnant, then those fluids will stagnate. If there is insufficient qi, by and by there will be insufficient nourishing fluids. The amount of blood flowing through the uterus (called the pulsitility index) plays an important role in fertility. In general, in the absence of other problematic issues, the greater the pulsitility index, the greater the likelihood of conception. This is why acupuncture is so good at supporting fertility. It encourages the movement of qi, and therefore blood, in and through the uterus, often resolving the stagnation and allowing conception to occur.

Linda was thirty-five, practiced an intensely vigorous form of yoga for hours a day, was thin as a rail, and had never been pregnant despite having unprotected sex her entire life. She assumed she was infertile. She came to me for treatment of scanty periods. On her first visit, we did a very simple acupuncture treatment that moved qi in the body, especially in the uterus. The next time I saw her, she was pregnant. Linda is one of many women I have seen become pregnant after beginning acupuncture. Moving and harmonizing qi is powerful medicine.

CALM YOUR SPIRIT

A second key maxim of Eastern medicine is that if the spirit is disturbed, qi will become disturbed. If the spirit stagnates, so will qi. If the spirit is scattered, qi will scatter and become weak. This means that to conceive, it is beneficial to get out of a rut if we are in one and to calm down if we are nervous. Once the spirit is calm, qi can flow easily through the body. When qi flows, blood will flow, the pulsitility index will improve, and the likelihood of conception will increase. To focus only on the quality of the eggs is to miss the forest for the trees. It is equally, if not more, important to consider the quality of the spirit and to ensure that it is content and peaceful.

In 2001, Judith Hanson Lasater wrote in *Yoga Journal* about a couple that tried unsuccessfully for five years to conceive a child. They finally succeeded after practicing yoga for seven months and focusing on becoming healthy, rather than on becoming parents.[35] Indeed, this is a very common story. The stress involved in trying to conceive decreases the flow of qi or *prana* that circulates in the body and mind, and it can actually hinder the physical process of conception.

There is an open secret among physicians and health-care practitioners who work with couples trying to conceive. These couples try and try, and their stress levels get higher and higher with each unsuccessful attempt, until one, the other, or both partners give up. They decide they'll wait, maybe adopt, maybe try again, but in any case take a break for a while. It is then that the woman finally conceives. This is not to minimize the couples' plight or to say that stress is the only cause for infertility and a woman can always conceive if she would "just relax," but this is an impressively common story.

Katie and her husband, Zach, both busy professionals, tried for four years to conceive, but to no avail. Katie's cycle was regular and Zach's sperm count was normal. Their doctors diagnosed infertility but couldn't find any physiological reason behind it. The couple began to feel desperate and turned to assisted reproductive technologies to support their endeavor. After five rounds of the prescription ovulatory stimulant Clomid, multiple trips to the doctor, and accumulated debt from the cost of treatment, Katie still wasn't pregnant. Stress and frustration was becoming a way of life and got cyclically worse with each ovulation that didn't produce a pregnancy. When stress began to take toll on Katie and Zach's relationship, they decided they needed to stop trying to conceive a child. They began to take a philosophical view that perhaps it wasn't meant to be. They scheduled a trip to Laguna Beach, California, where they could spend a week surfing, lying in the sun, and reconnecting in a way that had nothing to do with charts, planned sex, or ovulatory mucous. It was during this week that they conceived. Their daughter, Katlyn, is now a healthy six-year-old, and their son, Eli—also conceived without ART—is an energetic four.

Eastern medicine explains this phenomenon by understanding that stress causes us to clench, emotionally and physically. Clenching causes stagnation of qi or *prana*. Stagnation of qi is a decidedly poor condition if you want to conceive. It is essential that the qi move smoothly, so that blood can flow smoothly and irrigate the uterus and associated organs.

YOGA FOR CONCEPTION

One way to support a calm spirit and smooth-flowing qi is to practice slow and stretchy yoga poses that encourage the hips to open and qi to flow smoothly in the lower abdomen and reproductive organs. The physical exercise supports free-flowing qi and the calming, centering practice of yoga supports a calm spirit.

In November 2001, *Yoga Journal* reported that Rahul Sachdev, MD, a specialist in reproductive endocrinology and infertility at the Robert Wood Johnson Medical School in New Brunswick, New Jersey, suggests that a woman's chances of successfully conceiving may be vastly increased by incorporating stress-relieving yoga with traditional and medical intervention.[36] Dr. Sachdev supervised a program that showed remarkable results for couples who hadn't been able to conceive. Regardless of the woman's cause of infertility, 50 percent of couples who completed a program that incorporated yoga, meditation, and dietary changes conceived within the following year.[37] A similar Harvard study that incorporated yoga and relaxation found that participants were about three times more likely to conceive than were women who didn't participate.[38]

That same article recommended specific yoga poses that stimulate the smooth flow of energy through the reproductive organs and increase the circulation of energy and blood in the area.[39]

Jacklyn was thirty-two and her husband Frank, forty-three. Although their fertility doctor could find no physiological conditions that would preclude conception, they were unable to conceive for two years. They decided they were uncomfortable with pharmaceutical drugs or interventions as a solution, so they came to me to see if there was a different option. Both had strong constitutions and good baseline health. Frank had some deficiency of what Traditional Chinese Medicine calls Kidney qi, which relates to reproductive vitality. The onset of Jacklyn's periods fluctuated between twenty-five and thirty-two days and she experienced pain and cramping with her cycle. Her symptoms indicated stagnant qi in the reproductive organs. I recommended that they take three months off from trying to conceive and spend those months focusing on improving their own individual health and well-being. We came up with a plan. Frank began to include some qi gong—a qi-building exercise—for his Kidney qi into his daily routine. Jacklyn was more attracted to yoga, so she began some local classes and started a ten-minute daily yoga practice that included some poses called "hip openers" that encourage the free flow of *prana* through the reproductive organs. She also practiced five minutes a day of gentle, deep alternate-nostril breathing, a form of *pranayama* (breathing exercises) that helps balance hormones. She also applied castor oil packs three times a week (see Appendix E) except during her period, and she took a personally tailored herb formula for three months. These worked together to support smooth qi and blood flow through the uterus.

After three months, Jacklyn's periods were no longer painful and had shifted to a regular cycle of twenty-eight days. She no longer required herbs or castor oil packs but she continued her yoga practice. Frank reported having greater stamina. He continued his qi gong practice, as this would help ensure that his initial imbalances would be less likely to recur.

What Should I Do?

1. Follow the three pillars of health listed in Part III: appropriate diet, lifestyle, and stress management. (Suggestions for how to get started in these areas are listed in on pages 46–52.) These help prevent stagnation that might impede conception; they support free and easy movement of qi or *prana*, which in turn increases the chance of conception, and they encourage the hormonal balance necessary for conceiving.

2. Focus on getting healthy first. Then focus on conceiving.

3. Relax.

4. Be in good shape three months before you want to conceive.

5. Consult with a qualified Ayurvedic practitioner to determine whether doing *panchakarma* (ending three months before you want to conceive) is appropriate for you. Some *panchakarma* facilities are listed in Appendix A.

6. If possible, have your baby before age thirty-five—or as soon after age thirty-five as you can—and with the age of the father less than fifty.

7. Avoid smoking and breathing secondhand smoke.

8. Avoid chemicals and polluted water, air, and general environment, especially for the three months prior to conception, and during pregnancy and nursing.

9. If you are having trouble conceiving, read *Taking Charge of Your Fertility: The Definitive Guide to Natural Birth Control, Pregnancy Achievement, and Reproductive Health* by Toni Weschler, MPH. It's an essential guide to fertility awareness.

10. Consult with a qualified practitioner of TCM or Ayurveda if you are still having trouble conceiving.

২৩ 13 ৩৫

Breast Health

B reast cancer is the most common form of cancer in women.[1] As of 2001, the United States had one of the highest breast cancer rates of any country in the world.[2] From 1940 through the early 1990s, the incidence of breast cancer rose steadily there and, by 2001, was the second leading cause of death for U.S. women, second only to heart disease.[3] Breast cancer rates are higher in developed countries (especially North America and Europe) than in Asia.

As we've seen with other health problems, the risk factors for breast cancer include elements that are both within and outside our control. Genetic predisposition, exposure to ionizing radiation, not having babies (or having a late first pregnancy), and late menopause are all factors that increase a woman's risk. But if we lump together all the factors that we know increase the risk of breast cancer, including genetics, they explain only about *a third of all cases*.[4] What is causing the other two-thirds? We don't know the whole story, but several factors are highly suspect, some of which are within our control. These include exposure to pollutants, poor nutrition, poor exercise habits, and high stress. Reproductive organs, particularly breasts, ovaries, and the uterus, are highly sensitive to estrogen, whether it is good or bad estrogen.

Considering the Known Risk Factors

GENETICS

Genetic predisposition to cancer is a factor that's not within our control and, unfortunately, it does have a strong influence on breast health. You may have increased genetic risks associated with your race, or other genes that indicate higher risk. If your mother and sister both have had breast cancer, your chances of developing it are four to six times higher.[5] Genetic risk doesn't mean you will definitely develop it, though. It just means that it is that much more important for you to avoid other factors that increase the risk of breast cancer and to adopt lifestyle and dietary habits that are known to reduce your risk.

ENVIRONMENT

Estrogen-like pollutants, aptly called endocrine disruptors, have detrimental effects in the body. Breast tissue is particularly vulnerable to their toxic effects. Women in developed countries, which contribute high levels of toxic estrogenic chemicals to the environment, account for over 50 percent of all cases of breast cancer.[6] Because genetics may account for only 10 to 15 percent of breast cancer cases,[7] some scientists are looking at whether environmental factors are at the root of some of the others.

Two researchers, Devra Lee Davis from the Department of Health and Health and Human Services and H. Leon Bradlow from Cornell Cancer Research Laboratory, have proposed that environmental estrogenic substances may contribute to breast cancer in several ways. They can enhance production of "bad" estrogens (see Chapter 3), damage DNA, bind to estrogen receptors in breast tissue and relay signals that lead to abnormal cell growth, or support the generation of new blood vessels needed to feed tumors.[8]

Breast tissue is rife with estrogen receptors and so may be particularly vulnerable to the nasty effects of chemical pollutants. A 1993 study by Mary Wolff of New York's Mount Sinai School of Medicine revealed "unusual amounts" of DDE, a by-product of DDT, in the breast tissue of women with breast cancer.[9] Davis and Bradlow found that chemical pesticides and by-products greatly increase the amount of "bad" estrogen in cultured breast-cancer cells, whereas natural plant estrogens produced a positive effect.[10] They stated,

> If reducing avoidable exposures to xenoestrogens [by-products of industrial or chemical processing that have estrogen-like effects] were to make it possible to avert even 20 percent of breast cancers every year (four times more than are caused by inheritance of flawed genes), at least thirty-six thousand women— and those who care about them—would be spared this difficult disease.[11]

In Part III, we will look at these estrogen-like chemicals in detail and see how they make their way into the body from the environment. Although it is unclear exactly how much environmental estrogens contribute to the prevalence of breast cancer today, this factor, unlike congenital factors, represents one we can avoid.

DIET

Changes in diet may prevent 30 to 40 percent of cancer cases, or 3 to 4 million cases annually.[12] In a study widely reported in April 2008, women with the highest levels of trans fats in their blood were found to have about twice the risk of breast cancer compared to women with the lowest levels.[13] These results are similar to those released in 1997 after a fourteen-year study of eighty thousand nurses.[14] Trans fats are not found in nature. They are the result of food processing, and although food manufacturers are phasing them out, they are still present in many baked goods, snack crackers, stick margarines, salad dressings, and microwave popcorn. Check the Nutrition Facts label on processed foods to see if they contain trans fats. Also note that foods that list "partially hydrogenated vegetable oil" on the label contain trans fat.

Eating lots of fruits and veggies might be one of the most important dietary factors that we can change. They protect against many types of cancer by enhancing cancer-protective capacity, deactivating carcinogens, and blocking tumor development.[15] Many vegetables, such as broccoli, and beans like soy contain phytoestrogens that can have a protective effect against breast cancer. We'll look more at phytoestrogens in Part III.

ALCOHOL

In 2009, the National Cancer Institute reported the results of the Million Women Study. Conducted in the Great Britain and reported in the *Journal of the National Cancer Institute*, it followed over a million women for an average of seven years. It is the largest study yet undertaken. The results were clear: The possible beneficial effects of moderate alcohol consumption on cardiovascular health were outweighed by the increased risk of various kinds of cancers. For each additional daily drink—no matter what type of alcohol—there were eleven additional breast cancers per thousand women up to age seventy-five.[16]

In April 2008, a study of more than 184,000 women was reported to show that having one or two small drinks a day—again regardless of the type of alcohol consumed—raised a woman's risk of developing a hormone-sensitive tumor (the most common type of breast cancer, comprising 70 percent of all cases) to 32 percent higher than that of nondrinkers. In addition, the study found, having three or more drinks a day raised the risk to 51 percent higher than that of nondrinkers.[17]

Apparently at least one of the ways that alcohol leads to an increased cancer risk is that it interferes with estrogen metabolism. Healthy kidneys and liver (which is taxed by alcohol consumption) are vital to maintain a proper estrogen balance. A healthy liver breaks down excess estrogen in the blood and sends it to the kidneys, which flush it from the body. If alcohol compromises liver health, the liver may not break down excess estrogen efficiently. Instead, the excess estrogen will get reabsorbed into the blood and continue to circulate.[18]

In February 2007, twenty-six scientists from fifteen countries met in Lyon, France, at the International Agency for Research on Cancer to reassess the connection between alcohol and cancer. In April 2007, Britain's prestigious *Lancet Oncology* journal reported the results of this gathering.[19] These results are in line with those of the 2008 study and also explore the link to other types of cancer. The scientists estimated that people who drank fifty grams of alcohol a day—roughly five standard drinks—had a 40 percent greater risk of colorectal cancer than did nondrinkers and that the women within that group had a 50 percent greater risk of breast cancer. Even if they drank only eighteen grams a day—less than two drinks—their risk was significantly higher than that of nondrinkers.[20]

RADIATION (MAMMOGRAMS VS. PHYSICAL BREAST EXAMS)

Radiation has been proven to increase the risk of cancer. Radiation comes in many forms. It can come from radioactive fallout, radiation accidents, or X-rays. A major risk factor of breast cancer is irradiation of the chest with high doses of X-rays, as was common in the past.[21] One study revealed that women with scoliosis who were given multiple chest X-rays during puberty were more likely to develop and die of breast cancer than were women without this history.[22]

This may cause us to ask about the radiation involved in mammograms. A mammogram is an X-ray of the breast. On one hand, high-risk women are usually encouraged to get mammograms more often. But if you have a greater risk, we might question the practice of increasing the exposure of your breast tissue to radiation, a known carcinogen.

While it is indisputable that mammography delivers radiation, the level of radiation in today's mammography is reported to be quite low, compared to that associated with older, high-dose radiation equipment. The number of rads (the units used to measure radiation absorbed from X-rays) a woman receives in one mammogram today has been compared to what she would be exposed to during a commercial flight from New York to California (due to being closer to the sun and other stars). One mammogram picture delivers a dose of about 0.1 to 0.2 rads and most mammograms require two pictures per breast.[23] It seems to me that the difference here would be that the radiation a woman would be exposed to on the flight may be evenly distributed, compared to a mammogram, which would concentrate the dose in the breast tissue. There is some evidence that, especially in premenopausal women, breast tissue is highly sensitive to the effects of radiation.

Whether or not the radiation dose that mammography delivers is a problem, there is also the question of how much mammography actually works to decrease mortality from breast cancer. From 1990 to 2006, the death rate due to breast cancer decreased about 2 percent per year, a drop that has been attributed to better treatment and earlier detection.[24] Mammograms are promoted to increase the chance of early detection of breast cancer, and early detection is said to increase the chances of successful treatment. Some evidence suggests, however, that although mammography may increase early detection, it doesn't affect the overall mortality rate, because the tumors that mammograms detect are either so slow growing they would never threaten the woman's life or could be detected by a vigilant woman doing breast self-exam before it reached a dangerous stage, or they are so rapid-growing that even early detection by a mammogram will be too late to catch it early.

In a 2009 letter to the *Times* of London (as reported by the *New York Times*), experts complained that handouts on mammograms exaggerate the benefits of screening and omit crucial information about the potential downsides, thereby misguiding women.[25] They cited a 2006 analysis by the Nordic Cochrane Center collaborative, an independent research and information center based in Copenhagen, that found that for every woman's life saved by screening, up to ten are subjected to overtreatment that unnecessarily disrupts their lives. The experts complained that women are often diagnosed and surgically treated for cancers that are so slow growing that they would never have threatened the women's lives. The same *New York Times* article also reported that not everybody agrees that these statistics accurately reflect the situation. Not all experts agree that the risks of mammograms might outweigh the benefits.

One issue is that slow growing cancers do not look any different under a microscope than fast-growing cancers, so it is difficult to know when to aggressively treat and when to take a more relaxed approach. In the final analysis, the article promotes women's educating themselves as much as possible and making the final decision themselves about whether to have mammograms, and how often to have them.

Veronica was a vibrant, active engineer with a busy life that involved national and international travel. She ate a diet of mostly whole foods and favored organic produce and regular exercise, but since her late twenties, she had had a history of breast lumps that would come and go. These were both fibrocystic lumps and benign tumors. Her doctors were concerned that she was at risk for breast cancer and kept a vigilant watch over her breast health. Veronica had had mammograms every six months since she was thirty-five years old. When she was diagnosed with breast cancer at age fifty-three, three months after her last mammogram (which did not detect it), it was an aggressive form that had already spread to her lymph nodes. Veronica underwent chemotherapy and surgery. She saw an acupuncturist weekly, to support her as she went through these rigorous treatments. She felt the Western treatments were essential but said that the visits to the acupuncturist were the only hours of the week when she felt better. Veronica used the wisdom and practices of Eastern medicine to support her return to strength after the Western treatment regimen was over.

It is certainly difficult to meet the challenges present today in how best to monitor our breast health. Dr. Otis Brawley, a cancer researcher from Emory University, told the *New York Times* in 2002, "Mammogram screening, at best, prevents one breast cancer death per year out of every 17,000 women over age 50 who are screened. The figure is even lower for women in their 40's—one out of every 25,000. Yet doctors and public health officials have said mammograms are vitally important in the fight against breast cancer."[26]

The U.S. Preventive Services Task Force is an independent panel of experts that analyzes data and then advises the medical community on appropriate medical protocol. From 2002 until November 2009, they encouraged women to have yearly mammograms beginning at age forty. Their message was heavy on the "early detection saves lives" line. In November 2009, after analyzing the most current data available, they reversed their recommendations. Now regular mammograms are recommended only for women fifty and over, and even then, only every other year instead of annually.[27] The task force concluded that although these new recommendations would provide nearly the same protective benefits as the old ones, the negative effects would be roughly halved. The negative effects cited are the increased risk of unnecessary treatments, such as biopsies and treatment of cancers that are so slow growing they would never threaten a woman's life, and the significant anxiety and physical discomfort related to such procedures and treatments. Members of the task force found themselves in the middle of an emotionally charged political maelstrom as a result of announcing this reversal. However, the task force, appointed by Republican president George W. Bush,[28] revealed their findings under Democratic president Barack Obama, and profess to be unbiased and apolitical. This is simply an emotionally charged issue for many people.

Samuel S. Epstein, MD, the founder and chairman of the Cancer Prevention Coalition, who shares the concern about radiation exposure from mammograms, suggests the use of breast self-exam as a safe alternative to mammograms. On his Web site, he cites a September 2000 publication based on a large-scale screening study at the University of Toronto that concluded that a monthly breast self-examination (BSE) following brief training, coupled with annual clinical breast examination by a trained health-care professional is a safe alternative to mammograms and is at least as effective in detecting early tumors.[29]

This may sound like a good idea, but upon further analysis, it is not clear that the BSE method is particularly helpful. In fact, it may present more problems than solutions. In a trial in China, conducted over about ten years, 266,000 women were randomly assigned to one of two groups. One group received regular, periodic instruction in the BSE method and frequent reminders to practice it. The control group received no instruction or reminders. After ten years, the number of deaths due to breast cancer was almost identical. The group that practiced BSE had more women who had benign breast biopsies.[30] This would seem to show that women did find more lumps, but the lumps were benign and it might have been preferable not to find them in the first place than be subjected to the subsequent, sometimes costly, and ultimately unnecessary fear-inducing procedures that determined their benign status. Another problem with this approach is the expense involved to effectively and accurately teach women the BSE method and to provide follow-up care to ensure they do the self-exams.

There is some evidence that when BSE or clinical breast examination is being practiced accurately by trained health-care practitioners, it can be as effective as mammography and can reduce mortality as well. The challenge is making sure that the exams are practiced accurately. The logistical and financial challenges inherent in training all women or health-care practitioners to practice excellent breast examination methods currently seem insurmountable.[31]

Other Tools for Detection

Aside from mammograms and breast exams, there are other tools to increase the possibility of early detection. Although the American Cancer Society maintains that thermal imaging, or thermography, is not an effective method of early detection, some health-care practitioners feel that when it is practiced and interpreted correctly, it is an effective alternative or complementary technique to mammography, BSE, and clinical breast examination, especially for women under age fifty (for whom mammography is less effective). Thermal imaging is a noninvasive, comfortable, and simple procedure that involves no radiation. It measures the skin temperature of the breast, looking for places where the temperature is higher, possibly indicating the presence of tumors, which have increased temperature due to increased blood flow. But finding someone well trained in thermal imaging is not easy, and I am not aware of any studies that show long-term success in both increasing life expectancy and in not subjecting women to undue, unnecessary procedures in the cases of early detection. Thermal imaging can detect thermal changes so early that it is detecting precancerous rises in temperature—or conditions that may predispose a woman to developing cancer, and so she can then choose to change her diet and lifestyle to avoid getting it in the first place.

It is up to each of us to assess the methods available for breast-cancer detection and decide on a course of action for ourselves. For myself, I feel that combining a monthly self-examination with a thorough, near daily massage of the breasts and surrounding tissues is the most beneficial for preventive care. It also seems to me that, if we start out with a healthy diet and lifestyle, rather than waiting for diagnosis or thermal differentials in our breasts or some other warning sign, we may often be able to avoid more difficult choices altogether.

Synthetic Hormones and Breast Health

As we discussed earlier, synthetic progesterone in the form of Depo-Provera causes the rapid proliferation of breast cancer cells. It has been shown that after less than a year of using synthetic progesterone–only supplementation, there is a 60 percent increase in risk of breast cancer. Another study found that "all of the women diagnosed with breast cancer under twenty-five years of age and nearly all of those diagnosed under forty-four years of age had used combined oral contraceptives,"[32] that is, ones that combine estrogen and progestin. The prestigious medical journal the *Lancet* published the results of a large study on oral contraception showing that use of birth-control pills before age twenty doubled the risk of breast cancer.[33] As already noted, in 2005 the World Health Organization's cancer research group reclassified the Pill from "possibly carcinogenic to humans" to "carcinogenic to humans.[34]

For most women, the most important risk factor for breast cancer is lifetime exposure to estrogen. With each menstrual cycle, a woman is exposed to a surge in estradiol, the most potent of the three main types of estrogen. Therefore, the more cycles she has in her lifetime, the greater her overall exposure to estradiol.[35] This means that the later a woman's menarche, the earlier her menopause, the more pregnancies she has, and the more she nurses, the less she is exposed to the surges in estradiol that accompany her cycle. Indeed, less breast cancer is seen in these women than their sisters with early menarche, late menopause, fewer pregnancies, and less nursing.[36]

Some literature suggests that only women who have babies before the age of thirty-five reduce their risk of breast cancer, but at least one study showed that, regardless of a woman's age, her age at her first birth, her country of origin or ethnic origin, and even without her breastfeeding, her risk decreased by 7 percent with each birth.[37]

We have seen that there is a movement to pharmaceutically induce fewer periods to reduce a woman's chances of breast cancer. But we have also explored the potential problems with this line of thinking as well.

One concern with taking synthetic hormones is that some synthetic hormonal prescriptions are linked with increased risk of breast cancer or abnormal mammograms. In 2002, a study published in the *Journal of the American Medical Association* found a 60 to 85 percent increased incidence of all histologic types of breast cancer combined when women used either long-term estrogen therapy, either alone or with combined estrogen and progestin therapy.[38] (*Histology* refers to the study of the cellular structure of tissues and, in the case of breast cancers, it commonly includes lobular or ductal cell cancers, though there are other rare types.)

Other studies show that unopposed synthetic estrogen (that is, estrogen without progestin) is associated with a 34 percent increased risk of breast cancer,[39] but the picture is not entirely clear. A 2006 study published in the *Journal of the American Medical Association* found that in 10,700 women without a uterus (women who had had prior hysterectomies), taking estrogen supplementation alone did not increase the risk of breast cancer, but did increase the risk of more abnormal mammograms ("usually requiring that the test be repeated, and more breast biopsies").[40] This, like the false alarms created by mammograms, breast self-exam, and clinical breast examination methods, causes unnecessary stress, which we know is a main culprit when it comes to hormonal imbalance. It also is costly and time consuming. This same study was halted in February 2004 because the estrogen supplementation increased the risk for strokes, blood clots in the legs, and dementia in women over age sixty-five.[41] Although the study was halted in 2004, the women will continue to be studied for the next seven years to see the follow-up effects of estrogen on breast cancer. Of course, it is not known yet what the longer-term effects of estrogen exposure are. If it increases the risk of abnormal mammograms, is it likely that over a longer period of time it would increase the real risk of breast cancer?

In 2009, an *Archives of Internal Medicine* follow-up study on seventeen thousand WHI participants revealed that postmenopausal women who experience breast tenderness when they go on combination hormone therapy may face increased risk of breast cancer. Women with this new-onset symptom after being on HRT for twelve months were about 50 percent more likely than were women without breast tenderness to be diagnosed with breast cancer over the next 5.6 years. This association was not seen with women in the placebo group.[42]

Whether or not unopposed estrogen increases the risk of breast cancer, or simply false alarms, the risk is not mitigated by the presence of progestins, the way that it is with uterine cancer. In fact, the presence of a progestin may even increase the risk of breast cancer. The large-scale NIH study we discussed in Chapter 6 showed a 29 percent increased risk of breast cancer over five years of use of combined estrogen and progestin. Some science suggests a 53 percent increased risk of breast cancer compared with women not taking hormones and that the longer a woman takes HRT, the greater her risk of breast cancer.[43]

In October 2010, a follow-up of 12,788 participants in the Women's Health Initiative study revealed that not only did HRT use increase the incidence of breast cancer, it also increased the risk of the cancer being deadly.[44]

Dr. Peter B. Bach, a physician at Memorial Sloan-Kettering Cancer Center, said in an interview, "If you care about preventing this disease and keeping women from suffering and dying from it, then it's hard to look at these drugs and not have serious concerns about them being used, even for what are intended to be relatively short periods of time."[45]

What Does Eastern Medicine Do for Breast Health?

I find myself looking to Traditional Chinese Medicine and Ayurveda for a greater understanding of how to promote breast health and why conditions such as fibrocystic breasts, benign cysts, and breast cancer arise. Over the years I have come to believe that there are two main factors that foster breast disorders: the accumulation in breast tissue of toxic sludge (which Ayurveda calls *ama*) and stagnation, which keeps the sludge in place.

TOXIC SLUDGE (*AMA*)

Ama is a sticky, toxic sludge created from poorly digested matter. It is also a by-product of exposure to pollutants. We will discus *ama* more extensively in Part III, but in terms of breast health there are a couple of things to know. *Ama* arises from toxic external chemicals that have an affinity with breast tissue, from ingested chemicals that have the same affinity, from poor-quality food, or from poorly digested food. In each case, *ama* circulates in the bloodstream and lodges in the breasts if there is stagnation in the chest area.

Diet and digestion are inextricably linked in Eastern medicine. I recommend reading Chapter 21 and following those recommendations under the guidance of your health-care practitioner to ensure that you are eating a diet that is appropriate for you and one that you can digest. However, there are some points specifically related to breast health that are worth a minute or two here.

Healthy digestion and elimination reduces the amount of *ama* that circulates in the bloodstream, and hence the levels of *ama* that are available to pollute breast tissue. We see this connection between diet and breast health talked about in Western medicine, too. A high-fiber diet—one that includes a lot of vegetables, fruits, and whole grains, and very little processed food, white flour, and white sugar foods—causes less fecal bacteria. Having less fecal bacteria is a good thing because it means less excess or bad estrogen in the blood is reabsorbed into the body and more of it is eliminated through stool.[46] We also know that too much estrogen in the blood is unhealthy for breast tissue, so there is a direct connection here between diet and breast cancer. Results of one Canadian study of fifty-six thousand women indicated that those who followed a high-fiber diet had 30 percent less breast cancer risk than did women on a low-fiber diet.[47]

Trans fats act just like *ama*. We have seen, in studies from 1997[48] and 2008,[49] that women with the highest levels of trans fats in their blood had about twice the risk of breast cancer compared to women with the lowest levels.

Soy is often touted as a food that helps prevent breast cancer. The question of soy is one that's been prevalent recently; we'll discuss this further in Chapter 24. We will see that Asian populations, which consume easily digestible forms of soy, enjoy a decreased risk of breast cancer. [50] Eastern medicine says that soy is easier to digest if it is cooked well, consumed as warm soy milk, tamari, tofu, miso, or tempeh, and, preferably, eaten with fresh ginger.

STAGNATION

According to Eastern medicine, there can be stagnation of qi, or of nourishing fluids—manifestations of yang and yin, respectively. Stagnation in the breast tissue of both qi and nourishing fluids is a common malady for modern women. We encourage stagnation by holding our breath, breathing shallowly, and not having physical movement of our breast tissue. We breathe shallowly or even hold our breath when we are stressed out. This, Eastern medicine says, contributes to stagnation of energy in the chest, lungs, heart, and breasts. The concept of stagnation is covered more in depth in exercise section of Chapter 25, but in relation to breast health, it is important to know that stagnation of energy or substance in the breast tissue fosters an environment where *ama* can lodge and fester, rendering the breast more vulnerable to disease or disorder.

We rarely get cancer of the biceps, the heart, or other muscles. Eastern medicine would explain this by observing that energy and blood get pumped through muscles on a regular basis, bringing nutrition and acting as an efficient waste removal system. For example, even if we are not bench-pressing weights, the muscles in our arms get used multiple times every day and blood pumps through them, bringing nutrition and removing waste debris. This self-cleaning system is not as efficient in breast tissue, which has less blood flow because, unlike muscles, our breasts are mostly comprised of the more passive adipose (fat) tissue.

Throughout our lives, breast tissue remains relatively stagnant compared to muscles. To further ensure a lack of healthy flow of *prana* through our breasts, we hold our breath, pack our breasts into bras (often underwire—which serves to hinder the flow of *prana* to them), apply antiperspirants that hinder the flow of *prana* and sweat, and we get massaged by masseurs who avoid touching our breasts. We rarely perform the tidy, finger-tipped breast self-exams we are taught and, when we do, they are hardly stimulating. Aside from a little foreplay, our breasts may never see much action. With one notable exception: breastfeeding.

There seems to be a reduced risk of breast and ovarian cancer in mothers who breastfeed their babies.[51] Generally, the longer she breastfeeds, the more a woman decreases her risk of breast cancer.[52] One study showed the risk decreased by 4.3 percent for each year of breastfeeding.[53] (By the way, scientists have found evidence babies who are breastfed have a reduced risk of developing heart disease as adults.[54])

Some of my favorite moments in teaching are when women put theory into practice immediately. In two separate seminars, when we were discussing the role of underwire bras in breast stagnation (they encourage it), two women maneuvered out of their expensive underwire bras without removing their shirt, whipped them around like lassoes, then stuffed them into their handbags for use on "special occasions" only.

HOW TO GET RID OF ACCUMULATED AND STAGNANT SLUDGE

There are two ways to rid the body of accumulated *ama*. The more drastic way is through *panchakarma*, the detoxification regimen I mentioned in the previous chapter. One study showed that, within a few days, *panchakarma* effected about a 50 percent reduction in fat-soluble toxins associated with chemical pollutants, without negative side effects. Fats and lipids in the body store fat-soluble

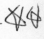

lipophilic toxins, whose half-lives may be several years, but *panchakarma* practices use healthy fats in such a manner as to loosen and remove those toxins.[55]

Although *panchakarma* may be effective, it is important that it be supervised by a skilled, experienced Ayurvedic practitioner. This, combined with the fact that it is not generally covered by insurance, makes it an option that is not easily accessible to everybody.

The second method we can employ to rid the body of *ama* is perhaps the most important, and is accessible for most of us. It is to ensure that diet, lifestyle, and stress levels are appropriate for each of us, so that digestive fire is strong. Then further *ama* formation is not fostered and any ama is eliminated from the body, little by little, over time.

What Should I Do?

1. Follow the three pillars of health listed at the end of Part III: appropriate diet, lifestyle, and stress management. (Suggestions for how to get started in these areas are listed in Chapter 8, pages 46–52.) Yoga and meditation both encourage the free flow of qi or *prana*, which helps to eliminate stagnation.

2. Avoid wearing underwire bras. Although they give support and provide shaping, they hinder the free movement of energy and encourage stagnation in the area. Whenever something leaves a mark on tissue, we can guess that there has been stagnation. It is common for women accustomed to underwire bras to have a permanent line of discoloration under their breasts, where the wire sits. Don't worry; with a little searching, you can find nonunderwire bras that are shapely and don't create the dreaded "uni-boob" effect.

3. Avoid use of antiperspirants. Deodorants may be fine, but antiperspirants discourage toxins from exiting the skin in the armpits, thereby causing an undue concentration of toxic material near the breasts. This is not something you want to encourage if you are already experiencing stagnation in that area. Also check to be sure your deodorant doesn't contain triclosan or pthalates. ("Fragrance" or "parfum" is often code for pthalate. When in doubt, call the manufacturer.) They are nasty for the environment and act as endocrine disruptors, which may increase the risk of breast cancer. More about that in Part III.

4. Avoid caffeine, especially coffee. This is not a popular recommendation. I hope we can still be friends. If you have to have coffee, make sure it is organic and try to limit it to one cup daily made with half decaf. Coffee is grown in places outside the United States that use very strong pesticides and chemicals, which are estrogenic in nature and so are not good for a women's reproductive and breast health. Coffee itself, even organic coffee, tends to have an affinity with breast tissue and often has a negative effect on it and other reproductive tissue. When you couple this natural affinity with the malefic effects of the chemical residue associated with nonorganic coffee, it is likely to be an unhealthy brew.

5. Exercise. Read Chapter 25 to help decide which exercise is most appropriate for you. An appropriate exercise routine is an important factor in maintaining optimum weight, as well as for reducing the risk of stagnation. (Postmenopausal obesity appears to increase a woman's risk of breast cancer.[56]) But it is easy to go overboard. Remember that too much exercise can be just as damaging as too little. Both can severely affect hormone balance, which is essential to a woman's health. In addition, more is not always better. Running a few miles every day may be very good for one person, but could damage another who may benefit more from a gentle yoga practice. *Yoga Journal* reported in September 2001 that yoga can help prevent breast cancer in three important ways: by helping balance the hormones, by supporting the immune system (mostly by stimulating lymph flow), and by helping support a healthy relationship for women with their bodies and environments. That article suggests specific poses that may be especially beneficial.[57]

6. Massage your breasts. Because breasts are mostly adipose tissue, they do not have the quantity of blood flow available in many other parts of our bodies where there is more muscle tissue with blood pumping through. So the *ama* that has collected in the tissue over time is allowed to stagnate and putrefy, or the tissue simply becomes denser. I have come to believe that it is time to take the gloves off and really move breast tissue. I often advise my patients to do a daily, or at least weekly, loving and brisk breast self-massage in the following manner.

- Keep a bottle of castor oil, Banyan Botanical's Breast Balm, untoasted sesame oil, or other appropriate massage oil in your shower. (Discuss with your health-care practitioner which of these is best for you). Each time you take a shower, warm some oil or balm in your hands and massage it vigorously into the breast tissue and around the area of the breasts, including the armpits. In general, if your breasts are lumpy, castor oil is better. If they are not, Breast Balm is particularly pleasant.

- If you have any breast lumps, it is best to avoid massaging them until you determine with your health-care practitioner that it is safe to do so.

- Then follow up with a self-exam of the breasts, as taught by a qualified health-care practitioner. This works in the oil further, as well as allows you to become familiar with the feel of your breast tissue at different times of the month.

- Then let the hot water of the shower or bath rinse off the oil. Don't use soap. Ayurveda teaches that it is good to leave a little oil on the skin. When you get out of the bath, towel dry. Keep this towel separate from others because it will get oil on it over time, which will eventually ruin the towel. But your breast health is worth it.

7. Have babies, if you are inclined toward motherhood. The more you have, the better, as far as breast health is concerned.

8. Breastfeed. For each year a woman breastfeeds, her risk of breast cancer is cut by 4.3 percent. As I joke with a friend who is mother of one, "Just breastfeed

him until he's about twenty-three and then you'll have a zero chance of breast cancer."

9. Breathe deeply. Take full breaths. This helps circulate qi or *prana*.

10. Be sure to only eat organic dairy and meat, if you eat meat. Dairy concentrates pollutants that act as estrogens and that are carcinogenic. Meat does this even more.

11. Eat organic and/or locally grown food, when possible. Food that is imported from countries with lower herbicide/pesticide standards may be using more toxic chemicals in the production of their food. Although fruits, veggies, grains, and beans don't harbor estrogen-like pollutants as much as dairy and meat do, they still count. If your food is not organic, wash it well, and peel waxed fruits and vegetables.

12. Consume soy, in easily digestible forms, daily and in moderation. Soy sauce, tempeh, or tofu cooked well with fresh ginger; miso; and warm spiced soy milk are good examples.

13. Have *panchakarma,* if you are strong enough and can find an experienced, qualified practitioner to supervise it (see Appendix A for places that offer *panchakarma* treatments).

14. Avoid environmental pollutants. More about this in Part III.

ॐ 14 ॐ

Perimenopause
and Menopause

The Russian novelist Fyodor Dostoevsky once said, "The second half of a man's life is made up of nothing but the habits he has acquired during the first half." Very insightful. We can have a much smoother menopause if we have established healthy habits earlier. That's why this chapter is for women of *every* age: young, older, and in between.

Audrey, a forty-year-old friend of mine, received a call from a fifty-five-year-old friend—Eileen—a few months ago. It was a delicate call, because Eileen was sensitive about offering unsolicited advice. She told Audrey that she wished she knew when she was forty, what she now knows at fifty-five. It would have changed how she made choices in her forties that would have enhanced her experience; not only her menopausal experience, but her life in the decade leading to it. She had a few books Audrey might find helpful in this regard at her stage of life.

Audrey was receptive and brought the books home. The only thing was, she told me through laughter, that she found it a little embarrassing to have books about menopause lying around. Like, "Oh my. Here's what's coming: old and shriveled." And her husband who, by the way, is one of the most women-sensitive (in a good way) men I've ever met, felt a bit funny about it, too. They both noticed their resistance and laughed about it, and Audrey started reading them. She called me a few days ago and told me how much she was enjoying them, how they were validating impulses that she was having and gave her bearings. Even though she is smack in the middle of a seemingly different life stage—she has a two-and-a-half-year-old who is sleeping poorly these days from teething—she is getting educated, learning the importance and ramifications of the choices she is making now, not only on her current health, but on her future life stages and strength. And she and her husband are laughing as they learn about the new subject.

Starting to think about menopause only when it hits is a little like trying to dig a well only when you get thirsty. Better to dig little by little so the water is available when you need it.

Perimenopause and Menopause: From Brawn to Brains

> At her first period a girl meets her wisdom. Through her menstruating years she practices her wisdom, and at menopause she becomes her wisdom.[1]
> —NATIVE AMERICAN SAYING

At first glance, we might dismiss this Native American saying as nothing more than a poetic way of viewing what has become increasingly seen as a bothersome monthly event. If we look at it another way, it reflects the reality that often not until menopause does a woman really get how to maneuver through life smoothly. Modern-day Traditional Chinese Medicine teaches that a woman is born with a certain amount of "life essence," sort of a concentrated form of yin. She uses it up little by little throughout her life, and when it is finished, so is her life. I find this to be a bit of a dismal picture. I prefer a point of view attributed to more ancient philosophy: A woman is born with a certain amount of "life essence" and, as she ages, it transforms into wisdom. That is to say, her life culminates in wisdom, not emptiness.

In the beginning of her life, with ample life essence to spare, a woman is young and headstrong. She often goes about life the hard way—bulldozing her way through schools, jobs, opposition, having children, relationships, and goals, all but ignoring the rhythms and cycles of nature—a practice that may generate more resistance than necessary and consume her life essence at a brisk pace.

As she ages, she gains sagacity and insight that provide her better maps and equipment for navigating the turns and curves that life offers. Although real or perceived obstacles do not stop presenting themselves, she maneuvers through them with more ease and consumes her life essence more slowly. Instead of squandering it by muscling through life, she preserves it by cooperating with the flow of reality, so she doesn't require as much muscle.

Eastern tradition teaches that, if a woman studies the laws and patterns of nature, she may begin to take her cues from what these patterns reveal and surrender to that reality. Flexibility is not to be confused with weakness or subservience.

A woman can learn to recognize signs that she is running contrary to the natural direction in which events are moving, recognize her own position within this flow, and find joy in cooperating with reality. For example, she may start out in one direction and find that many obvious or subtle obstacles present themselves. In her younger years, she may attempt to plow through them, regardless of whose feelings she may shred or what is in the way. As she gains wisdom, however, she learns to quickly detect resistance to her direction, and may approach this in various ways. She may wait for the obstruction to dissolve, may encourage its transformation, or may simply move around it. Any of these choices preserve her life essence. If her relationship with life is built on awareness and experience rather than ambition and desire, she can move through life easier. She won't require the physical stamina that the extra yin of youth once afforded her.

It is convenient that when we are young and headstrong and often creating more stress for ourselves than necessary, that we have a greater reservoir of yin—higher levels of sex hormones—than we do when we are older. When we are older, we have less yin with which to balance stress, so by the time we reach menopause, it is important that we have either reduced our external and internal stressors or learned how to navigate them in a way that requires less strain.

Menopause, itself, is not a problem. Most of us don't worry about our menstrual cycles stopping. Our popular culture has caught on that menopause is not a disease, it's a natural process. But we still worry. We worry that our bones will turn to dust before we die; we worry about heart disease and breast cancer, about hot flashes and night sweats, vaginal dryness, insomnia, and other supposed "side effects" of menopause. Many of us have been told these things are due to a deficiency of estrogen (yin) that can be remedied by taking hormones.

As we saw in Part I, however, this is not necessary. If we do not have a lot of stress, we have plenty of yin after menopause. It's true that our yin sex hormones naturally begin to decline at age thirty-five and drop significantly at menopause. This means that if yang activity and stress do not drop as well, or if we do not learn how better to tolerate it, we can use up the lower level of yin we do have and wind up out of balance.

Perimenopause is this period of transition from normal cycles and levels of sex hormones to menopause. Menopause is when it has been a year since our last period, and it is driven and accompanied by more dramatic changes with our sex hormones. Perimenopause is considered to last anywhere from a couple years to twelve or more before menopause and, although this is not implicitly stated, the term tends to be applied more to women who are experiencing discomfort with the transition. As we know that progesterone starts dropping at age thirty-five, we could argue that most women enter perimenopause at that time and that it progresses as our sex hormones diminish. The more imbalanced our hormones, the more likely it is that perimenopause will be difficult. If our hormones are balanced, it is possible to go from age thirty-five to fifty-five without any discomfort.

At menopause there is a more drastic change in our levels of sex hormones, but this isn't necessarily a problem. Since we no longer make and bear babies, we no longer need to maintain the potential to nourish another being. We still require nourishment ourselves, however, and, provided we have not consumed too much yin in our earlier years by plowing through life's obstacles, our bodies can still provide us with what we need. In Part I, we saw that postmenopausal women still produce 40 to 60 percent of their premenopausal levels of hormones, that estrogen falls only 40 to 50 percent at menopause, and that we have the ability to synthesize sex hormones sufficient for our natural postmenopausal needs via the adrenal glands and our various bodily tissues. We have also seen that to make estrogen, we need estrogen precursors and aromatase—the enzyme necessary to convert precursors into estrogen—and we have both of these just about everywhere in our bodies, even after menopause. So we have great potential to synthesize sufficient estrogen.

This is why not all older woman have osteoporosis or deficient estrogen or progesterone. Many women navigate menopause with minimal discomfort and have never had hormone replacement therapy of any sort. They hike, bike, swim, garden, and walk up a storm, and have healthy hearts and strong bones—even if they are otherwise genetically predisposed. Other women have no family history of osteoporosis or heart disease, yet they develop heart and bone problems, experience hot flashes and night sweats, and experience a generally difficult menopause.

Estrogen deficiency may simply be due to a long-term excess of stress hormones draining our sex hormones. Adding more estrogen via hormone replacement therapy without calming the stress in our lives is like pouring water into a bucket with a hole in it. We learned how this pattern works generally in Part I, but it's helpful to look at it as it specifically relates to menopause.

Stress renders us less responsive to normal amounts of hormones and pretty much ensures hormonal imbalance. For example, a woman with excess cortisol but normal amounts of estrogen may get hot flashes or other symptoms typically associated with estrogen deficiency. If this woman were to treat these symptoms with estrogen replacement therapy, she would possibly then develop estrogen-dominant symptoms such as weight gain, water retention, and mood swings. This is also the case with other sex hormones (or thyroid hormone), and if this goes unchecked long enough, it creates a general resistance to our own hormones.[2]

The main problem is, by the time we reach menopause, many of us have already drained our reserves of yin sex hormones in the service of our yang stress hormones. Now when our ovaries are producing a smaller quantity of sex hormones, our adrenal glands are supposed to kick in and produce more of the hormones and hormone precursors we need. But what if these glands are already burnt out from producing lots of stress hormones to manage our stressful lives over the last twenty or more years, and by producing the DHEA required to assuage the effects of excess cortisol? Answer: They will be tapped and tired out and be unable to deliver our postmenopausal hormonal requirements.

In Western terminology, this can translate as high or low cortisol levels (low, when they've been high too long and crash), a deficiency of sex hormones, thyroid problems, adrenal burnout, and a host of other imbalances. From an Eastern medical perspective, we say that we no longer have enough yin to continue smoothly into our second life. If yin is deficient, we may not have enough nourishing qualities to keep us grounded, cool, calm, and lubricated. We may also have overused our yang and no longer have enough of that, either. The result can be a menopause accompanied by insomnia, hot flashes, mood swings, compromised immune systems, and eventually osteoporosis and heart disease.

Hot flashes are a good indicator of hormonal imbalance. About 80 percent of menopausal women will experience at least one hot flash, making this a significant symptom accompanying menopause.[3] Generally, the more intense the symptoms of menopause, the more out of balance the hormones are. Hot flashes are one of the major reasons that women turn to estrogen-replacement therapy or hormone replacement therapy, which is a combination of estrogen and progestin (a synthetic progesterone-like hormone). There is little doubt that these therapies help. A report published in 2001 suggests that ERT may provide relief for more than 80 percent of women who suffer from hot flashes. But the same article went on to say that most women cannot tolerate HRT and will stop taking it within a year.[4] Let's take a closer look.

Synthetic Hormone Replacement Therapy

The most important cures for the discomforts of menopause, if our hormonal balance has been thrown off due to a history of overwork and excess stress, are found in the three pillars of health: appropriate diet, lifestyle, and stress management. Although these three habits may sound simple, they can be hard to establish, especially if we haven't done so earlier in life. It may take time to bring healthy change to these areas of our life and it may be necessary to lean on some supplementation as we make the changes we need to make. There are several options we can look to. Hormone replacement therapy (HRT) and estrogen re-placement therapy (ERT) have been widely prescribed for menopausal women. There are also options for bioidentical hormones and herbal preparations, which we'll discuss a little later.

Until 2002, if you were a woman in or nearing menopause, and you still had your uterus, you would routinely be directed toward HRT, now commonly called hormone therapy, and instructed to take it for years—or even for the rest of your life. This protocol, it turns out, was not based on sound scientific evidence. It appears to have originated in the charismatic preaching of one man, backed by one drug company, and perpetuated by physicians and women who may not have understood the big picture.

The history of HRT use dates back to 1966 and the success of Dr. Robert Wilson's best-selling book *Feminine Forever*, which he promoted vigorously. The premise of the book was that it was as natural and necessary for a menopausal woman to replace estrogen as it was for a diabetic to replace insulin. Dr. Wilson preached that doing so would keep a woman young, healthy, and attractive. He went so far as to declare that the lack of eggs and decline of reproductive hor-mones in a menopausal woman was a "galloping catastrophe"[5] that could only be averted by taking estrogen supplements. He explained that with estrogen sup-plements, "Breasts and genital organs will not shrivel. Such women will be much more pleasant to live with and will not become dull and unattractive." According to Dr. Wilson's son, Ronald, all of his father's expenses to write *Feminine Forever* were paid for by Wyeth-Ayerst, the maker of the synthetic estrogen supplement Premarin. He also said that Wyeth-Ayerst financed his father's organization, the Wilson Research Foundation, which had offices on Park Avenue in Manhattan.[6]

Within just a few years of the publication of *Feminine Forever*, ob/gyn text-books even stated that a woman's life "could be destroyed" if she didn't go on es-trogen replacement therapy, according to Nadine F. Marks, an associate professor at the University of Wisconsin. What woman would choose to be dull, unattrac-tive and have her life destroyed? Apparently fear sells. By 1975, Premarin was the fifth-leading prescription drug in the United States.

By and by, some not very scientifically strenuous studies began to suggest that women could keep their minds sharp, vaginas lubricated, bones strong, hearts healthy, and risk of strokes lower by taking HRT for years—even if it did increase their chances of breast cancer, which had by then been documented. Millions of women took HRT or ERT indefinitely because of such health claims. I have had patients who told me they actually felt guilty when they refused HRT because their doctors felt they were refusing something that could save their lives.

As it turns out, the medical literature that did support the safety and effectiveness of HRT may have been suspect. In August 2009, the *New York Times* reported on court documents that had just been released for public scrutiny. The documents described a relationship between ghostwriters and Wyeth, the pharmaceutical company that produces Premarin and Prempro, the most commonly prescribed hormonal drugs. Wyeth had paid a medical communications firm to produce twenty-six scientific papers in favor of HRT use. The papers, published between 1998 and 2005, in medical journals, emphasized HRT's benefits and downplayed their risks—and almost certainly contributed to significant financial gain for Wyeth.[7]

"Scientific papers" like these were one reason that sales of Premarin and Prempro reached almost $2 billion by 2001[8] and that, by early 2002, an estimated 6 million women in the United States were taking some form of HRT. Another reason for these impressive numbers was advertising. Between April and June 2002 alone, 22.4 million HRT prescriptions were dispensed and $71 million was spent on promotion. HRT was one of the most heavily promoted medications on the market.[9]

Then, in the summer of that year, the picture changed radically. I first learned the news when I walked into the women's health class I was teaching and one of my students handed me the July 9 issue of the *New York Times*. On page one was an article headlined STUDY IS HALTED OVER RISE SEEN IN CANCER RISK by Gina Kolata, a staff science reporter who covered (and still covers) women's health issues.

Kolata's article related what was probably the most shocking news in the Western medical community in my lifetime.[10] Dr. Wolf Utian, executive director of the North American Menopause Society, called it "the biggest bombshell that ever hit in my 30-something years in the menopause area."[11] The article explained that after too many unsubstantiated claims about the benefits of HRT, the National Institutes of Health (NIH) had been given a grant to study the effects of HRT compared with placebos in healthy women. This massive study, called the Women's Health Initiative, involved sixteen thousand women aged fifty to seventy-nine. It studied the effects of taking synthetic estrogen and progestin (a synthetic hormone designed to mimic the effect of progesterone) supplements. The study had been scheduled to last until 2005, but was halted in the summer of 2002 when its authors found that the women in the study who were taking the estrogen-progestin supplement had a significantly increased risk of breast cancer, heart attacks, blood clots, and strokes. After an average of five years on the estrogen-progestin supplement, the women had a 29 percent higher risk of breast cancer, a 26 percent higher risk of heart disease, and a 41 percent higher risk of stroke.[12] Given in absolute percentages, these numbers sound very scary. Because the world of scientific research expresses numbers in ways that make the minds of anyone outside that world bend, it is useful to look at these numbers in a more concrete way. What these numbers really mean is that, from a pool of ten thousand initially healthy women, up to thirty-one more adverse incidents per year occurred, as a result of HRT. Of these thirty-one, seven were coronary heart disease; eight were strokes; eight, pulmonary embolisms; and eight, more invasive breast cancers.[13] This might be a less scary way to view the numbers, but no less dramatic to the scientific community. Because of these findings, the study was halted and millions of women were advised to get off HRT. Millions of them did. Within nine months of the NIH report, HRT prescriptions declined by 32 percent and pharmaceutical advertising dollars declined similarly.[14]

The startling negative results of the NIH study did not even include "all the women who suffered from weight gain, fatigue, depression, irritability, headaches, insomnia, bloating, low thyroid, low libido, and gallbladder disease" as a result of being on HRT.[15]

The most commonly prescribed form of HRT at the time was a combination called Prempro, which combined Premarin, a synthetic estrogen derived from pregnant mare's urine, and Provera, a synthetic progestin that was designed to act like progesterone by supporting the health of the uterus and balancing the unwanted effects of estrogen. Within a few months of stopping the Women's Health Initiative study and advising women to use HRT only as a short-term, stopgap measure—and with caution, if at all—the number of women taking Prempro dropped from 2.7 million to 1.5 million.[16] By 2003, the rate of visits to physicians during which HRT was prescribed plunged by 44 percent from its 2001 level.[17]

This was a radical drop, but it is equally remarkable that the number did not drop to zero, considering the health risks involved with HRT. Reversing the momentum of physicians' and patients' beliefs in HRT overnight may simply have been too drastic an expectation. "We have had a real love affair with hormone therapy . . . it [the news from the study] was like telling someone they have an ugly baby," said Dr. Susan L. Hendrix, a study investigator and gynecologist at Wayne State University in Detroit.[18] It must have been easier to cling to the belief that HRT was still justifiable in some cases. For example, it was still hoped that HRT would help prevent Alzheimer's.

In 2003, another NIH study, which followed 4,500 women who used Prempro for an average of more than four years, revealed that *the reverse was true*.[19] The women in the study actually increased their risk of Alzheimer's and other types of dementia by taking HRT.

Around this time, Wyeth's own Dr. Victoria Kusiak agreed that HRT should be used to treat uncomfortable symptoms of menopause "for the shortest duration and the lowest dose."[20] This is also the FDA's recommendation.[21] Using HRT as a stopgap measure to help women through uncomfortable symptoms became a more ethically comfortable position to take. Presumably this recommendation is based on the idea that short-term exposure to HRT does not carry the same risks as long-term use. Unfortunately, this may not be a prudent assumption. In October 2002, researchers said that taking HRT for an abbreviated time held the same increased risk of breast cancer as did taking it for years, and that the risk did not disappear when the drugs were stopped.[22] Today, some feel that it is okay to pursue HRT if a woman has a low risk of breast cancer, but other experts say that there is no reliable way to identify these women to begin with.[23] With these facts in mind, it is not surprising that some physicians recommend not taking HRT at all. Physicians such as Dr. Deborah Grady, director of the University of California at San Francisco/Mount Zion Women's Health Clinical Research Center, labels HRT supplementation "dangerous."[24] Cardiologist Nannette Wenger flatly states, "I would not tell anyone to start taking it."[25]

In late 2006, it was found that in the seventeen months following the news of the link between synthetic hormones and breast cancer—when more than a million women stopped using HRT—the most common form of breast cancer decreased by 15 percent. This indicates a significant link between HRT use and breast cancer.[26] These findings were supported by a comparable county-by-county study in California that found the incidence of breast cancer correlating to the number of women who had quit HRT. The more women who had quit hormone therapy, the greater decrease in breast cancers. Breast cancers decreased by 22.6 percent in those counties with the most women reducing their hormone therapy.[27] More recently, in February 2009, the *New England Journal of Medicine* reported a clear correlation between discontinuing HRT and reducing the risk of breast cancer.[28] There had been some speculation that what was causing the increased breast cancer risk was not HRT but the number of mammograms women were having. This study ruled out mammogram frequency as a cause and placed the blame squarely on HRT. The finding was that women's risk of breast cancer clearly increases within five years of starting HRT and their risk drops back to about normal within a year of stopping it.[29] This is at odds with the 2002 report

I cited, that some risk remains even after stopping HRT. It is unclear to me which numbers to trust, but the message remains clear. In October 2010, as we saw in Chapter 13, a follow-up Women's Health Initiative study showed not only an increase in breast cancer, but in the chance that it will be deadly. It also showed that, for women who had breast cancer and took HRT, they were also more likely to die of other causes.[30] So my take-home message is to err on the side of caution and avoid the use of HRT, if possible.

With the increased risk of breast cancer, stroke, heart disease, and dementia associated with HRT, why do many women still take it and physicians still prescribe it? The answer might possibly be skin deep. Dr. Margaret M. Polaneczky, a gynecologist at the Iris Cantor Women's Health Center in New York, said, "You wouldn't believe how many women want to stay on estrogen for their skin."[31] This is indisputable. HRT does make a woman's skin softer. But at what cost? Eastern medicine will use diet, with sufficient good-quality yin and good sleep, appropriate exercise, and topical use of natural oils to keep the skin healthy. (See Appendix A for more about facial care and oils.)

The current NIH studies on the effects of EST (estrogen-only therapy, without the added progestin in HRT) are not showing all the same risks as HRT, so far. A 2009 study has shown that estrogen only supplementation did not, as previously speculated, reduce the incidence of congestive heart disease. Rather, it increased the risk of thromboembolic events and gallbladder disease over an average follow-up time of 4.1 years.[32]

In addition to these risks, the risks of uterine cancer with estrogen-only supplementation are substantial enough that it not recommended for any women with a uterus, in any case. In addition, in early 2001 the *Journal of the American Medical Association* reported a study showing that ERT causes a significantly increased risk of ovarian cancer.[33]

To recap the current situation: If you have a uterus you shouldn't take ERT, and whether you have a uterus or not, you shouldn't take HRT. In both, the risks of taking them are greater than their benefits. Ultimately it seems there is really no safe synthetic hormone replacement option. What about the new "bioidentical" hormones?

Bioidentical Hormone Replacement Therapy

The Women's Health Initiative study was examining the effects of synthetic estrogen and synthetic progesterone. Because they are not identical to our naturally occurring hormones, they don't act *exactly* the same way, and that they are a little different may, in fact, be the cause of the side effects that we have seen with synthetic hormones. Bioidentical hormones are identical to our naturally occurring ones. We discussed their use and risks on pages 36–38. Although we saw that there are reasons to use even bioidentical hormones cautiously, they may serve as a stopgap measure while we regain our natural balance of yin and yang.

It seems that more modern physicians than ever currently advocate use of bioidentical progesterone to help with hormonal imbalance and its symptoms, such as hot flashes, and studies are showing their efficacy.[34]

I still feel cautious about the use of bioidentical hormones. I approach putting any highly processed substance in the body as a last resort, as it can have a very powerful effect. Many bioidentical hormones come in the forms of creams that you apply to your skin. I am cautious about this delivery system, as it circumvents the body's digestive system, which is then not given the chance to do its job, which is to transform what we ingest into the most refined, biologically useful substance possible. We need more comprehensive research and studies on the effects of bioidentical hormones. As discussed in Part I, it may be best to have extensive studies on medicines that rely on isolated active ingredients for their efficacy. Unlike herbal remedies, these highly manipulated substances do not have nature's balancing touch regulating their effects.

Menopause is a natural passage in life, yet it is also the Great Unveiler. Whatever maladies were lurking under the surface before menopause will be revealed, the way a bright light reveals dust in corners of a room. It's a time when either we refuse to change what is problematic in our diets and lifestyles and thus the lurking maladies grow bigger, or we make those long-awaited changes and the maladies can resolve. Let's see what Eastern medicine proposes for dealing with the problems that the Great Unveiler brings to light.

What Does Eastern Medicine Do for Perimenopause and Menopause?

If, during perimenopause, a woman has heavy or scanty bleeding or any of the problems we've looked at in the previous chapters of Part II, we would address those things in the ways we have described in those chapters. Beyond this, we would address the signs of hormonal imbalance associated with either perimenopause or menopause the same way.

Ayurveda addresses the symptoms of perimenopause and menopause first with changes in lifestyle and diet. If this doesn't alleviate a woman's symptoms, it offers herbal remedies. You can talk to an herbalist, Ayurvedic consultant, or

Chinese medical herbalist about appropriate herbal supplements. Some studies have shown herbal remedies and acupuncture to be effective.[35] In my experience, they are effective if the right remedy is matched to the individual.

While there are myriad natural remedies for the specific symptoms of imbalanced hormones, such as insomnia or hot flashes, I find that balancing hormones through lifestyle and diet changes will usually heal the problem, not just its symptoms. If you focus on treating insomnia, for example, without addressing its cause (hormonal imbalance due to excess stress), you will have to treat it forever.

We have seen that as we age, our yin hormones decrease. Menopause marks the most dramatic drop. From this point onward, a woman has less of a buffer against physical or emotional stress. This is a physiological indication that a change has occurred. This is why menopausal women often feel they no longer are the women they once were. They aren't. This isn't a problem. The problem comes when we do not adjust our behaviors to reflect this reality.

In Ayurveda we would consider that one cause of excess stress is poor diet, another is inappropriate lifestyle, and a third is going against the nature of things. Throughout perimenopause and menopause, if we continue to try to employ the "full-steam-ahead" habits, tactics, and strategies we used in our twenties and thirties, we may well find that, not only do they not work anymore (if they even worked in the first place), but they make us feel physically tired, emotionally stressed, and spiritually exhausted.

The inherent strength of a woman's constitution dictates how well she can tolerate a stressful lifestyle and poor nutrition. If her constitution is weak, she may never have been able to tolerate poor habits without her body complaining loudly. She may have had to be very conscious of her diet and lifestyle and learned to tailor them according to what her body could handle. If her constitution has always been strong, she might have been able to tolerate poor habits longer without too much complaint from her body. She may have been able to drink three or four glasses of wine a day and smoke a half pack of cigarettes and still have received a clean bill of health from her Western medical checkups her entire life. However, in her early to midfifties, she may find her tolerance plummets. Health problems begin to surface that clearly demonstrate all is not well. For example, she may suddenly test positive for high cholesterol, high blood pressure, breast cancer, adrenal burnout, emotional disorders, or a host of other possible diagnoses. Or maybe she gets colds and flu that are more severe and last longer than ever before.

Ayurveda considers that menopause marks a major turning point for a woman. It's a time of transition when she is naturally suited to begin an inner journey.

Up to now in her life, it was natural for her to educate herself, raise a family, develop her profession, and engage fully in the world. Menopause is the time to reverse the momentum of her involvement in the activities of the world, turn this energy inward, and begin to plumb the depths of her soul. It helps if she has explored this territory already, but one way or another—by force of circumstances or by choice—she now needs to become as comfortable with her inner world as she has been with the world around her. If she hasn't done so before, now is the time to read books written by saints, elders, teachers, and disciples of truth (some titles are suggested in Appendix A) and to go on retreats (alone or with others) designed to support her growing discovery of her own true nature. Which spiritual tradition she pursues may not matter, as long as it resonates with her deepest inclinations and inspires her to a deeper relationship with her true nature.

What Should I Do?

This is the time to finally keep all those New Year's resolutions: Eat well. Live well. Let go of stress. Move your body. It is most important now to consider the lifestyle and dietary changes we will discuss in detail in Part III. Spiritual issues may also require your attention.

- *Whether you are on hormones or not*, take the steps listed below.

1. Follow the three pillars of health described at the end of Part III: appropriate diet, lifestyle, and stress management. (Suggestions for how to get started in these areas are listed on pages 46–52.) If you don't know what an appropriate diet and lifestyle is for your basic genetic constitution and your current emotional and physical condition, consult Appendix A to learn how to find an Ayurvedic lifestyle and diet counselor and to find books to help you. *Make this a priority.* Because it takes time to make these changes, you may need other support, in the form of herbs or, if they aren't sufficient, you may need to use bioidentical hormones for a while if you are having symptoms of hormonal imbalance. If you have hot flashes, especially avoid alcohol, spicy foods; hot, cold or stimulating beverages; tobacco; marijuana; and hot baths.

2. Learn how to do gentle alternate-nostril breathing, which is a type of *pranayama*. *Pranayama* is the name for breathing exercises that are designed to encourage the free flow of *prana* (qi) in the body. It is best to learn alternate-nostril breathing from a yoga teacher who has practiced it herself and knows how to instruct you, though I do include some instruction in Chapter 26. Do 15 to 20 minutes of gentle, alternate-nostril breathing every day. This helps to balance yin and yang hormones in the body.

3. Do *abhyanga* (a form of self-massage) if you and your Ayurvedic diet and lifestyle consultant feel this is appropriate for you. (See Chapter 26 for details.)

4. Be sure to include more time for personal retreats and daily time for meditation. (See Appendix A.)

5. Take herbal supplements if needed. If you need more help with the symptoms of menopause than lifestyle and diet are providing, you can try herbal supplements. Either an experienced Ayurvedic herbalist or a practitioner of TCM can advise you. He or she can tailor a formula for your unique situation.

The following is the basic formula of Ayurvedic and Chinese herbs that I have given to many menopausal women. These are raw powdered herbs, mixed together in varying proportions, depending on your needs. In Eastern medicine, each individual is unique and has unique needs. One size does not fit all. I modify the amounts and add other herbs, or subtract some, depending on the woman's basic constitution and her current condition. This is an example formula. Your practitioner can help you determine if these or other herbs may be beneficial for you. The usual dose is a half teaspoon on the tongue, washed down with warm water, a half hour before meals, three times a day. The herbs are: *shatavari*, 3 to 5 parts (unless you have uterine fibroids or fibrocystic changes in your breasts, in which case I would omit it); *vidari*, 3 to 5 parts; *dang gui*, 3 to 5 parts; *shan yao*, 3 to 5 parts; licorice, 2 to 3 parts (unless the woman has high blood pressure), and *sheng ma*, 1 to 3 parts.

If your practitioner doesn't mix their own herbs, you may together consider Banyan Botanical's Women's Support pills (see Appendix A), provided you don't have fibrocystic changes in your breasts or uterine fibroids. The usual dose is two pills with a cup of warm water, taken 30 minutes before meals, two or three times a day. If you have a slight constitution or are sensitive to herbs, use the lower dose. If insomnia is one of your symptoms, try taking two tablets of Banyan Botanical's I Sleep Soundly an hour before bed. All these herbs should have only beneficial effects. If you have any uncomfortable or negative effects whatsoever, you should stop them. Always use any herbs with the consideration and partnership of your health-care practitioners.

6. When diet, lifestyle, stress management, and herbs aren't enough: If you don't feel considerably better within about three months of establishing an appropriate lifestyle and diet and taking herbal support, it might be time to find a nurse practitioner (see Appendix A) who is qualified to help you find tailored bioidentical hormonal support. You might need to lean on this for a couple years, until your lifestyle, diet, and herbs can have time to restore your balance. As bioidentical hormones have not yet been extensively studied, however, I would recommend the lowest efficacious dose for the shortest duration.

- *If you are currently taking synthetic hormones*, don't stop cold turkey without consulting with your health-care practitioners. Quitting HRT cold can be very disturbing to your system if there is no replacement therapy in the wings. Consider consulting with a nurse practitioner who is qualified to recommend and monitor bioidentical hormones. You may want to first switch to bioidentical hormones before taking other steps.

- *If you are currently taking bioidentical hormones,* I think it is best to get your diet and lifestyle in order with the help of an Ayurvedic diet and lifestyle consultant, before attempting to wean off bioidentical hormones. Then consult with the practitioner who prescribes the hormones for you and determine if you are ready. If you have uncomfortable symptoms when you come off bioidentical hormones, you may take Ayurvedic or TCM herbs (with the help of a qualified practitioner) for a few months before quitting the hormones, and then continue to take the herbs as long as you feel you need them. This should all be done with the cooperation of your various qualified practitioners. It may well be necessary to continue to take bioidentical hormonal support for months, or years, depending on how out of balance your hormones have been and for how long, how stressful your life is, and how healthy your lifestyle and diet are.

- *If insomnia is one of your symptoms,* follow the suggestions on pages 222–223.

15

Heart Health

The English word *rhythm* comes from the Sanskrit word *hrdayam*, meaning the heart. Our heart sets the rhythms of our lives. The heart is the first organ to form and the last to quit, and it plays a remarkable role throughout our lives. For some women, it is also in trouble.

Heart and blood vessel disease is responsible for more worldwide deaths than every other cause combined.[1] In 2006, Americans spent over $100 billion on bypass operations and angioplasty (surgery to clear blocked blood vessels) to address heart disease that is largely preventable and usually reversible through natural measures when we take responsibility for our own health. In fact, the 2004 INTERHEART study found that lifestyle changes can prevent 90 percent of all heart disease.[2]

According to the American Heart Association, heart disease remains the number one cause of death in the United States. It has become associated with menopause because women have more heart disease after menopause. This has been believed to be due to a decrease in estrogen, as estrogen is thought to increase HDL, the good cholesterol. Based on this belief, women were commonly recommended to take synthetic estrogen to ward off heart disease. Sadly, it turns out that women on combined (estrogen and progestin) synthetic hormones actually have an *increased* chance of heart disease, and that estrogen replacement therapy alone does not reduce the incidence of congestive heart disease. In fact, it increases the risk of gallbladder disease and clot-related problems such as stroke and pulmonary embolism.[3] It is also not clear that drugs that increase HDL are entirely beneficial. In late 2006, Pfizer had to discontinue its HDL-raising trial drug Torcetrapib because it significantly increased the death rate in users. It was known to raise blood pressure, which is not good for cardiac patients, but it was hoped that this side effect would be outweighed by the drug's ability to raise HDL. Pfizer's reversal, however, also opened up the debate on whether drugs that raise HDL are in fact beneficial. When this story came out, the *New York Times* reported, "Some scientists worry that the drugs cause the body to produce a form of HDL that may actually be harmful."[4]

In Chapter 14, we looked at the problems associated with women taking synthetic hormones, and throughout Part I we looked at the more likely underlying cause of hormone imbalance: excess stress. Indeed, stress and depression not only cause hormonal imbalance, but they come with a sometimes fatal side effect. They can almost triple the risk of a heart attack.[5] Until Western medicine can come up with a pill that has no dangerous side effects (like increased heart attacks and death), it may be best for us to commit to the remedies that everybody agrees are most vital to heart health: diet, exercise, and relaxation.

With this in mind, let us look at some various factors relating to heart health for women.

Women's Heart Health vs. Men's Heart Health

Heart disease is the leading cause of premature death for women. In her book *Women Are Not Small Men*, Dr. Nieca Goldberg explains how the symptoms of a heart attack differ greatly between men and women. Whereas men suffer from the so-called classic symptoms of a gripping feeling in the chest, sweating, and radiating pain down the left arm, women may not have any of these symptoms when they have a heart attack. One study found that the top six signs of a heart attack in women are unexplained or debilitating fatigue that doesn't go away with sleep, difficulty sleeping, shortness of breath, indigestion, nausea, and tightness and pain in the back, arms, jaw, or neck. Often the pain is felt lower in the torso than it is in men and is mistaken for simple indigestion.[6] The "classic" symptoms of heart attack recognized by most people, including many physicians, are classic for men, not women. These differences can cause women's heart disease to be misdiagnosed.

My friend and colleague, Dr. Jane Schauer, a prominent cardiologist, explains that there are other reasons why heart disease in women is not diagnosed quickly. She says that women who are having chest pain receive emergency care on average about twenty minutes later than do men. She says that when women first feel these disturbing signs, they tend not to call emergency services or get to emergency care until they have made sure their family is taken care of.

Perhaps it is not so surprising that the symptoms we women experience are different, as there are significant differences in the causes of heart attacks between the sexes. Some of this information is only recently becoming clear. In 2006, the *New York Times* reported a study that found that although about three-quarters of men with heart symptoms suffer from blocked arteries, only about a third of women do.[7] Whether these numbers are accurate across the board is not entirely clear, but the study does at least illustrate that women's heart disease is often different from men's. Women can be more likely, for example, to have clear coronary arteries but have microvascular disease, where there is a constriction or stiffening of the smaller arteries that nourish the heart, leading to oxygen deprivation to the heart muscle.[8]

Dr. Schauer illustrated this difference with a story: "A woman gets a phone call saying her husband was killed in car accident. Her family is gathered around her as she receives this news. She hangs up the phone and gets heart pain and pressure, sweating, and shortness of breath. Her family immediately takes her to the emergency room and her EKG shows she's having a heart attack. She is taken to the cardiac catheterization lab, where it is discovered that although her coronary arteries are perfectly normal, a portion of her heart is dead. *We do not see this in men.*" In men, we would likely see some blockage of the coronary arteries that would have caused the problem. But in women the coronary arteries can be perfectly clear. So what causes the death of a portion of the woman's heart? Dr. Schauer explained that it could be caused either by the big arteries' spasming or microvascular spasm or occlusion. She reiterated, "We do not see this in men. Men externalize things. Women take them to heart."

The cause of the constriction or stiffening in microvascular disease is not plaque, but the inability of the vessels to dilate. Modern medicine does not know why women are more likely to suffer from microvascular disease than are men.[9] High blood pressure, cholesterol, inflammation, and hormonal fluctuation remain the usual suspects, and women are advised to exercise, not smoke, and maintain a good body weight. But the fact remains, Dr. Schauer told me, Western medicine does not know for sure how to treat it. There have been no trials of what works and what doesn't work for this sort of heart condition. She explained that Western medicine would tend to treat it the same way they treat male heart disease, with vasodilators and other drugs that serve to change the hormonal milieu of blood vessels.

Statins are a popular choice because they affect free radical formation, have an anti-inflammatory effect, and curb the liver's production of cholesterol, something which we're not positive is as much a culprit as is sometimes thought.[10] Although it may be common practice to prescribe statins to prevent heart disease, Dr. Schauer said, 'We don't really know if statins work on this type of microvascular disease."

Statins have not been Western medicine's only attempt to address women's heart disease. For many years it was thought that HRT—that is, synthetic hormone therapy—would support women's heart health. But, as we saw in Chapter 14, the 2002 NIH study provided indisputable evidence that the opposite is true. It was shown that women who took an estrogen-progestin supplement had a 26 percent higher risk of heart disease. And, as we have also seen, estrogen replacement therapy alone, instead of reducing the incidence of congestive heart disease as hoped, increases the risk of gallbladder disease and clot-related problems such as stroke and pulmonary embolism.[11]

Eastern medicine would look to the possibility that stress and overstrain may be the root causes of microvascular constriction.

Nancy had it all. She was slim, ran five miles a day, never smoked, had "perfect" blood pressure, a family history of longevity, watched her diet, and was only thirty-nine, yet she developed microvascular disease and was prescribed four heart medications. Her symptoms began during her third pregnancy, were accompanied by night sweats and chest pains, and prevented her from running, but she could walk and practice yoga without a problem.

Eastern medicine would say that Nancy not only had it all, but had too much. Too much ambition, too much pushing beyond her natural limits. In general, she had too much activity that depleted her yin, the nourishing element in life. Pregnancy, birth, and raising children, although not necessarily damaging in themselves, certainly have the potential to drain yin, especially if other factors in life are stressful and the woman is overexercising or overworking, further depleting her yin. To begin with, running is one of the exercises that, as we will see in Chapter 25, can deplete yin, and she was already a thin woman, without a lot of excess yin to waste.

We may want to enjoy healthy diets and lifestyles, but it is possible to fret about it or to even overdo it to the point where that would outweigh any benefits. In fact, instead of worrying, if you are a woman like Nancy, with too little yin, one good way of building more of yin is to nap. Western science supports this. A 2006 analysis of healthy individuals found that more frequent nappers suffered fatal heart disease less than did non-napping folks. Occasional napping carried a 12 percent lower mortality rate, whereas regular nappers enjoyed a 37 percent decreased risk.[12] Eastern medicine would suggest that napping may not be appropriate for a heavy, sedentary individual but may do wonders for thin, driven types.

How could yin deficiency lead to microvascular stiffness? Generally, insufficient yin in the body can lead to a reduction in the flexibility of blood vessels, increased heat that dries and stiffens vessels, or constriction of vessels. Consider a rubber hose. If left too long in the desert sun, it dry out, stiffen, and eventually crack. However, the hose would also stiffen if we poured glue through it long enough that the glue built up. Too much yin acts as glue, especially if it is of poor quality or if the body doesn't transform it into a refined form that is biologically useful. This can result in plaque buildup and lead to one form of stiffness and risk of heart disease.

According to Ayurvedic medicine, it is also possible that inflammation causes stiffening of the vessels. The heat of the inflammation causes the natural intelligence of the body to come to the rescue with some sort of buffering material. The resulting buffering material can lead to the stiffening of the vessels. This is a scenario that is gaining a good deal of attention in Western medicine.

Inflammation and Heart Health

Persistent underlying inflammation in the body is seen with increasing certainty as a major trigger of heart attacks, provided some heart disease is present to begin with. Although inflammation alone won't trigger a heart attack, if there is plaque buildup, inflammation seems to increase the likelihood that the buildup will rupture and cause one.[13] In 2002, a Boston Brigham and Women's Hospital study based on about twenty-eight thousand women found there was strong evidence that "simmering, painless inflammation deep within the body is the single most powerful trigger of heart attacks."[14] For reasons not entirely clear to Western medicine, it appears that the danger of persistent inflammation in the body is greater for women than men.

Inflammation occurs when the body detects infection and dispatches white blood cells to the site. For example, white blood cells may respond to deposits on blood vessel walls as a threat and arrive on the scene to remove them. Inflammation is a natural defense mechanism of the body, but is not meant to be on the job 24/7. For some of us, unfortunately, this is exactly what happens. Factors that may serve to increase the risk of chronic inflammation include:

- Stress
- Genetic predisposition
- Ongoing low-level inflammation in the body, and use of substances or engaging in activities that increase it, such as using birth control pills, smoking, eating a diet high in sugars and poor-quality fats, excess weight, and too little exercise.
- Exposure to environmental toxins

STRESS

As we know, when we experience physical or emotional stress, stress hormones are increased in the body and the sympathetic nervous system is overstimulated. When this happens, hormone-like substances called eicosanoids also become imbalanced. Their imbalance is associated with tissue inflammation.[15] It is not a stretch to see, once again, the crucial role that stress and hormone balance plays in the role of women's health.

GENETIC PREDISPOSITION

Our genetic predisposition to chronic inflammation, or to some of the disorders that are commonly associated with chronic inflammation, is not a factor within our control, but many of the other factors are. For example, as we saw with breast cancer, not everybody with a genetic predisposition to a given condition goes on to develop it. Our diets and lifestyles may be the most important contributing factors for whether genetic dispositions become our reality.

ONGOING LOW-LEVEL INFLAMMATION

If you suspect an underlying infection in your body and you know you have heart disease, there is a simple and relatively inexpensive test that can serve as a marker for the presence of inflammation. This test checks for C-reactive protein (CRP), a protein not found in the blood under normal circumstances. The liver produces CRP when it detects inflammation in the system.[16] Chronic low-grade infections associated with such conditions as gum disease, hypertension, rheumatoid arthritis, chronic tissue injuries, or colitis increase CRP. It may also be present in women taking oral contraceptives or in late-stage pregnancy, and in people who have suffered exposure to chemical irritants, which cause inflammation.[17] "In women, CRP seems to be a better predictor of cardiovascular disease, including heart attacks and strokes, than LDL ("bad") cholesterol. Persistent inflammation may lead not only to heart attacks but possibly to colon cancer, Alzheimer's, and many other diseases as well.

A CRP test can predict risk fifteen to twenty-five years in the future.[18] If the test shows that you do have a risky level of inflammation, this gives you ample time to make changes in those factors that could be contributing to the inflammation. Dr. Paul Ridker of Boston's Brigham and Women's Hospital said that these changes don't have to be huge. He suggests modest exercise, modest weight loss, and stopping smoking.[19] Perhaps we don't need to test our CRP level before beginning to make these changes, changes that will benefit not only the heart but the entire physiology.

ENVIRONMENTAL TOXINS

In our environment, exposure to heavy metals such as lead, mercury, and arsenic can trigger inflammation in the body. The process of coal combustion releases such heavy metals. These and other pollutants then enter our bodies via the air, water, and food we take in. As they are practically odorless, colorless, and tasteless, it may be difficult to avoid exposure. If you are aware of pollutants in your environment, you can reduce your exposure to toxic airborne dust by living and working "in tight buildings in which the fresh air enters and re-circulates through high-efficiency air filters."[20] But nothing can serve as a substitute for fresh, clean air when possible. One of my teachers, in fact, maintained that fresh air is the single most important factor in good nutrition.

One substance that has been shown to block the body's inflammatory process is delta-9-tetrahydrocannabinol (THC), which is found in marijuana.[21] But before you run out to score some weed to protect your heart, it is important to know that the study was on mice that were *fed* THC. Smoking cannabis may actually damage the heart.[22]

Diet, Walking, Stretching, and Heart Health

Several studies on heart disease, when looked at together, reveal very helpful facts related to heart health. Between them, they examined two generations of men and women and followed their diets, levels of exercise, as well as health conditions and mineral absorption rates.

DIET

The first study was the most extensive long-term dietary survey ever conducted. It was the Nurses' Health Study begun by Harvard Medical School professor Frank Speizer in 1976. Its data was collected from questionnaires that were completed by 121,700 female nurses, 48,400 of whom were finally included in the study.[23] Dr. Walter Willett, chairman of the department of nutrition at the Harvard School of Public Health, and several colleagues conducted the second study, called the Health Professionals Follow-Up Study, which included 52,000 men. Dr. Willett concluded that it is beneficial to have a daily diet that includes "abundant fruits, vegetables, whole grains, and vegetable oils, as well as optional portions of fish and chicken." He also recommended consuming alcohol in moderation and taking a daily multivitamin to cover nutritional gaps. He advised that daily exercise is essential and advocated walking as the optimal choice for many people.[24]

Dr. Willett's dietary advice is similar to that of Dr. Dean Ornish, author of *Dr. Dean Ornish's Program for Reversing Heart Disease* and other books, that use diet as an important element in treating heart disease. He recommends avoiding animal fat, sugar, refined carbohydrates, highly processed food, excess salt and trans fats, and increasing fiber in the diet. Dr. John Lee suggests we make sure our levels of magnesium and/or potassium are adequate and that we eat antioxidant-rich foods or take supplements such as vitamins C, E, A, beta-carotene, and selenium.[25] Most of these prominent physicians also attribute stress as a major factor in heart disease. We looked at the effect of stress on the body earlier in this book and it would be difficult to disagree with this assessment.

Regarding fats, Dr. Willett found that the quality of the fat that women consumed was an important factor. Women who ate more unsaturated fats had fewer heart problems. These include vegetable oils, like olive oil. (Note: Cold-pressed vegetable oils have not been exposed to the damaging effects of high heat and are worth the extra you pay for them.) Saturated fats such as animal proteins and butter were less problematic than hydrogenated fats (lard, shortening, and margarine), but because pesticides, insecticides, and other environmental pollutants are found in concentrated amounts in dairy products and in even higher levels in meat, be sure to eat organic dairy and meats. Dr Willett recommended regular use of omega-3 fatty acids (found in fish oil) to support heart health. And remember, consume trans fats at your peril. Even at low levels they can be detrimental to your health.

EXERCISE

When we consider what types of exercise are most beneficial for heart health, walking leads the pack. The Nurses' Health Study revealed a "very strong link" between walking and protection against heart disease. Women in the study who walked an average of three hours a week were 35 percent less likely to have a heart attack over an eight-year period than did those who walked less.[26]

Along with walking, stretching is emerging as a useful support for heart health. A study conducted at the University of North Texas and a few Japanese universities, and published in 2009 in the journal *Heart and Circulatory Physiology*, proposes a test that you can easily conduct—but perhaps not easily pass—on your own rug. Sit with your legs stretched out in front of you, feet flexed. Reach forward without bending your knees. Can you touch your toes? If you can, your cardiac arteries are likely more flexible than those of someone who can't. Why would that matter? Because supple arteries allow blood to move more freely through the body than do stiff ones, which require the heart to work much harder, possibly leading to a greater risk for heart attack and stroke.

The researchers studied 526 healthy adults between the ages of twenty and eighty-three. The participants did the touch-your-toes test and, using precise measuring devices, were sorted into groups of high and poor flexibility with their age and gender taken into account. No correlations between artery and body flexibility were found in people under forty, but there was a clear correlation between people with flexible arteries and a flexible bodies in participants older than forty, and stiff arteries correlated with inflexible bodies. Stiff arteries tax your heart.

Why do stiff muscles have anything to do with stiff heart vessels? Although it's not totally clear, the guess is that, because heart vessel walls and tissues are made of the same kinds of tissues as muscles in your body, including your back and legs, the health of one kind of tissue is likely to reflect or correlate with the health of the others. In a small 2008 study at the University of Texas at Austin, it was accidentally discovered that people who stretched could increase the flexibility of their arteries by over 20 percent in just thirteen weeks.[27]

The take-home message of these studies seems to be, if you can't touch your toes, you might want to go to your doctor and determine your chances of heart disease. Here's another take-home message, which lands the responsibility for heart health more squarely in our corners. If we can't touch our toes, add stretch-ing or yoga to our daily or weekly routines. If we can increase flexibility, we may benefit our blood vessels.

Smoking and Heart Health

The fact that smoking significantly increases the risk of heart disease is scientifically undisputed. There is little need to elaborate here. Whether your smoking is active or passive, if you are exposed to smoke, you need to quit if you want to have a healthy heart. A case in point: In the eighteen months following a Pueblo, Colorado, smoking ban in public indoor places, the number of heart attacks fell 27 percent among its residents. In the three years following this ban, there was a 41 percent reduction in heart attacks in Pueblo. Although that number is so impressive that we have to wonder if some of it is due to a decrease in smoking, researchers from Colorado and the Centers for Disease Control and Prevention concluded that this drop in heart attacks was due primarily to the reduction of exposure to secondhand smoke.[28]

Emotions and Heart Health

In 2009, an analysis of forty-four studies confirmed a strong link between anger and coronary heart disease. The results, reported in the *Journal of the American College of Cardiology*, showed that both the onset and outcome of heart disease are affected by anger. In fact, 1.5 percent of heart attacks are brought on by fits of intense anger.[29] Heart rate variability (HRV) is a pattern that governs the pace of the respiratory system and the brain. Just one fearful or angry thought can change the HRV pattern.[30] When we are in the middle of rage, these HRV patterns become agitated and disorderly. When a person returns to a loving, calm mood, they become coherent and regular.[31] Both blood pressure and heart rate fall when someone remembers and discusses the things he or she loves most in life.[32]

This is not news to Traditional Chinese Medicine, where the connection between anger and the heart has always been understood. Anger is said to increase heat in the body, and the rising fire affects the already heat-prone heart. If anger is part of our lives and heart health is a concern, finding ways to cool the anger and calm the heart may be life-saving strategies. In Ayurveda, we recognize the heart as the seat of the mind and we realize that whatever emotions saturate the heart will affect the entire body.

The heart is a remarkable organ. Modern medicine is only beginning to realize its importance and relationship to stress and emotions. In 1983, the heart was reclassified as an endocrine organ because it produces and releases a number of mood-altering hormones, including dopamine, oxytocin, norepinephrine, and atrial natriuretic factor (ANF), which affects blood vessels, the kidneys, adrenal glands, and the brain. We have already seen the stress-antidoting effects of oxytocin. Remarkably, we find oxytocin levels in the heart as high as concentrations in the brain. Our thoughts become biology as these hormones have far-reaching effects in physiology.

Consider "broken heart syndrome," the vernacular term for stress-induced heart failure. This occurs when there are high levels of stress hormones, which are toxic to the heart. Research has found thirty times more adrenaline in people suffering from broken heart syndrome than in healthy people.[33] The stress hormones increase heart rate and constrict arteries that can be otherwise clot free and healthy. Broken heart syndrome can even hit women who eat the right stuff, exercise, and appear successful in every way (except they are stressed). Curiously, broken heart syndrome is more common in women than in men.[34]

The heart is the first organ to form and the last to stop functioning. Emotions and stress affect the heart, which then irrigates our brains and bodies with the flavor of these experiences and the hormonal responses, for good or for ill.

Synthetic Hormones and Heart Health

We have seen that major studies have linked HRT with a significant increase in heart disease.[35] Some studies indicate there may be a small window of opportunity, before a woman is sixty, when she can use HRT without significantly increasing her risk of heart disease, but the jury is still out on that. If there is a window of safety, it is unclear exactly when that might be.

We have also seen there is concern that any hormone use, whether for menopause, fertility, or contraception, may bear the same risks.[36] We know that birth control pills and other forms of synthetic hormonal contraception use the same hormones as HRT. There is solid evidence that synthetic hormonal birth control increases the risk of stroke and heart disease. The University of Ghent measured plaque in the arteries of 2,500 healthy men and women and found that women who had used contraceptive pills had a 20 to 30 percent increase in plaque—a major contributing factor to heart disease—in their carotid and femoral arteries by the time they reached late middle age.[37] We know that higher levels of CRP are associated both with women taking oral contraceptives and an increased risk of heart disease.[38]

Alcohol and Heart Health

There is a connection between alcohol consumption and decreased risk of heart disease. On first glance, this sounds like great news to those of us who enjoy a glass of wine at the end of the day. Many of us would like to tack on the "happily ever after" line to the tale and leave it at that. But this is not the whole story. First, there is the question of what is good for men versus what is good for women, because of the differences in their sizes, the ways they respond to stress, and how their physiology in general and heart health specifically differs. A 2006 Danish study including twenty-seven thousand men and nearly thirty thousand women determined that although men reduced their chances of heart disease with one drink daily, women did better with one drink weekly.[39]

It may be prudent to consider the effects of alcohol on the rest of the body, not just its effect on the heart. Then we can make more informed choices. Regular consumption of any kind of alcohol has been demonstrated to play a role in causing many types of cancer, including larynx, esophagus, liver, breast, and colorectal cancers. Breast and colorectal cancers are two of the most common cancers worldwide.[40]

We have already seen the trouble with excess estrogen circulating in the bloodstream. As we saw in Chapter 13, one factor associated with excess estrogen is an overworked or sluggish liver, a potential result of alcohol consumption. If the liver's health is compromised because of alcohol consumption, it may not be able to break down the excess estrogen. Instead, the excess estrogen gets reabsorbed into the blood, and the body continues to have excess circulating estrogen, which is associated with an increased risk of breast cancer.[41]

Over my years in practice, I've seen women using heart health as justification for drinking. I find this a bit dismaying because it is an incomplete perspective and a poor reason to make alcohol a daily part of life. I asked Dr. Schauer her opinion. She pointed out that there is no substitute for controlling what is within our control, that is, the lifestyle choices that make a far more significant and certain impact on heart health. These factors include diet, exercise, and reduction in stress. Consuming alcohol daily increases sugar and calories, plus it can aggravate diabetes and influence our life choices, often leading to undesirable consequences. But the notion that a glass of red wine a day is good for heart health remains for many an attractive idea—even more attractive than the idea that a daily pill could ensure the health of our heart—because it gives us a green light to use a substance we think gives us some respite from stress.

But does alcohol really reduce stress? Dr. Schauer suggests it can do just the opposite if it serves to impair our judgment and cause us to respond to our environment in ways we might regret in the morning. Even if we don't get intoxicated to the point of impaired judgment, we can question the benefit from an Eastern medicine point of view.

In Chinese medicine, alcohol affects the Liver system, responsible for the free and easy circulation of energy and emotions in the body and mind. When our energy and emotions circulate easily, we feel good. While alcohol jump-starts this function, it ultimately weakens it. In a vicious circle, it requires more and more alcohol to move energy—and thereby feel better—and the natural ability of this system to help us feel good suffers more and more. This is one reason alcohol is addictive.

In Ayurvedic medicine, it is understood that many forms of alcohol, including red wine, may increase heat in the body. In susceptible individuals, this increase in internal heat may increase inflammation in the body, manifesting as acid reflux, full-blown gastroesophageal reflux disease (GERD), or gingivitis (inflammation of the gums). We have already seen how inflammation can have a negative impact on heart health. The increased possibility of inflammation may outweigh any positive effects of alcohol on the body.

The two leading causes of death for women are heart disease and breast cancer. Although very moderate alcohol consumption may improve a woman's heart health, even moderate drinking may significantly increase her risk of breast cancer. A woman may consider that her risk of heart disease outweighs her risk of breast cancer, and may therefore choose to consume alcohol to support her heart. This is a risky gamble, however, because it is difficult to accurately assess any woman's risk of breast cancer when all the known risk factors account for only about a third of breast cancer cases. It seems an especially risky gamble when some lifestyle and dietary practices are guaranteed to benefit the heart without compromising other aspects of health.

Because of the widespread misuse of alcohol—approximately 14 million people are addicted to or abuse alcohol in the United States, where it is the third-leading cause of preventable deaths[42]—it is irresponsible to promote its use for health. Dr. Schauer agrees: "We simply cannot endorse alcohol use in women for decreasing their risk for heart disease." Instead, she suggests including grape juice, which has the same beneficial flavanoids as red wine, in our daily diets, and—first and foremost—to engage in the three pillars of health: healthy diet, exercise, and stress reduction.

What Does Eastern Medicine Do for Heart Health?

In Traditional Chinese Medicine and Ayurvedic medicine, we consider many different causes and corresponding treatments for heart disease. For example, excess stress can cause qi or *prana* to stagnate and the heart's large or small vessels to constrict or spasm, robbing it of vitalizing energy. The treatment? Breathing exercises (*pranayama*) and moderate physical exercise like yoga or walking. If deficient yin or excess yang is causing inflammation or heat and narrowing the blood vessels, the treatment includes a nourishing diet, plus breathing exercises to calm the mind and decrease anger, thereby protecting the heart. Exposure to toxins can lead to heat and inflammation as well, and this we would address with herbs, breathing exercises, a diet that is easily digestible, and minimizing exposure to pollutants. Accumulated sludge from poorly digested food—poor-quality yin—can cause blockages. In this case, too, we would need to alter our diets.

An experienced Eastern medicine physician can determine what the problem is by taking a health history, feeling the pulse, and looking at the person. Treatments include tailored diets, herbs, exercises, and meditation, but there are certain things each of us can include in our daily routines that can help support good heart health.

What Should I Do?

1. Follow the three pillars of health described in Part III: appropriate diet, lifestyle, and stress management. (Suggestions for how to get started in these areas are listed on pages 46–52.) Pay special attention to getting daily exercise. Walking is great.

2. Minimize stress. Stress makes qi stagnate. That predisposes heart vessels to constrict.

3. Minimize anger. One of my mentors used to suggest drinking a tall glass of cool water and going for a walk when anger strikes. Only after cooling off is it appropriate to address whatever issue we found aggravating. Also useful are counseling, alternate-nostril breathing (which we will address in Part III), and meditation. Use whatever works. A happy heart is more likely to be a healthy heart.

4. Eat good-quality fats like cold-pressed olive oil, flaxseed oil, and hemp seed oil.

5. If you eat saturated fats (meat and dairy fat), be sure they are organic. Dairy products and especially meat concentrate large amounts of pollutants.

6. Do not eat hydrogenated fats (lard, shortening, margarine) and do not ever eat trans fats.

7. Don't smoke or breathe secondhand smoke.

8. If you drink alcohol for your heart health, consider replacing some of that alcohol with some other substance or behavior that will relax you without the side effects. Try to keep alcohol intake to one drink a week.

9. Address the issue of inflammation. Check with your health-care practitioners to see if you have hidden inflammation or heat in your body. Your doctor can do this with a CRP blood test, but Traditional Chinese Medicine and Ayurvedic diet and lifestyle consultants have methods of discovering underlying heat as well. Treat any gum inflammation or chronic irritation that you have been ignoring.

10. Avoid exposure to heavy metals like lead, mercury and arsenic by encouraging a fresh-air or filtered-air environment.

Osteoporosis

A mericans spend about $5 billion a year on drugs to protect bone health, roughly 50 percent more than they spent for this just five years ago. Thinning of the bones is a natural process and not in itself a problem. The problem arises when bone porosity increases to the point where we start fracturing hips, something that about 15 percent of older Americans do, and which often triggers a decline in health.

Although we lean heavily on results of bone density scans to alert us to potential problems, these tests do not always provide conclusive results. It is possible to have normal scores on these tests yet still be at risk, or to have poor scores and be pretty much in the safe zone. A bone density scan is not the only measurable aspect of bone health. Your history of bone fractures; whether you drink alcohol, smoke, or use steroids; your height, weight, agility; even your vision and your mother's skeletal history are all telling signs. A woman's risk increases if she has vision problems (especially with depth perception), if she is tall or weighs less in her fifties than she did at age twenty-five, or if she has had broken any bones (wrists, ankles, hips) after age twenty. Her risk also increases if her mother experienced broken bones. (If a woman has a hip fracture before she turns eighty, chances that her daughter may suffer a similar fate increase roughly threefold.) Naturally, the more of these risk factors you have, the higher your risk of fracture. On the other hand, if a woman can get out of a chair without using her arms, she has less than half the risk of fracture than do women who can't.[1]

Bone Quantity and Quality

Every tissue in the body is constantly engaged in a building and dissolution process that leads to healthy tissue. New cells come in and build healthy new tissue while old, tired, dirty cells are eliminated to make room for the new cells. This is the case with bones. As yin relates to building-up functions and yang is a lighter force, we can see that yin sex hormones would serve more to build and maintain bone density, whereas the overproduction of yang stress hormones contributes to thinning of the bones.

According to Miriam E. Nelson and Sarah Wernick, of *Strong Women Stay Young*, the most critical time to prevent bone loss is during the first five years after menopause. This is the time in a woman's life when she will lose bone mass most quickly, between 1 and 2 percent per year.[2] In general, women gain bone mass until they are twenty-five years old, level off until age thirty-five, then lose about a half a percent per year until menopause. After the five-year post menopausal drop, bone loss slows down to about 1 percent per year and back to half a percent again after age seventy. These are useful numbers to know, so we don't freak out if we see our bone density drop from fifty to fifty-five years old, faster than it had when we were younger. This is a common picture, and loss of bone mass is not necessarily a problem unless it reaches the point where bone fractures increase.

There are two major reasons for excessive bone loss. The first involves a process whereby specialized cells called osteoclasts dissolve the old bone cells too fast. This process is catalyzed by too much yang, which occurs when the body is marinated in stress hormones. The second is an insufficient number of fresh, healthy bone cells—osteoblasts—coming in to rebuild the bones. Eastern medicine would say that this is a result of not enough yin, or substance (i.e., bone mass), relative to yang.

Quantity of yin is not the only important factor when it comes to bone health. Quality of yin is important, too. If the quality of the available yin is poor, then the quality of tissue will be poor. Suppose bone-building and bone-dissolving are in balance, but the building-material quality is poor. Then bone density could be good, but bone quality poor. This is an area of bone health that Eastern medicine may be more interested in than is Western medicine.

Several factors can lead to osteoporosis. You have an increased risk if you have a strong family history of it, no children, poor nutrition, poor exercise habits, depression, stress, or too many refined carbohydrates in your diet. Not surprisingly, hormone imbalance, poor diet, and lack of exercise could be argued to be the biggest culprits. Happily, these areas are often within our control.

Hormones and Bone Loss

Earlier, we saw how yin is affected by stress levels. A 2007 study related premenopausal depression with high levels of the stress hormone cortisol and showed that when cortisol is high, bone density drops. Women with high levels of cortisol were likely to have depression and had significantly lower bone density and a higher risk of osteoporosis.[3]

Stress hormones are crucial for survival; however, in excess they promote the breakdown of all yin in the body, that is, all structural material including the bones, skin, muscles, and brain.[4] This leads to a double assault on bone health. First, bone mass is decreased by high levels of cortisol. Second, many tissues that produce estrogen are depleted, resulting in decreased production of estrogen. Estrogen slows the development of osteoporosis, and it has been common for doctors to prescribe synthetic estrogen (balanced with a progestin if the woman has a uterus) to combat osteoporosis. Aside from the problems that we have already seen with the use of synthetic hormones, other arguments suggest this is a flawed approach to supporting bone health.

Although estrogen replacement therapy does slow osteoporosis, it does not prevent or reverse it.[5] In fact, bone loss begins to occur in women at age thirty-five, the same age when progesterone begins to decline, but a time when estrogen levels are fairly stable. Progesterone helps support bone-rebuilding activity; estrogen simply retards bone-dissolving activity. One study shows:

- If a woman uses estrogen replacement therapy, she will not lose any bone mass.
- If she uses bioidentical progesterone replacement therapy, she will enjoy a 15 percent gain in bone mass over a three-year period, as long as she is not on thyroid medication and has an adequate amount of hydrochloric acid in her stomach juices.

Although there is a case for natural progesterone supporting bone density, it is not clear that the impressive bone mass increase seen in this study was related solely to progesterone supplementation. Results may have reflected other factors as well. For example, the women in the study were also given dietary supplements, exercised, and made changes in their diets.[6] It is possible that diet and lifestyle play equally, or more important, roles when it comes to building bone mass.

In the final analysis, I would use bioidentical progesterone supplementation only after it became clear that lifestyle and dietary factors were insufficient to maintain bone health. We discussed the role of stress in hormone imbalance and will look at diet and lifestyle in detail later, but a few points of interest in these areas directly relate to bone health.

Calcium, Diet, and Exercise

It is a common practice to turn to calcium supplementation or increased dairy consumption to boost our calcium levels and support bone health. But to have healthy bones, is it really necessary to consume lots of dairy? No. The origin of calcium is not in milk, it's in the soil and it gets taken up through the root systems of plants, which are then eaten by dairy cows. So, to get enough calcium, what we really need to eat are plants.

Walter Willett, chairman of the department of nutrition at the Harvard School of Public Health, agrees. He advises that dairy products are not necessarily our best source of calcium because they also deliver saturated fats and concentrated calories. His advice is that the recommended daily dose of 1,200 mg a day for women over age fifty is excessive, and it is best to include high-calcium vegetables, such as dark leafy greens, into your daily diet; take a calcium supplement; and exercise, which offers considerable protection against fractures.[7]

Some sources show that increased protein hinders calcium absorption.[8] Consider the popular Atkins diet, which has high protein intake as its basis. Consider, too, that women often commit to diet regimens like this during the five years after menopause, when they may have gained weight due to hormonal imbalance. This is a time when we want calcium absorption to be optimal, but we may be hindering its absorption with a high protein intake.

Another time when we would like to be supporting bone health is during the first twenty-five years of life, when we should be building bone mass yearly. The bone mass we build in these years of life becomes our foundation of bone health for life. Now consider the fact that soda pop leaches calcium out of our bones. If we grow up drinking soda pop every day and get through the demands of high school and college with the help of caffeinated and carbonated beverages, we risk weakening our foundation, as we will see in Part III.

It is hard to tease apart diet and exercise, when we look at what is important for bone health. They each seem to support the good effects of the other. For example, we need hydrochloric acid and vitamin D to get calcium from the stomach into the bloodstream. Then we need micronutrients, progesterone or testosterone, and exercise to get it from the blood into our bones. If nutrients are available but don't get circulated via the bloodstream and absorbed into the body and its deeper tissues, they are wasted. On the other hand, if we have good exercise but poor nutrition, there won't be enough nutrients to get into our bloodstream, let alone into our bones. This is another example of how yin (structural material, like nutrients) and yang (movement and exercise) support each other.

In *Strong Women Stay Young*, Nelson and Wernick report on their experiments at Tufts University with postmenopausal women who were not taking hormone replacement therapy or an unusually high amount of daily calcium. When these women engaged in simple strength-training exercises designed by the Tufts scientists, they gained about 1 percent bone density in their hips and spine over the course of a year, their balance improved, and bone fractures were prevented. These results are comparable to those from hormone replacement therapy, but without the negative side effects. Over the course of the same year, the control group of sedentary women lost between 2 and 2.5 percent of bone mass.[9]

We have seen that balance is a key to health. Yin balances yang, and yang balances yin. Too much of either disrupts the balance. Here's a case in point that relates to bone health. Although we need to exercise for nutrients to get into our bones, too much exercise during our menstrual years leads to irregular menstrual cycles, alteration of the amount or quality of blood flow, and imbalanced hormones, which lead to increased risk of bone loss and fractures after menopause.[10]

How much is too much exercise and how much is too little? This is an important question that we will look at in the exercise section of Chapter 25.

Breastfeeding

Nursing your baby not only helps the health of your child, but supports your own bone health in years to come, decreasing the risk of postmenopausal hip fractures. It also decreases your risk of ovarian cancer and premenopausal breast cancer.[11]

Antidepressants

Drugs like Prozac, Seroxat, and other antidepressants that are serotonin reuptake inhibitors (SSRIs) have been implicated in an up to 4 percent increase in bone loss and about double the number of falls, as compared with people not taking the drugs. A study at McGill University in Montreal followed five thousand people over age fifty for more than five years and found that the risk increased as the drug dose increased, but researchers in the United States feel the findings are still uncertain.[12] Rather than wait for this link to be confirmed in future studies, we need to consider the importance of lifting the spirit as much as we can through stress reduction, lifestyle, and dietary choices. When a thirty-minute walk or jogging three times a week can give comparable results to taking antidepressants, without the side effects,[13] it is worth the effort.

This is not to say that it is never appropriate to take antidepressants. It is possible that we need extra support at certain times in our lives, but it is also possible that antidepressants are too often the first choice—instead of a last resort—when diet, lifestyle, and meditation might work instead.

Osteoporosis Drugs

Fosomax is a widely prescribed drug designed to prevent bone loss. It belongs to a class of drugs called bisphosphonates, which also includes Actonel and Boniva. Millions of patients have taken these types of drugs over the past decade or so to help prevent or treat osteoporosis. Although it is appealing to turn to a pill to heal bone loss, I feel at least as cautious about bisphosphonates as I do about synthetic hormone replacement therapy. In 2008, the FDA issued an alert that warned against the "possibility of severe and sometimes incapacitating bone, joint, and/or muscle (musculoskeletal) pain in patients taking bisphosphonates."[14] Even the common side effects of bisphosphonates concern me, and the rare ones are downright macabre.

For example, when taking a bisphosphonate pill, it is important to drink a full glass of water and to sit or stand for a while afterward so the medication doesn't irritate, ulcerate, or otherwise damage the esophagus. Esophageal troubles caused by bisphosphonates may lead to other problems and end up all but incapacitating women who had been otherwise active and healthy. When we are elderly, we can be especially vulnerable to a pattern where initial harmful events trigger a whole series of negative reactions.

Consider Mary, the sixty-seven-year-old mother of a patient of mine. Mary had led an active life and was in excellent health, but was experiencing a slightly increased rate of bone loss for her age. Her doctor recommended she take Fosomax. Although she took the medication as directed, sitting up for at least an hour after taking it, she developed ulceration of the esophagus anyway. This led her to change her diet to applesauce, yogurt, and other soothing foods that wouldn't aggravate the ulceration. But this diet didn't give her the nourishment that her usual diet did and she began to feel weak. Her weakness led her to stop her regular exercise routine. Exercising less led to constipation, which led to headaches. She even began to develop depression because the quality of her life had changed so dramatically. Within months of starting Fosomax, Mary's life went from active and pleasant to depressed and sedentary. And, as we noted earlier, depression and lack of exercise lead to increased bone loss.

From the point of view of Eastern medicine, if a substance has qualities that could irritate and ulcerate esophageal tissue, then it has hot, sharp qualities, and these could lead to irritation of other gastrointestinal tissues, too. This may disturb digestion and consequently the quality of nutritional substance (yin) that circulates and nourishes the tissues of the body. Certain individuals are particularly susceptible to hot, sharp qualities aggravating their state of balance and could be particularly vulnerable to the negative effects of bisphosphonates. But the drug has the potential to affect anyone's digestion in a negative way, leading to poor-quality yin in the body. If poor-quality yin feeds the bones, the resulting bone quality will be inferior as well.

Years ago, I remember reading of concerns in Europe about taking bisphosphonates for longer than five years, as they seemed to cause poor-quality bones if taken long term. This was about the same time period when I was seeing more and more women in the United States taking them to prevent fractures. Although it may be appropriate to take bisphosphonates in certain severe cases of osteoporosis, they may be widely overprescribed. Now we seem to be slowly catching up to our European cousins, and there are now questions in the United States about whether taking bisphosphonates for longer than five years can actually weaken bones.[15]

There have been reports of a rare type of fracture of the femur that occurs without any external injury and is associated with women who take bisphosphonates for longer than five years. This type of fracture is otherwise seen due only to car accidents or in the elderly. The woman's thigh may ache for a few weeks or months and then just snap when she is standing or walking. It is not certain whether this effect is due to accumulation of micro damage in the bones of women who take bisphosphonates or due to something else; and the risk of it may not show up in X-rays or scans.

Although not common, there is also a dramatic condition associated with bisphosphonate use that has everything to do with very poor-quality bone. This side effect is called osteonecrosis (death of bone tissue) of the jaw. It is a painful, apparently untreatable condition that leaves exposed jawbone in the mouth. The bone appears moth-eaten and doesn't respond well to surgery, scraping, or filing of the bone. Cancer patients with metastases to the bones are sometimes prescribed bisphosphonates to avoid bone fractures, but the National Cancer Institute warns that they will then have a more significant risk of osteonecrosis of the jaw. In June 2006, Gina Kolata of the *New York Times* reported that this has been seen in 1 to 10 percent of cancer patients who take bisphosphonates. Kolata wrote that even after the women discontinued taking them, "Bisphosphonates remain in bone for years, and no one knows how long the osteonecrosis risk remains."[16]

More recently, in January 2009, a study reported in the *Journal of the American Dental Association* found that even short term use of Fosomax can lead to osteonecrosis of the jaw. One in twenty-three patients who received oral Fosomax developed the condition.[17] After about a year on the drug, they may get dental work, which then triggers this sinister side effect. As of September 2009, Merck, the manufacturer of Fosomax, was facing about nine hundred federal and state court cases about Fosomax and osteonecrosis of the jaw.[18]

Even if rare, such serious side effects are noteworthy. Considering there are studies that suggest there is little extra benefit in taking the bone drugs for longer than five years, it may be that this is a class of drugs best used for those with severe risk of fracture and, in any case, they should be taken for no longer than five years without serious consideration.

Bisphosphonates may well increase the quantity of bone mass, but even in less extreme cases they may also decrease its quality over time. I always advise my patients to discuss the pros and cons of bisphosphonate use with their physicians and to come to their own decisions, but never to take these drugs in place of appropriate diet, exercise, and stress management.

What Does Eastern Medicine Do About Osteoporosis?

Good-quality yin and smooth-flowing qi or *prana* lay the foundation for healthy bones. We can have good-quality yin if we consume moderate amounts of high-quality food and drink and digest it properly. If we live on fast food and junk food, we create poor-quality yin and eventually our tissues, including our bone tissue, will become diseased.

We can ensure our qi flows smoothly if we breathe deeply, feel relaxed, and engage in moderate exercise. If our qi flows smoothly, our blood will, too, and it will adequately nourish our bone tissue. Smooth flow of qi also ensures that waste will be carried away from bone tissue and disposed of appropriately.

What Should I Do?

1. Follow the three pillars of health described in Part III: appropriate diet, lifestyle and stress management. (Suggestions for how to get started in these areas are listed on pages 46–52.) Eat well. Digest well. Address digestive issues, if you have any, to ensure you are getting good-quality yin. Exercise moderately. If it is the right kind of exercise for you, it will support smooth flow of qi. And, as a nice side effect, it will also increase muscle mass, which indirectly serves to increase bone density as well.[19] Minimize stress in your life. This will minimize release of cortisol, which is important because cortisol is very detrimental to bone health.

2. Practice *abhyanga* (for details, see Chapter 26). Warm oil self-massage calms the nervous system. When the nervous system is calm, we are less likely to freak out about small things. Less freaking out means fewer surges of cortisol.

3. Do what you can to address hormonal health during your menstrual years if your period is interrupted, irregular, very light, or very heavy, because these are indications of hormonal imbalance. Restoring hormonal balance before menopause means a smoother menopause and more balanced hormones for the first five years after menopause, the time when we naturally lose the most bone mass.

4. Breastfeed your babies.

5. Don't smoke or hang around smoke. Smokers lose bone mass more quickly after age forty and have lower bone density in general.

6. Drinking alcohol increases the risk of osteoporosis. In any case, don't have more than two drinks a day, lest they interfere with calcium metabolism.

7. Avoid steroid use.

8. Avoid chemical and heavy metals exposure.

9. Eat regular amounts of soy products cooked well, with fresh ginger. (We'll address this more in Part III.) Enjoy dairy products if you can tolerate them, plus cooked collards, broccoli, spinach, and beans.

10. Consider following Dr. John Lee's osteoporosis treatment program in his book *What Your Doctor May Not Tell You About Menopause.*[20]

ৰঙ 17 ঙৰ

Alzheimer's Disease
and Dementia

lthough modern science does not know what causes Alzheimer's disease, it does know that people with Alzheimer's have protein deposits in the spaces between their nerve cells (called "plaque") or within the nerve cells (called "tangles"). Plaque or tangles may hinder free communication between nerve cells or directly affect their health. Recent evidence suggests that plaque and tangles may be protecting the body against more damaging factors.[1] This is a familiar concept in Eastern medicine, where it is generally understood that the body, in its innate wisdom, will routinely create masses or buffer material to protect its delicate tissues from assault from inflammation or pathogens.

Heart health and brain health are strongly linked. They share the plaque factor and there is a growing body of evidence that they also share risk factors and preventive steps. Much of the advice that applies to heart health applies to the brain as well. Having a healthy diet and lifestyle, limiting tobacco and alcohol use, and engaging in mental activities have all been shown to have a protective effect against Alzheimer's.

Western medicine does not have a cure for Alzheimer's and is forever on the lookout for potentially effective medicines. This eagerness originally led the Western medical community to use hormone replacement therapy as preventive medicine for Alzheimer's. But as we saw earlier, this did not work. The 2003 Women's Health Initiative Memory Study by the National Institutes of Health followed 4,500 women who used the hormone replacement Prempro for an average of more than four years. Results showed that using the synthetic estrogen-progestin drug approximately *doubled* a woman's risk of Alzheimer's and other kinds of dementia, compared with placebo groups. Furthermore, Prempro did not protect women from memory loss or other milder mental conditions.[2] In 2009, the journal

Neurology reported that taking hormone replacements causes brain atrophy in postmenopausal women, especially if they already have some mental impairment before beginning to take it.[3]

This is not to say that hormone balance does not play a part in Alzheimer's. Once again, stress hormones seem to have an important role. Even in the short term, the presence of cortisol, one of our major stress hormones, can affect memory. One study showed that volunteers injected with cortisol had trouble recalling a story that they had just been told, but that their memory was restored to normal within a week of stopping the injections.[4] I particularly love that part of the story: that memory returned within a short time after shutting off the cortisol faucet. If we change our behavior, our bodies and minds change, too.

Even if the cortisol faucet is not turned off and stress hormones remain with us long term, there may be things we can do to support balance. In Chapter 15, we saw that increased stress hormones lead first to an overstimulated sympathetic nervous system and then to an imbalance of cellular messengers called eicosanoids, which are associated with tissue inflammation. Long-term inflammation may contribute to Alzheimer's, Preliminary research suggests that low-dose aspirin or fish oil, both of which are anti-inflammatory, seem to reduce the risk of Alzheimer's if they are used regularly before any mental problems begin.[5] If these do prove beneficial, other anti-inflammatory substances may also be useful. There are diets and herbs that suppress inflammation in the body, but why not use a treatment that will help address the root of the problem? We might turn to meditation, yoga, tai chi, chats with girlfriends, tending children (remember the "tend and befriend" behavior we discussed in Chapter 4?), or other stress-reducing activities, like exercise. Many of us have experienced stress reduction as one of the main and immediate rewards of regular exercise.

Just as the body needs its workout, the mind also may benefit from both physical and mental exercise. Thanks to recent discoveries in the field of neuroplasticity, we now know that the brain is a "plastic" organ that morphs according to what we do and how we do it. We know that we can repattern our brain and stimulate changes in it. For example, physical exercise actually creates new neurons in the brain. And, by "physical exercise," we are not talking about running marathons. Walking at a brisk pace will do fine. Regular normal, natural movement of the limbs is sufficient to stimulate the growth of these neurons.[6] And, while physical exercise stimulates production of new neurons in the brain, mental exercise—or learning—prolongs their survival.

Studies have long linked regular mental workouts to a decreased risk of Alzheimer's. In 2006, the most convincing study yet came out of the University of New South Wales in Sydney, Australia. This paper integrated data from twenty-two studies and twenty-nine thousand individuals across the world and found that complex mental activity cuts the incidence of dementia by almost half.[7]

It may be, then, that doing crossword puzzles or sudoku, playing cards, and trying new things are all mental exercises that may be beneficial. A common concern among women approaching menopause is that they are becoming too fixed in their ways and less open minded. They sense that this is not healthy. In an attempt to counteract this rigidity, some branch out and try new things, expose themselves to new experiences, languages, music, therapies, studies, or countries. As long as exposure to new ideas and practices does not lead to stress, it may be beneficial as well as fun. If it leads to stress, it may take a little searching to find a healthy balance.

What Does Eastern Medicine Do for Alzheimer's and Dementia?

Like Western medicine, Eastern medicine also considers that the brain and the heart are intimately connected. What affects one is likely to affect the other. So it is not a surprise to us that those who are free from heart disease are less likely to contract some form of dementia.

Eastern medicine pays close attention to stress, diet, and digestion to prevent dementia. If it has already begun, Ayurveda considers how advanced it is. If the disease is not too advanced and the patient is strong enough, Ayurveda would recommend she undergo *panchakarma*, the cleansing routine I discussed in Chapter 12. Practically speaking, this option is not accessible to many of us, due to its cost and the difficulty in finding a qualified local practitioner and facility. Instead, most of us will want to focus on prevention.

Eastern medicine recognizes at least two major causes for buildup of plaque or tangles (which Ayurveda would include under the umbrella term *ama*, or toxic sludge in the body). One cause is underlying heat or inflammation, which causes the body to create a buffer to protect its tissues from being affected. This buffer can be *ama*. Another cause is the inefficient digestion of all that we ingest—food, drink, and environmental pollutants such as insecticides and pesticides. The resulting *ama* circulates in the body and lodges in the heart, brain, and other vulnerable tissues. In either case, the *ama* can manifest as plaque, tangles, or other sticky material. As we saw at the beginning of this chapter, Western medicine is beginning to suspect that plaques and tangles exist in response to other factors.

It is also possible to create mental *ama*. Eastern medicine counsels that just as we need to fully digest food and drink to receive the best nourishment from them, we need to mentally and emotionally digest our experiences in life, otherwise we will create mental waste in the same way that poorly digested food becomes *ama*. Emotional and physical digestion affect each other. Consider how when you are upset, it is almost impossible to efficiently digest even nourishing and otherwise easily digestible food. Likewise, when you have physical indigestion, it is more difficult to concentrate and learn new information.

Because healthy physical and emotional digestion are necessary to avoid *ama* production, an appropriate diet, attention to good digestion, and attention to emotional health are all concerns that Eastern medicine addresses first and foremost in regard to preventing the various forms of dementia.

Both the quantity and quality of diet have an influence on the mind, and these influences vary from person to person. After eating a large meal, one person may feel logy and thick, whereas another feels energized and grounded. A little caffeine might make one person alert, and another frazzled. Eastern medicine looks at the current requirements of an individual and recommends a diet that supports an equally calm and energized outlook. We will also want to avoid too much highly processed or gluey foods, like pastries, cookies, and breads or other wheat flour products, fast foods, and frozen or canned foods, to support good physical digestion and avoid production of *ama*. As I mentioned earlier, in Eastern medicine we say, "Like increases like." Too much sticky, heavy, dense, highly processed food can increase *ama*—plaque, sticky masses or sludge—anywhere in the body.

We will also want to favor whole grains, beans, and cooked fresh vegetables and fruits as the mainstays of our diets. Western medicine is beginning to recognize the value of unprocessed, unrefined foods. Consider this 2006 study of fruit juice, reported in the *American Journal of Medicine*. It followed about two thousand people for up to ten years and found those who drank juice more than three times a week had a 76 percent lower risk of Alzheimer's than did people who drank it less than once a week, *provided it was unrefined juice*.[8] This would include most of the juices sold in a health food store, which do not have sugar, corn syrup, or any added sweeteners, and whose pulp has not been removed. These are just juices made from fresh fruit, juices that might be pasteurized but not made from concentrate. They are usually a bit cloudy. This study was on juices. It is possible that raw fruit might be just as beneficial, or more so. It is also possible that the amount of juice and nutrients delivered in a glass of juice is significantly more than you would get from a piece of fruit.

And just as physical exercise supports proper digestion of food, mental exercises appear to support mental health. We have seen that mental stimulation can help prevent Alzheimer's.

The best medicine? Keeping our stress hormones to a minimum, making sure our diets are appropriate, and engaging in appropriate physical and mental exercise.

What Should I Do?

1. Follow the three pillars of health described in Part III: appropriate diet, lifestyle, and stress management. (Suggestions for how to get started in these areas are listed on pages 46–52.)
2. Drink cloudy (unprocessed) juice at least three times a week.
3. Engage in mentally stimulating but nonstressful activities.
4. Discuss possible anti-inflammatory supplements with your health-care practitioner.

PART III

USING THE THREE PILLARS OF HEALTH TO RESTORE HORMONAL BALANCE

৺ৡ 18 ৡ৺

The Importance of Diet and Lifestyle
AN OVERVIEW

Disease Care vs. Disease Prevention

The doctor of the future will give no medication, but will interest his patients in the care of the human frame, diet, and in the cause and prevention of disease.
—THOMAS EDISON

Western health care emphasizes disease care over disease prevention or health maintenance. In the United States alone in 2008, we spent 16.5 percent of our gross national product on medical care. Of that *$2.1 trillion*, we spent 95 percent treating diagnosed diseases. About three-quarters of those diseases were chronic conditions such as diabetes, osteoporosis, breast cancer, obesity, or heart disease, all of which are usually preventable or reversible through lifestyle and dietary changes.[1] Sometimes it seems we are confused between catching something early and preventing it in the first place. Early detection does not equal disease prevention.

In the West, we ignore the fundamental causes of ill health and pay for it three times over. First, we suffer the immediate effects of living a stressful life and eating poor-quality foods. Second, we suffer the long-term effects on our health. Finally, we have to pay for medications and procedures we wouldn't require if we addressed the core causes of ill health in the first place.

Eastern medicine emphasizes health maintenance as preventative medicine. The word *doctor* comes from the Latin *docere*, meaning "to teach." The word *physician* comes from *physickos*, meaning "nature" or "natural." In Eastern medicine, the role of doctors is to educate their patients about how to cooperate with nature. This encourages self-awareness and places the lion's share of the responsibility for health maintenance on each individual's shoulders. It is then up to the patients to maintain lifestyles and diets that serve to balance them.

Many of us confuse energy with urgency and constant movement, and nourishment with ballast, and we have wound up finding our own perverted states of balance. We live our lives on the go, favoring ambition and drive over peace and contentment. When we find ourselves exhausted, spent, or spacey, we reach for fast carbs, highly processed and overrefined foods, and other quick fixes to fuel us so that we may proceed full speed ahead. In this book, we have seen that stress stimulates the release of yang hormones, disrupting our balance of yin and yang. This eventually leads to adrenal exhaustion, panic attacks, diabetes, heart disease, and more. If these conditions do not bother us, there's not much motivation to change. But if we are not happy, it might be time to do something different, like beginning to include good quality and quantity of yin and yang in our lives and diets.

We can see good-quality yang as clean, centered qi or *prana* in our bodies and minds, while poor-quality yang can lead to stagnant qi, causing excess ambition, irritability and stress. Yin is nourishment. There is physical nourishment, food, drink, and sleep, and there is emotional nourishment: love, contentment, and peace. There is also spiritual nourishment, found in reading works of inspiration, knowing what our purpose is, and living accordingly. Each of these forms of nourishment is a source of high-quality yin. We need to have a sufficient quantity of these forms of nourishment, that is, enough food, enough sleep, enough clean air, enough love, enough contentment. A little pill, no matter how great it is or how few side effects it has, can never make up for what we put in our mouths and minds and how we live our lives.

Many of us suffer from feeling crummy, or worse. No single factor is the culprit. The problem isn't only due to hormones or pollution or processed food or stress. It's all of them. To make soup, you need more than one ingredient. To have arrived at the complicated problems facing us now, there has to have been more than one factor that got us here. To solve the problem, there is more than one solution. Lifestyle, diet, which drugs or herbs to take or avoid, the environment in which we live—all these are factors we need to address if we are going to change the "soup" of life.

In the following chapters we will look at ways to restore and support balance in our lives in general. By following these practices in ways that are tailored to our current needs, we will address the root causes of most of women's health conditions. In my practice, I recommend to most women suffering from any women's health disorders, that they first adjust their diets and lifestyles, and learn to manage their stress levels. Usually my main task is that of cheerleader. If they can make the necessary changes stick, they often need no further medicine. If they do, herbs and natural remedies are the next supportive measures in line, to address the root causes of specific disorders. I find the vast majority of women find a comfortable balance with these tools. As Hippocrates said, "Leave your drugs in the chemist's pot if you can heal the patient with food."

Occasionally a woman continues to experience hot flashes, insomnia, or some other symptoms. Only then will I refer the woman to a specialist in bioidentical hormones for hormonal supplementation as a stopgap measure. These women often have a history of adrenal burnout. Sometimes they are living a life that their hormonal or adrenal reserves are insufficient to support.

Changing our lives often constitutes a major challenge. It may require a reorganization of perspective and priorities. If we have been focused on prioritizing ambition and stretching our resources, it may take some convincing to realize that this is not promoting our well-being. The convincing doesn't necessarily need to come from a book or practitioner. It often comes from our own body's grumbling—or screeching—its discomfort distinctly enough to reach our conscious awareness.

It may seem simplistic to relegate the causes of women's health problems to the domain of diet, lifestyle, and stress management. After all, many women's issues are associated with severe conditions, such as breast cancer, uterine fibroids, osteoporosis, and heart disease. However complicated the picture has become, though, the root causes usually remain simple and treatments are often straightforward. Hormonal imbalance contributes to each of these and, as we now know, the cause of hormonal imbalance is usually excess stress. We can drastically reduce our stress by adjusting our lifestyle so that we are engaged in a life we want to be living and we are neither under- nor overworked, either emotionally or physically. Appropriate exercise and diet can treat a host of ailments and whatever side effects we can expect from this kind of medicine will likely be positive: weight loss, improved muscle tone, a better sense of humor, and a deeper spiritual connection, to name a few.

A recent study of the effect of lifestyle and diet on longevity revealed an interesting connection with an enzyme called telomerase, which guards against age-related cellular damage. Telomerase repairs and lengthens the protective ends (called telomeres) of our chromosomes. If these caplike ends shorten, they leave our chromosomes more susceptible to damage or death, which quickens the aging process. Factors like smoking, obesity, and sedentary lifestyles are known to be associated with shorter telomeres, and evidence suggests that shorter telomeres and lower telomerase levels are risk factors for heart disease and cancer. Appropriate diet and lifestyle appears to increase telomerase levels by about 29 percent.[2]

Studies confirming the benefits of appropriate lifestyle and diet on health intrigue us, but they are not necessary for most of us, because they confirm what we already know. They do offer extra incentive, though, to put that knowledge into practice.

Not only will we live longer with good nutrition, we will live better, if a healthy diet is introduced as early as possible. Science has revealed a link between poor nutrition in utero, childhood, and even into early adulthood, and chronic health conditions, like osteoarthritis, for example.[3] Once thought to be a result of wear and tear on bones, substantial evidence is mounting that poor nutrition in early development is the larger culprit. It is as likely to be caused by *what* we eat as it as by how much or little we consume. Although it is too late to correct how we were fed in utero or childhood, we still have time to turn things around by changing our diets.

A study published in the Proceedings of the National Academy of Sciences found that lifestyle and diet changes transform us from the inside out. They actually alter hundreds of genes within months. Protective genes were activated and those associated with diseases like cancer and heart disease were deactivated.[4] Genes are not dictators. As Dr. David Barker, an expert on early development and nutrition at Oregon Health and Science University, says, "What they do, how they're expressed, is conditional on the rest of the body. The human being is a product of a general recipe, and the specific nutrients you get or don't get."[5]

Awareness

I remember a student in one of my Ayurvedic classes. After some in-depth discussion of the effects of certain foods and certain activities, she exclaimed with exasperation, "Ayurveda has to analyze *every* little thing!" She added, pretty conclusively, "I'm not sure I like Ayurveda." I don't remember what I answered, but I drove home that night fussing to myself. Maybe she was right. Maybe I'd been teaching rigid, analytical, spontaneity-sucking tedium. Then a clear voice piped up from inside with one word: *awareness*.

Ayurveda is about choosing to live life with awareness. What we eat and how we spend our time are two very time-consuming aspects of life, and each and everything we do and ingest affects us. If we learn specifically how our diet and lifestyle affect our bodies and minds, we can make better-informed choices about whether to change or to continue in the direction we are headed. This requires that we pay attention to how we feel immediately after ingesting something, how we feel a few hours later, once we have digested it, and how we feel a few days later, once it has established itself in our tissues. Generally, we feel good if we are consuming things that are high quality to begin with and that we can digest and assimilate well. We tend to feel poorly if we consume poor-quality food and drink or if we cannot digest or assimilate them properly.

If we are running ourselves ragged, squandering our qi or *prana*, we will be more likely to look to quick food—often poor-quality yin—for ballast just to keep us going. And then, like "fat Charlie the archangel" from Paul Simon's song, we may ask, "Why am I soft in the middle when the rest of my life is so hard?" Like Charlie, we complain we're overweight and have low energy, high stress, and high responsibility. But we don't take care in preparing nourishing meals for ourselves, engaging in appropriate exercise, or addressing our causes of stress, all of which have been proven (hands down) to improve our health.

Three Steps to Get Started

1. Make a commitment to learn how to identify your current state and requirements, and the appropriate dietary and lifestyle choices to support them. Part III of this book should help you learn how to get a good start on this. For further assistance and direction, check out Appendix A.
2. Pay attention to how different foods make you feel. After you eat do you feel tired? Energized? Heavy? Inspired? Depressed? Cold? Hot? This is the first step in learning how various foods affect your body, mind, and spirit.
3. Focus on getting healthy instead of treating specific symptoms. Do this by following the three pillars of health described in this section: appropriate diet, lifestyle, and stress management. These are discussed in detail in the pages that follow.

৭৯ 19 ৭৯

Quality and
Quantity of Food

Quality

Let thy food be thy medicine and thy medicine be thy food.
—HIPPOCRATES

Both Ayurveda and Traditional Chinese Medicine recognize the truth of the maxim, "One man's meat is another's poison." We have probably all experienced this. We may know someone, for example, who loves spicy food and seems to digest it easily, whereas we ourselves are unable to eat it without experiencing heartburn, stomach pain, or diarrhea. Or perhaps we can enjoy bread, but our neighbor can't touch it without getting enough gas and bloating to keep the Goodyear blimp aloft for months.

Yin or yang qualities of foods are responsible for the beneficial effects one person may reap and the troublesome ones that another experiences. Even Western medicine is finding that nutrition is an individualized picture, due to such factors as differences in bodily composition and intestinal microbes.[1]

TCM theories are sometimes a little sketchy or confusing when it comes to exactly how to tailor a diet according to a person's individual requirements. In Ayurveda, some guidelines apply to everybody and many are more individual-specific. Although there are very refined, specified theories as to how to create an individualized diet, they can quickly get confusing, and are not always necessary. Analyzing food from the dual perspective of yin and yang is easier and often is a more practical starting point.

Eastern medicine teaches that there are specific qualities inherent in everything we consume. For example, ice cream is heavy, wet, and cold and will have a more building effect on a person than will popcorn, which is light, warm, and dry.

It is possible to analyze every food, drink, and substance we ingest by using pairs of opposite qualities. Is it more hot or cold? Oily or dry? More or less dense? Does it promote more stability or more movement in the body and mind? Is it dull or sharp? Is it sticky or clear? These various qualities combine to yield foods that are overall more nourishing and building (yin), or more reducing, motivating, or lightening (yang).

The way Ayurveda categorizes yin or yang foods is very elegant. (Note for students of Traditional Chinese Medicine: My labeling of food as yin or yang is not exactly how it's taught in TCM schools, as I find Ayurveda to be more practical in this application. Remember, from Chapter 1, that Ayurveda calls yin and yang *brmhana* and *langhana*, respectively. I will continue to use *yin* and *yang*, as we are more familiar now with those terms, but I will categorize foods more according to Ayurvedic theory than TCM's.)

Quick Overview of Examples of Nourishing vs. Lightening Foods

Nourishing, Building, Grounding (yin)	Reducing, Lightening, Energizing, Motivating (yang)
Dairy	Greens
Meat	Broccoli, cauliflower, brussel sprouts
Potatoes mashed with milk and butter	Roasted potatoes with a little olive oil and black pepper
Oatmeal	Fruit salad
Buttered bread	Dry toast
Oily food	Dry food

In Chapter 2, we learned "like increases like." Because this is true, we can use opposites as medicine. We can assess our current condition (too much yin or too much yang) and balance it with the opposite qualities. However, we all need to eat some of both kinds of foods even if we choose predominantly from one category. If we have too much yang or stress in our lives—if we are too mobile, thin, dry, and scattered—we may want to promote more yin by eating more nourishing foods. On the other hand, most spices, chile peppers, or caffeinated drinks promote more light, mobile, sharp qualities—yang ones that motivate the system—so we would eat those when we are feeling dull, depressed, heavy, or stagnant.

USING OPPOSITES AS MEDICINE

**Let nothing which can be treated by diet
be treated by other means.**
—MAIMONIDES

In Eastern medicine, we consider that each food has its own inherent qualities, including temperature. Each food is inherently cooling or warming to the body, to some degree or another. For example, cilantro, watermelon, and avocado are cooling; chile pepper, sharp cheese, and onion are warming, no matter at what physical temperature they are consumed. This inherent temperature—as opposed to the physical temperature—of a substance is sometimes called its "energetic."

Although each food has some degree of cooling or heating influence, most whole vegetables, fruits, grains, beans, and dairy are only slightly cooling or slightly heating. So when we eat a balanced diet of whole foods, avoiding extreme flavors, such as ingredients that are excessively sweet, sour, salty, spicy, or bitter, the cumulative effect is usually fairly neutral.

One problem arises. Suppose our lives are stressful and we determine that we need to promote more nourishing, yin foods in our diet. These foods tend to be a little too heavy or cool to easily digest.

Fortunately, there is a solution. We can balance the heavy qualities of some foods that make them difficult to digest by adding a small amount of spices, such as turmeric, ginger, or black pepper, to lighten and warm them, which renders them easier to digest. We can also consume them freshly cooked and in small amounts. Warm food (whether inherently warm or physically warm) is easier to digest. Whether we are looking to nourish and ground ourselves (yin) or to energize and motivate ourselves (yang), we want to eat most foods right after they have been cooked.

The effect of energetics becomes more important the more imbalanced someone is, when we are considering what medicine to use or how to make certain foods more digestible. Herbs and spices tend to have more pronounced hot or cold energetics, which is one of the factors that distinguish them as medicine instead of food. *Neem*, for example, is a bitter herb used in Ayurveda. It is a very cooling and highly effective medicine if someone is suffering from certain conditions, like hot rashes, that reflect excess heat in the body. *Pippali*, a common herb in Ayurveda, related to the black pepper we use in cooking, is warming and supports digestive function if there isn't enough heat in the body.

Remember that there is always a little yin within yang and a little yang within yin? This should be reflected in our diet. It is useful to consume a little bit of yang spice, for example, with heavy foods, to warm and lighten them, and it is good to consume light foods with something heavy, like a little oil, to maintain balance.

Here are some good-quality nourishing and grounding yin foods that are freshly cooked and minimally processed, and balanced with the use of a little spice, to help them digest easier:

- Mashed yams with a little ground cinnamon
- Warm milk spiced with ground cinnamon, nutmeg, ginger, or saffron
- Cooked, lightly spiced squashes (any kind you like)
- Cooked root vegetables with organic butter, ghee (clarified butter, available at health food stores or Indian grocery stores), or extra-virgin olive oil and black pepper
- Guacamole with black pepper in it
- Most cooked whole grains or whole-grain pasta, with some olive oil, ghee, and a little black pepper, turmeric, or ginger. (See Appendix D.)
- Toasted fresh bread or freshly baked whole-grain breads. When they are warm, they are lighter and easier to digest.
- Cakes made with natural sweeteners and consumed with a little ginger tea, to help digest them. (Steep 1 cup of boiling water with ½ teaspoon of ground ginger or 1 teaspoon of freshly grated ginger for 3 minutes. Add natural sweetener to taste.)
- If you eat meat, eat only small amounts, cooked in stews, with black pepper or ginger.
- Sautéed tofu, tempeh, or seitan (wheat gluten, a common meat substitute) with fresh ginger, turmeric, and black pepper
- Oatmeal and other warm breakfast cereals, with ground cinnamon, nutmeg, and cardamom
- Dairy products consumed with ground spices such as black pepper, ginger, cumin, coriander, paprika, or, if it is a sweet dish, with ground cinnamon, cardamom, cloves, or saffron
- High-quality fats such as cold-pressed olive oil, flaxseed oil, and hemp seed oil.

Good-quality yang—energizing, lightening, and motivating foods—are light, sharp, warm, dry, and rough. Although these are generally easier to digest than are heavier, more building foods, they often have cooling energetics and so can also benefit from being cooked with some moderate amount of gentle spices such as ground coriander, ginger, turmeric, and so on. It is also good to add a little oil, so they are not excessively lightening. Here are some examples:

- Steamed or sautéed greens such as kale, chard, collards, and spinach with a drizzle of olive oil and lemon juice
- Broccoli, cauliflower, Brussels sprouts, and cabbage with a drizzle of olive oil and black pepper
- Salads with olive oil, black pepper, and lemon juice to taste, and eaten in the middle of the day in warm weather, when the heat of the environment supports the digestion of raw foods, which can be hard to digest otherwise
- Small amounts of beans, depending on the way you cook them. Many people find beans gas-producing. But if you soak them overnight in room-temperature water and then cook or pressure-cook them with a stick of kombu, and a couple of pinches of asafetida powder (found in many health food or Indian grocery stores, where you might find it by its Hindi name, *hing*) until they are very soft, they are often much easier to digest.
- Spices, such as ground cumin, coriander, fennel, black pepper, and fresh or ground ginger are all lightening and can be used to make other foods lighter and easier to digest, too. (See also page 185.)
- Whole-grain crackers with very few ingredients, ones recognizable as food (like whole wheat flour, oil, and salt or whole popped grain and salt) and popcorn
- Green tea

Generally, if you need more grounding and nourishment, you would choose more grounding and nourishing foods, and if you need stimulation, lightening, and motivating, you would choose foods with those qualities.

These are general guidelines based on Ayurvedic yin and yang theory. If you find you are still confused or that you need more specific modifications according to your constitution or current requirements, it is helpful either to have a consultation with someone familiar with the basic principles of Ayurvedic medicine or to become familiar with them yourself. (See Appendix A for information on how to find, choose, and use an Ayurvedic consultant.) Each system of medicine has its own strengths and weaknesses. In my experience, Ayurveda offers a truly elegant and understandable model for constitution-specific, individualized lifestyle and dietary considerations.

Certain dietary parameters are beneficial for most people. If you begin by making sure, for example, that you are eating mostly whole, freshly cooked, minimally processed or refined foods in the right quantity for you, you will have a good foundation upon which to build. Then you and your health-care practitioner can design more specific and refined dietary choices specifically for your constitution and current requirements.

Quantity

If we look at food from the viewpoint of what is building—yin—and what is lightening—yang—we want to consider not only the qualities of food, but also quantity. In general, the less we eat, the more lightening the effect; and the more we eat, the more building the effect. Eating too much or too little can cause imbalance and have a negative impact on digestion.

In Ayurveda, digestive capacity and strength (or "fire") is called *agni* and is very yang. Although specific foods can be more yin or more yang, food in general is fundamentally yin because it is substance. Just as a campfire consumes the logs we add to it, digestive fire consumes the food and drink that we put into our stomachs, transforming them into biologically useable energy. And just as too much fuel can smother a campfire and too little will not allow the fire to thrive, the quantity of food we consume is an important factor in our digestive fire's health.

The general idea is, we shouldn't eat too much or too little, we should eat only when we're truly hungry, and we shouldn't drink much during a meal. Moderate sipping of room-temperature water during a meal is okay, but more may hinder our natural ability to digest food. Digestive fire is yang. Water, especially cold water, has yin properties and will smother the digestive fire if you drink too much when your digestive fire needs to be active.

Eating too much at one time or drinking too much of anything during a meal pretty much guarantees the food will not be digested well and will result in toxic sludge (*ama*). We wind up feeling heavy and lethargic. Our brains feel foggy.

On the other hand, eating too little food denies our digestive fire sufficient fuel and our body sufficient yin. This can also negatively affect digestion. After voluntarily or involuntarily fasting for too long, for example, the digestive system becomes too weak to handle much food at all. People often develop troubled digestion after fasting (or coming off fasts) in inappropriate ways. I once did a then popular lemonade with cayenne fast for a fortnight just before going off to China for a month or so. I was unable to come off the fast appropriately and wound up nearly ruining my digestion for months.

Ayurveda teaches that suppression of natural urges, including the urge to eat, creates disease. If we eat without being hungry or overeat when we are, it is likely that food will be poorly digested and *ama* will result. It is best then to eat only when hungry and drink when thirsty—preferably not much during a meal—and to do neither to the full capacity of your stomach. This usually means to stop eating just a little before we feel completely full. If we eat or drink too much at one time, it is too taxing on the digestive fire. Just as fire requires oxygen to burn, so our digestive fires require a little space.

Appetite has gotten a bad rap in the Western world. Women and many of their health-care practitioners are convinced that a good appetite is a bad thing. The concern is that if we have a good appetite, we will eat too much and gain weight. Ayurveda says that it is desirable to have a good appetite because that means our digestive fire is strong enough to transform what we eat into the energy and re-fined biological substances that our body needs to maintain health. Poor appetite indicates low digestive fire, which means that when we do eat, our food will not be well digested and will become *ama* and excess, poor-quality fat.

Having a healthy appetite, however, is different from emotional grazing. A healthy appetite is assuaged by eating a meal and then slowly builds until our next meal, when it should again be strong. With emotional grazing, we aren't truly hungry. We are either bored or eating for emotional reasons and this food won't be digested well, and so will create *ama* or unwanted fat.

If you feel that you never have a good appetite, increasing exercise may help. Exercising first thing in the morning until you warm up, then bathing and resting a bit helps build a true appetite. There is also an Ayurvedic remedy to increase the digestive fire and create true appetite: Take a slice of fresh ginger about an eighth of an inch thick. Put a pinch of rock salt on it, with a few drops of lime juice. Chew this about thirty minutes before meals.

Food, Medicine, and Poison

He that takes medicine and neglects diet
wastes the skill of the physician.
—CHINESE PROVERB

In Eastern medicine, it is believed that most diseases find their roots in disorders of the digestive tract, so the ability to properly digest what we consume, physically or emotionally, is of considerable importance. Ayurveda teaches us that food—or nourishment—is anything we ingest that is digested well, nourishes us, and passes through the body without any negative effects. Medicine is that which enhances digestive ability, and poison is that which hinders it. If we can't digest what we are eating, even if it is the organically sprouted and juiced nectar of the gods, then it is considered poison for us.

If a certain food is difficult to digest, it can have a negative effect on our health. If it is easy for us to digest well, it can be beneficial to our health. We could apply this concept to anything we consume. According to Eastern medicine, each individual has unique requirements that determine whether something is agreeable. What one person digests easily can cause disturbance in another. Hippocrates said (and Eastern medicine agrees), "It is more important to know what sort of person has a disease than to know what sort of disease a person has."

To know which foods are good for you, the first consideration is which foods you can digest well. You may need to start by learning to recognize whether you are digesting something appropriately or not. We know we are digesting food well if we feel energized after eating, have no significant burping, intestinal noise, gas, or bloating, and we have one or two well-formed bowel movements every day. We may suspect difficulty with our digestion if we feel tired or lethargic after eating, have intestinal gurgling, gas, bloating, heartburn, diarrhea, constipation, and/or sticky, incomplete, or malodorous stools.

Judging by the aisles of digestive aids that we find in every drugstore, it is fair to assume that many, many people are experiencing poor digestion, along with its effects.

Ama, or Toxic Sludge

Ama is either the end product of poor digestion or the result of exposure to toxic pollutants and pharmaceutical or recreational drugs. *Ama* is considered toxic because its presence creates a hospitable environment for diseases ranging from stiff joints and arthritis to high cholesterol, heart disease, and cancer.

We've talked about *ama* already, but I want to cover this ground in more detail now because it's a vital concept in digestion. How does poor digestion lead to the formation of *ama* and subsequently to disease? Ayurveda paints the following picture (only in more archaic and more formal language): We ingest stuff. It gets broken down into smaller and smaller particles, is absorbed into the bloodstream, and goes to nourish and build our tissues. If what we ingest is digested well and completely, the molecules absorbed are high-quality, refined, biologically useful building material for strong, healthy tissues. If either what or how we eat is problematic, the foodstuff will be poorly digested and the resulting molecules are sticky, toxic sludge molecules, which Ayurveda calls *ama*.

Ama circulates around the body. Everybody wants to belong and toxic sludge is no exception. It goes from tissue to tissue, reaching every nook and cranny, inquiring, "May I live here? How about here?" not unlike that baby bird in the child's book that goes around asking, "Are you my mommy?" The reply it gets will determine where the *ama* lodges. All the strong, healthy tissue cells in the body stand up, flex their (little) muscles, and say, "No way!" But when the *ama* finds a weak or challenged neighborhood of the body, it can sometimes muscle its way into the mix and take up residence. These vulnerable areas of the body are called *khavaigunyas* in Ayurveda. They are the weakest links.

These challenged areas in our bodies may be weak due to genetics. If my father had a weak heart despite leading a healthy life, then I may inherit a weakness in the heart, even if I am otherwise the picture of health. We may inherit a weak link created by a parent's behavior. For example, if a mother drinks alcohol during pregnancy, her child may have a weakened capacity for certain kinds of learning, which we associate with fetal alcohol syndrome. Of course, our own behavior can cause weak links as well. If I smoked in the past, my lungs may be weak now, even if I no longer smoke. If I drank alcohol to excess, my liver might be my weak link.

If there are no weak links, *ama* may collect in the body's joints, especially in the extremities, because joints—especially the small ones—are inherently more vulnerable than are other tissues like long bones or vital organs, so it is possible for sludge molecules to find lodging there. At first, it's no big deal. A little sludge here, a little sludge there. The body's cleanup crew and elimination team tends to it and regularly sends it packing. But if more and more sludge builds up in the weak spots and if the cleanup and elimination systems are unhealthy, sluggish, or backed up, the sludge will be able to stay. Eventually, wherever it is lodged will become overloaded and diseased. It's like a weak, overly compassionate, or distracted landlord who allows gang members to take over his apartment house. The gang winds up covering the place in graffiti, pissing off the neighbors, creating mayhem, and eventually ruining the place.

Manifestation of disease is a gradual process. We don't, for example, wake up one day in our sixties and discover we have arthritis. Poor digestion or toxic exposure over many, many days, months, and years allows sludge to build up in our joints. They start out feeling fine. Then they are a little stiff now and then, maybe just in cold weather. Then they are stiff all the time, but it's only a little bothersome. By and by, they hurt constantly, requiring medication that could cause digestive problems and ultimately lead to new sludge sticking to the sludge already in our joints. We wind up with arthritis. The same process applies to many diseases. Same process, different locations in the body.

This is not the only way that disease may arise in the body. But, according to Ayurveda—and my own experience compels me to agree—it is a common way for disease to be born, take root, and flourish.

Ayurveda teaches us that if digestion is weak, it affects not only the transformation process in the digestive tract, but also the transformation going on in other tissues in the body, such as the muscles, bones, and organs. Either our own digestive and transformative processes are strained due to a history of poor dietary or lifestyle choices, or we have been over exposed to toxic chemicals. One way or another, our transformational potential is compromised. This may affect important transformational processes in our bodies and determine whether substances transform into other good- or poor-quality substances.

For example, if the body's transformational processes are affected by a weak digestion, the transformational processes of the liver become distorted and it may wind up converting estradiol into "bad" estrogen instead of "good" estrogen, or making more "bad" cholesterol than "good" cholesterol. Another example is proteins. We all know they are good, but if they are poorly digested, proteins can transform into inflammation magnets, increasing the potential for heart trouble.

So, to recap: If you consume something but can't digest it, it becomes poison. If you consume something and can digest it, it's food. If you consume something that improves your digestive capability without causing other problems, it's medicine. If your digestive capacity becomes impaired, the resulting poorly digested material creates an environment conducive to disease itself and transfers its poor transformative powers to other organs and tissues in the body.

Considering the importance of digestion, we want to choose a diet that supports our digestive capacity.

Eat in a Calm Mood and Environment

Suppose you figure out exactly which foods suit your current requirements and, of those, which your body can digest. You've got the basics down and then consulted with twelve Ayurvedic diet and lifestyle consultants. They all agreed on the best diet for you, based on your basic constitution and current condition. Now suppose you are on Paradise Island and are spoon-fed meals prepared from these foods daily. But what if you can't digest them, if somehow you still get gas, bloating, or discomfort? As we just saw, even nectar of the gods will become poison in the body if you can't digest it. If you are eating the right stuff and still not digesting it well, chances are good that you need to look to your emotions.

How we eat is just as important as what we eat. So many of us eat on the go, in the car, in a noisy environment, or when we are sad, excited, fearful, or anxiety ridden. We may hurriedly throw a meal together and be off to our next event before we finish chewing and swallowing our last bite of food.

A full third of the nervous system is associated with the guts. It is impossible to digest our food well when we are stressed out. When we are calm, our digestive organs are relaxed. When relaxed, they are more likely to function optimally.

Eastern philosophy teaches us that we have awareness and we have choices about where to direct our attention. When we don't consciously choose where it will go, it scatters out of our sensory organs into our environment. If while we eat we make an attempt to minimize the amount of awareness scattered outside and direct some of our attention inward, we become more relaxed and still, and more energy is available for the digestive system because less of it is devoted to our outer senses. The more distraction or chaos there is around us when we eat, the less energy is left to facilitate efficient digestion.

Ideally, we want to eat in a quiet, calm environment without concurrently reading, watching television, trying to impress a date, engaging in stimulating conversation, feeling familial tension at the table, arguing, talking on the phone, driving, or working. Anyone who is a parent, especially of small children, probably just rolled his or her swollen and twitching eyes at this idea. Such an idyllic picture is near impossible to achieve. I'm just presenting the ideal here, and we need not to add more stress by reaching too hard for the ideal. But at least we have something to shoot for.

How to Reduce Food Intolerance

Often, if someone is intolerant to a food, it may be either that it does not suit that person's constitution or that individual is unable to digest it. Now, we can't change our constitution, but we can affect our ability to digest. In Chapter 19, we talked about the digestive fire (called *agni*) that transforms what we eat and drink into energy. If this digestive fire is strong enough, it will do its job efficiently. If not, we end up with poorly digested food. As we have seen, our bodies have unhappy reactions to poorly digested food, reactions that range from food allergies to arthritis and a host of other symptoms.

We can, however, alter a food's qualities and thereby render it acceptable to our digestive system. We will see this especially when we discuss soy. If cooked with some ginger, soy may be more digestible than if it is pulverized, concentrated, and cold, like soy powder in a shake.

Whereas Eastern medicine has learned through careful observation over centuries, that we can alter the nature of foods and drink by, for example, changing the temperature at which we consume them, Western medicine has a history of needing studies to prove things. When Western medicine does study something like the effects of temperature change in food, the results are not surprising to an Eastern mind. Here are a couple examples. In 2008 a study reported in the *Journal of Allergy and Clinical Immunology* demonstrated that a child's tolerance to milk increases significantly if it is heated. Three-quarters of the milk-intolerant children in the study became dairy-tolerant if their milk was heated.[1] And in December 2008, researchers at the Common Cold Center at Cardiff University found that hot beverages relieved common cold and flu symptoms far better than did room-temperature liquids.[2]

In general, consuming freshly cooked foods and drinking hot or room-temperature liquids supports healthy digestive fire far better than does consuming cold food and drinks.

Cravings and Choices

I saw an advertisement from the National Eating Disorders Association that carried the following advice: "Eat what you want—when you are truly hungry. Stop when you're full. And eat exactly what appeals to you. Do this instead of any diet, and you are unlikely to ever have a weight problem, let alone an eating disorder."[3] I like this advice and I fundamentally agree with it with one proviso: *As long as you are coming from a place of physical and emotional balance.* "Exactly what appeals to you" can change from person to person, as can the reasons something appeals to you. Here are some examples.

- Mary goes for a brisk walk for a half hour or so in perfect weather. Her blood is pumping, her mind is clear, and when she comes in the house around lunchtime, the idea of a salad appeals to her. She has one. It hits the spot. She feels great.
- Josie spends the morning reading and working at the computer and the idea of having a light soup for lunch appeals to her. She does so and she feels good.
- Nancy is addicted to heroin. She goes through sweaty, shaky withdrawal symptoms when she doesn't get it. Obviously, the idea of getting a fix appeals to her. When she finally does get one, she feels great. We know that this is not because the heroin is good for her, but we can't argue that satisfying her craving makes her feel much, much better.
- Jane forgot to eat breakfast, dropped three different kids off at three different places, and did errands at four different stores and before showing up at her job as marketing saleswoman at 8:00 AM. At 9:30, she walks by a plate of doughnuts. They appeal to her. She eats one and feels a little more grounded at first. Within a short time, however, she's slightly depressed and jittery.

All these women had cravings of one degree or another, but satisfying those cravings—ingesting what appealed to them—led to greater or lesser degrees of contentment. The objects we crave run the gamut from fresh apples to pizza, salad, soup, cigarettes, sugar, and heroin. Why do we sometimes crave what is good for us and sometimes what is not so good—or is downright damaging to our systems?

The body naturally craves what will maintain its status quo. It is used to its status quo and to what it needs to ingest, secrete, or excrete in order to maintain it. If its status quo changes, the body has to adjust accordingly. If we start out in a pretty healthy place, we will crave things that are going to support that state. The problem is, our status quo is not always healthy. If we start from an unhealthy place, we will crave unhealthy things that will maintain our perverted status quo.

So if our starting point is unhealthy, we can't trust our cravings. We need some rules or guidelines to follow until we return to a state of health (or achieve it for the first time in our lives) and learn or relearn what it feels like to be healthy in body and mind. After experiencing this for a while, our cravings start to become healthier because health becomes our new status quo. Once we reach our optimal health, and adjust to it, we can begin to trust our cravings. Until then, it takes effort and commitment to change our dietary and lifestyle habits. The further we are from optimal health, the more brave and tenacious we need to be to achieve it.

Ultimately it is ideal to know how anything we ingest is going to affect us, simply by looking at it or smelling it. As we have seen, anything we ingest is either inherently heating or cooling and has certain qualities, and that these qualities have particular, direct effects on our systems. This is quite a study but it has been my experience that we each have an innate ability to assess whether or not a food is good for us, once we are in a good state of health. At this point our cravings become trustworthy and all lists and rules can go out the window.

Until such a time as we reach optimal health and can trust our cravings, the guidelines in the next several chapters can help support healthy dietary choices. Once comfortable with these, it may be appropriate to get further, individualized guidance (I'd recommend a practitioner well-versed in Ayurvedic principles—see Appendix A for advice on how to find one) as to what is appropriate for you.

༼ 21 ༽

What to Eat
GENERAL GUIDELINES

When diet is wrong, medicine is of no use.
When diet is correct, medicine is of no need.
—AYURVEDIC PROVERB

Whole Foods

Eastern medicine considers our relationship to whole foods, rather than to the components of food, like vitamins, minerals, or carbohydrates. We consider which whole foods are most beneficial. However, the whole foods that one person thrives on, another may not tolerate. The way we provide ourselves with both nourishment and energy is to find a diet that we can digest well. If we digest well what we consume, we provide our bodies and minds with good-quality yin and yang.

Conventional nutritional advice often has a one-size-fits-all approach to diet, with the occasional trendy idea thrown into the mix. I am generally skeptical of fad diets or diets recommended by people or groups with personal interests at stake, such as the meat and dairy associations. The consensus that makes the most sense to me is taught in Eastern medicine and shared by many modern authorities from various medical traditions and backgrounds, including Drs. Dean Ornish, Andrew Weil, John Lee, Deepak Chopra, Vasant Lad, and Robert Svoboda; author Michael Pollan; and others.

The consensus basically goes like this: Eat lots of veggies, whole grains, beans, and fruits, some high-quality oils, and perhaps some dairy products. Some cultures add minimal meat, poultry, or fish to this list. Animal products, including dairy, should only be considered if your cultural, emotional, physical, and spiritual inclinations are tolerant of them and if you can digest them. Eastern medicine takes this a step further and considers which foods within these parameters are optimal for each person's current requirements.

Western and Eastern medicine agree that you will usually avoid what you need to avoid and get what you need if you eat real, recognizable food with straightforward, recognizable ingredients. (Often these are referred to as "whole foods." By definition, whole foods are as close to their natural state as possible: unprocessed, unrefined, and typically containing no added refined sugar, trans fats, hydrogenated or partially hydrogenated fats, chemical preservatives, flavorings, or colorings.) Steer clear of refined carbohydrates (like products made with white flour), sugars, too much saturated fat, and *all* trans fat. Eat mostly whole, mostly freshly cooked and minimally processed food grown without the aid of pesticides and insecticides. Do this and you've won way more than half the battle. As Michael Pollan, author of *The Omnivore's Dilemma* and *In Defense of Food*, succinctly puts it: "Eat food. Not too much. Mostly plants."[1]

Asians who long had a traditional diet along these lines had one of the lowest rates of many diseases, including cardiovascular disease, obesity, and diabetes. When they switched to a more traditionally Western diet, these rates jumped to some of the highest.[2] However, the opposite is also true. Dr. Dean Ornish, whose well-researched and well-conducted studies have appeared in books and prestigious, peer-reviewed journals, has proved that by making positive diet and lifestyle changes, people can not only maintain their health, but can stop or reverse the progression of heart disease.

Many of us know that whole foods are ideal but still go from one fad diet to another: We try high protein, high meat, high calcium, raw foods, low carb, low fat, or high fiber. Eastern medicine teaches that an extreme diet of any kind is unlikely to foster balance. Some of us look to pills to help restore or maintain health, but no pill can take the place of a simple healthy diet. It is not possible for a pill to counteract what we put in our bodies all day, 365 days a year.

I always find it slightly odd when various reports are hailed as discovering that this or that fruit, vegetable, or other simple product of nature is good for us. It seems so basic, so obvious. But apparently we need to see studies before we are convinced. And there are plenty of studies. They go on and on. They range from showing goji berries stimulate the secretion of human growth hormone (which is associated with a reduction in wrinkles and risk of disease) to the miraculous anticarcinogenic powers of broccoli sprouts; from the benefits of good oils to, thank God, those of dark chocolate. Because we are convinced by studies, I will cite some of them below, where appropriate. But, remember: Even a "superfood" should be incorporated into a balanced diet, rather than consumed exclusively or to excess.

Whole Grains and Beans

We have seen that the ability to digest what we eat is a crucial element of nutrition. Something might theoretically be an elixir for health, but if we can't digest it, it acts as poison. This aspect of nutrition is especially important when it comes to grains and beans.

It is common to have difficulty digesting certain beans or grains. For example, these days, many people are shying away from gluten, which is found in wheat, barley, and rye, among other grains. In my first seven years of practice, I encountered celiac disease only twice. Over the last five years, I hear about it so often, it feels like one of those top ten pop songs you can't get away from. In celiac disease, the body reacts to gluten by modifying it in a way that causes interference with nutrient absorption. Symptoms include vomiting, diarrhea, distension of the abdomen, and fatigue. Celiac patients are advised to avoid gluten.

We can understand the increasing incidence of celiac disease if we look at it from an Eastern perspective. When we significantly alter natural substances—whether they are hormones or whole foods—we run the risk of cheating evolution out of its well-earned rewards. Over millennia, the human body has evolved to efficiently digest whole foods, which in turn provide strength and sustenance. However, when we genetically modify—or otherwise adulterate—natural foods, our bodies no longer have the benefit of an evolved relationship with them, so our bodies may become less tolerant. In the same way that synthetic hormones, artificial sweeteners, and trans fats are aberrations of nature and come with serious side effects, modifying whole grains and beans may carry inconvenient consequences as well.

Celiac disease applies especially to wheat, which has been bred in modern times to contain more gluten than it carried naturally. From an Eastern point of view, it is not surprising that the body would find a way to reject this manipulated substance. What Western nutrition calls vitamins, minerals, proteins, carbohydrates, fats, and other isolated components of food, Eastern medicine describes with terms referring to their qualities, like heavy, light, hot, cold, slimy, dry, rough, smooth, and so on. Wheat, and especially gluten, for example, is described not according to the proteins and carbs it contains, but as a particular combination of predominantly sweet, heavy, sticky, and cooling qualities.

Our bodies evolved to digest, absorb, and assimilate certain qualities that historically have been associated with certain substances. In the case of wheat, the body evolved to digest the particular combination of qualities associated with wheat in its natural state. Then, within scarcely a decade, we were exposed to the same quantity of wheat having many times the amount of some of their qualities. It is not surprising that the body either had to evolve to handle this increase or find a way to reject it. It may be that the concentrated dose of gluten's qualities is too much for people with sensitive digestive systems, or that people with otherwise strong digestive systems consumed too much of this concentrated dose. Celiac disease may simply be the body's attempt to reject something it has either not evolved to deal with or has overdosed on.

An excess of wheat flour products may be an unintentional side effect of a busy life. They are quick, easy, and filling: toast or a bagel, English muffin, doughnut, or Danish for breakfast; cookies and crackers as snacks; sandwiches, pasta, or pizza for lunch or dinner; and cake or pie for dessert. Flour products are often present in every meal, dessert, and snack of the day. Superrefined, bleached white flour forms a sticky, heavy mass that is as tough for our digestive fires to transform into energy as it is for a match to ignite and transform pudding. Whole wheat flour is certainly more of a whole food and not *as* sticky, thanks to its higher fiber content (which translates in Ayurveda to having more rough quality). But it is possible, and common, to consume too much of that, too, overdosing ourselves with an excess of heavy, sweet, dense qualities.

Other grains, such as quinoa and millet are lighter, and less sticky, in nature and easier to digest, and most of us haven't oversaturated our system with their qualities, the way we have with wheat. Whole wheat flour products are nourishing and can usually make their way into a diet without much effort. It generally requires more effort to consume a variety of other whole grains like quinoa, millet, buckwheat, rice, and barley, all of which are tasty alternatives.

Whatever grains you choose, it is best to consume ones you can digest. If you know you have an intolerance to wheat or another grain, it is best to avoid it completely, at least until the intolerance resolves, as I have often seen it do after a period of eating a digestible whole foods diet.

As for rice, many people trying to improve their diets will switch from white rice to brown. It is my opinion that unpolished, unbleached, organic white and brown rice are both okay. Western science has shown brown rice to have higher protein levels and more iron and calcium than white rice, but both Ayurveda and Western science consider it more difficult to digest than white rice. Brown rice contains phytate phosphorus, which seems to interfere with absorption of calcium, zinc, and iron. Although it does slow down the body's absorption of carbohydrates, if you consume white rice with high-fiber vegetables and beans, the same effect will be achieved.[3] So it seems good-quality brown and white rice are both fine, provided you can digest them and that you eat them—especially white rice—with veggies and beans.

Like whole grains, beans can also pose digestive problems, although with beans, how digestible they are often depends on how they are prepared. People often complain they can't digest beans but, upon closer examination, we find that they are only consuming canned, leftover, or frozen beans, or even powdered, reconstituted beans. These are indeed difficult to digest. Beans prepared from scratch, however, are frequently much easier to digest. Taking tips from macrobiotic cooking, Ayurveda and Traditional Chinese Medicine, I have found the following method to result in the most digestible beans:

Easy, Digestible Beans

I CUP DRIED BEANS (SUCH AS BLACK, KIDNEY, LENTILS, OR ANY KIND YOU LIKE)
ENOUGH WATER TO COVER (2 TO 3 CUPS)
I TO 2 STICKS DRIED KOMBU
PINCH OF ASAFETIDA POWDER

Place the beans in a glass bowl with enough water to cover by a few inches. Soak in a cool place overnight (at least 8 hours).

The next day, rinse them and put them in a heavy-bottomed, 2-quart pot (or a pressure cooker, if you have one and know how to use it). Cover them with a few inches of fresh water, add the dried kombu and a pinch of asafetida powder, and cook until very soft, 35 to 90 minutes, depending on the variety of bean. (Kombu and asafetida make beans more digestible.)

Remove the kombu. The beans are now ready to add to a soup, sautéed onions and ginger, or any recipe calling for beans. (Note: Many kinds of beans will not get soft if you add salt before they are fully cooked, so I've found it best to salt them only after they are done.)

If you still have difficulty digesting beans, you may need to stick with only a couple that are generally the easiest to digest, such as split mung dal, available at Indian grocery stores and sometimes at health food stores. Cooking these with sautéed onions, black pepper, and ginger can make them more digestible.

Also, eating tofu made from organic, nongenetically modified soybeans is a common way to include beans in a diet. We'll look at soybeans in depth in Chapter 24 but, in brief, tofu is most digestible when cooked with warming spices such as ginger and black pepper. The same is true for tempeh, which is also made from soybeans.

Here is a list of whole grains, whole-grain products, and whole beans, plus examples of dishes that include them.

Whole grains: All kinds of unbleached, unpolished rice, quinoa, buckwheat, millet, barley, whole wheat, and rye.

Whole grain dishes: Any grain boiled and served plain with organic butter, ghee, or olive oil and tamari and black pepper; risotto, *kitcheri* (see recipe in Appendix D), plain rice, and rice salad; quinoa cooked with milk and ginger or with sautéed onions, celery, and carrots; buckwheat with kale and sautéed onions; millet and vegetable casserole; mushroom barley soup, and tabbouleh (made from bulgur, which is toasted, cracked wheat—one of the only ways I know to easily include whole wheat into the diet in a nonflour way). Including moderate amounts of bread made from whole-grain flour—like fresh whole wheat or rye bread—is not the end of the world, but ideally shouldn't be consumed as often as the whole grains themselves.

Whole beans: Aduki, pinto, lentil, split pea, chick pea, kidney bean, mung dal, toor dal, or any other dried bean.

Whole bean dishes: Aduki bean soup; pinto bean tacos; split pea soup; hummus, chili; Indian dal (a soupy, spiced bean dish) made from mung dal, toor dal, or other kinds of dal available at Indian grocery stores.

For recommendations of some cookbooks that include recipes for preparing whole grains and beans, see Appendix A.

DAIRY

It is not an accident that in India the cow is sacred. Ayurveda has always considered dairy to be wonderful. It is thought to have a calming, sweet effect on the mind and a very nourishing, building effect on the body. Thousands of years ago, however, milk was much different than it is today. There was no distinction between nonorganic and organic milk. All milk was organic.

Today, much of our dairy comes from cows that subsist on a genetically modified, pesticide-laced diet based on dried grain. This diet may be easier to deliver on the huge scale required for today's mass production of dairy products, but it's far from the natural foraging diet cows used to eat. It may also be a diet that today's cows have not evolved to tolerate as well as their ancestors, just as humans are having a hard time digesting genetically modified grains, artificial sweeteners, and other adulterated foods. Perhaps because of this, or due to their often overcrowded quarters, modern cows are more prone to sickness and they are regularly fed antibiotics to combat it. Their milk is then pasteurized and homogenized. Homogenization is a mechanical process whereby milk is passed through a tiny orifice under high pressure, which makes the fat globules in milk much smaller, with more surface area. This keeps the milk from separating and lengthens its shelf life, but—according to Ayurveda—would render the milk more difficult to digest. Sometimes the fat is removed or reduced, changing the milk's composition as well as its effects.

Modern-day milk is so different from what we evolved to digest that new terms have been developed to describe the milklike products of this industry. In one small town that I frequent in the summers, the first of way too many ingredients listed on the containers of all available ice creams and cream cheeses is the slightly unsettling, not very homey term "modified milk ingredients." Commercial sour cream typically has about seven ingredients that require more effort to pronounce than should really be necessary. Maybe lactose intolerance is not a surprising result of this tampering with nature. Dairy now joins wheat, soy, trans fats, and artificial sweeteners in the category of highly processed, manipulated foods, and, like them, often comes with troublesome side effects.

In the part of Chapter 12 that discusses the reproductive system, we looked at the results of the Nurses' Health Study, which followed eighteen thousand women to consider the effects of diet and other factors on ovulatory infertility.[4] The study found that one to two daily servings of whole milk (or foods made from it) were beneficial, but the same quantity of nonfat and low-fat milk was not. In fact, the more nonfat and low-fat milk a woman consumed, the more likely she was to have difficulty getting pregnant.

When we alter the naturally inherent qualities of milk, we are defeating its natural purpose. In Ayurveda, we say that whole, raw milk is sweet, heavy, cooling, stabilizing, calming, oily, and smooth—all yin qualities. In a rough and busy world, these qualities could be ambrosial as well as healthy for our hormonal balance, if only we could digest them.

Although it is against the laws of most states to sell unpasteurized milk for human consumption, it is still possible in some places to purchase whole, organic, nonhomogenized milk. I have found that many of my patients, and indeed myself, are able to digest this milk much easier than we can homogenized milk. When I can't find whole, organic, nonhomogenized milk, I either buy products as close to it as possible or avoid it altogether.

The heavy, cooling qualities of milk make it somewhat difficult to digest even in its natural state. In the centuries when Ayurvedic medicine was being codified, people without cars and supermarkets were likely more active than we are today.

As physical exercise supports a strong digestive system, it is possible that people back then could tolerate more dairy.

One thing we can do to make milk more digestible is to warm it up. For example, as we saw before, a child's tolerance to milk increases significantly if the milk is heated.[5] I have repeatedly seen this to be the case with adults as well. They are able to digest a small amount of warm, whole milk, even when they are unable to tolerate cold dairy.

Sheep or goat milk is considered, in Ayurveda, to be warmer, lighter, and easier to digest than cow's milk, while still offering a healthy dose of those wonderful grounding, oily yin qualities. Not everybody is a fan of the taste or smell, but fresh goat's dairy tends to come without this pungent side effect. The older the product, the stronger the scent and flavor.

In general, as long as our digestive systems can tolerate it, a little warm dairy or a serving or two of minimally processed dairy products is one way to include some good-quality yin in our daily diets.

SPICES

Not only in modern times have people had difficulty digesting dairy, legumes, or certain grains. Eastern medicine considers these foods to be heavy as a rule, and therefore more difficult to digest. In Eastern medicine, to improve digestibility, we use moderate amounts of spices that have a lightening, warming effect on heavy or cold food, making it easier to digest. Indian food almost always contains a mixture of spices, from cardamom, saffron, cloves, nutmeg, mace, and cinnamon in sweet fare or chai, to black pepper, cumin, coriander, curry leaves, turmeric, and many other spices in savory food. Rice is either spiced directly or consumed with a spiced legume or vegetable dish. *Kheer*, a sweet pudding made from rice and milk, is typically spiced with cardamom. Thai and Chinese food also use spices like ginger, galangal, or chiles, all of which serve to warm and lighten whatever heavier foods are being eaten.

Studies have shown that East Indians tend to have lower rates of cancer. This has caused scientists to study the possible beneficial effects of some of these spices. Because it is rare to have an Indian meal that does not include turmeric, this spice is a good example. Turmeric has anti-inflammatory qualities, causes cancer cells to take their own lives, and deters formation of new blood vessels that could support cancer growth. Good news.

Our modern tendency is to remove a substance from its naturally occurring habitat and expect it will deliver the same results. Then we are surprised when this doesn't work. We will see this in the story of soy (see page 206). When we divorce an ingredient from the manner and conditions in which it is naturally consumed—and from the foods or substances it has been traditionally consumed with—it is folly to expect it to have the same effect. Just as we can't take a panda or a child out of its natural environment and expect it to thrive, we would be shortsighted to expect anything different of food.

It is optimistic or misguided to think that isolating spices like turmeric, black pepper, or ginger, so that we can swallow them in capsules, will provide the same benefits as when they are cooked with whole grains and vegetables and consumed daily in freshly cooked food.

When they heard the good news about turmeric, researchers in Taiwan tried to treat cancer with turmeric capsules. But they found that, when consumed alone, it was poorly absorbed by the digestive system. Not so good. On they pioneered and found that when a pinch of black pepper or a little ginger—spices also commonly found in Indian food—was added to a quarter teaspoon of turmeric, the body's assimilation of turmeric was multiplied two thousandfold.[6]

In Ayurveda, we use spices in varying amounts, depending on someone's current requirements. (It is rarely appropriate to add more than a very small amount of very hot spices such as cayenne or jalapeño peppers.) Moderately spicing freshly cooked whole grains, legumes, and vegetables as part of a daily routine is far more effective than adding a capsule of one particular spice to a diet high in processed or fast food.

Too much spice can also be a problem, especially if someone already runs hot. For these individuals, the extra heat of the spices could serve to give them ulcers instead of good digestion. However, for almost any condition, a moderate amount of turmeric, ginger, and black pepper usually has a beneficial effect on digestion, as well as on other conditions, like cancer.

VEGGIES AND FRUITS

In short: Eat lots of them. You'll likely eat less of something else. And something else is not likely to be so good for you.

Although cooking veggies may reduce the levels of healthy compounds a little, it is not anywhere near enough to counteract all the benefits. Also, as we have seen, Eastern medicine teaches that freshly cooked food is easier to digest than cold food. It is not necessary to eat a raw foods diet if you can't digest it. If a raw foods diet causes you gas and bloating, then you are not digesting your food properly. I have heard that cooking broccoli actually allows the release of more good nutrients.

Regardless, veggies and fruits need to be well chewed. This begins the transformation process that turns the compounds in the food into become biologically useful material for us human beings.

Nutritional biochemists list the following enzymes and compounds in veggies and fruits:

- Phytochemicals, such as lutein, beta-carotene, allicin (in garlic), isoflavones (in soybeans), lycopene (in tomatoes), flavanoids (in green and black teas), sulforaphane glucosinolate (SGS; in broccoli and especially in broccoli sprouts), and lignans (in flaxseeds)
- Inducers (e.g., sulforaphane) of enzymes that do useful things like detoxifying carcinogens[7]
- Glucosinolates, which are found in cruciferous vegetables, especially broccoli sprouts, but also Brussels sprouts, cabbage, and cauliflower
- Vitamins
- Minerals
- Antioxidants
- High fiber, which may prevent colorectal cancer and cardiovascular disease.[8]

Eastern medicine focuses on whole foods rather than any particular component of that food. However, knowing what conventional medicine is saying about these components is intriguing and may offer inspiration to consume more of these veggies and fruits. Changes in diet may prevent 30 to 40 percent of cancer cases, or 3 to 4 million cases annually.[9] The most important change is increasing the amount of veggies we eat.

Here are some of the excellent effects that Western science associates with one or another of the above components:

- Helps antidote or counteract the inflammatory processes the body produces under stress
- Exerts an antibiotic activity against *Helicobacter pylori* (*H. pylori*), a bacteria that lives in the upper portion of the digestive tracts of more than 50 percent of the world's population, and which has been linked to peptic ulcers and stomach cancer.[10]
- Protects against many types of cancer by enhancing cancer-protective capacity, deactivating carcinogens, and blocking tumor development[11]
- Acts as a direct or indirect agent to neutralize free radicals[12]
- Stimulates the body's own antioxidant systems
- Supports the liver's ability to detoxify the body. The liver houses certain natural enzymes that help rid the body of toxic material generated by internal or externally generated pollution. Certain plant compounds support this process.[13]

Because we want to avoid the toxic load that insecticides and pesticides put on our bodies and our planet, it is ideal to eat organic fruits and veggies. Otherwise we may be counteracting some of their benefits.

JUICES

As we saw in Chapter 17, drinking cloudy (minimally processed) juice more than three times a week exerted a significant protective effect against developing Alzheimer's.[14]

It turns out that cloudy varieties of apple and berry juices contain up to four times as many polyphenols as do the clear, more processed varieties. Polyphenols are antioxidants found in red wine, berries, and yes (!), chocolate. It is interesting to note that more astringent varieties of apples have higher levels of polyphenols than do varieties that are bred to be sweeter.[15] Although it might be possible to breed the polyphenols back into juice we've stripped them out of, if we were to submit to Mother Nature a tad more humbly, situations like this may not have occurred in the first place. It is also possible that we have narrowed the field of the tastes we like down to a small postage-stamp size, and if we can open our minds to tastes other than extreme sweet, sour, and salty—the darlings of the modern world—we might find a new level of balance and new benefits from our diets not to mention a wider palate of acceptable, even enjoyable flavors.

OILS

The human brain is about 60 percent fat. Fat, though often demonized in modern culture, is important. It's hard to find a more yin, nourishing substance than good-quality fat. A lot is said about the quality of fats that we eat, and over the years we've had conflicting messages, such as in the flip-flop from "Margarine is better than butter" to, more recently, "Butter is better." Generally, the idea is to keep saturated fats to a minimum and eliminate trans fats altogether. They are the worst, acting exactly like *ama*—indigestible sludge that clogs and obstructs the various vessels and channels of our bodies.

In a widely reported study of April 2008, it was found that women with the highest levels of trans fats in their blood had about twice the risk of breast cancer, compared to women with the lowest levels.[16] This is not exactly new news. A fourteen-year study of eighty thousand nurses reported similar results in 1997.[17] But there is good news: trans fats are not found in nature. They are a construct of chemistry and are therefore only found in processed foods, which makes them easy to avoid.

Ayurveda is fond of vegetable oils. Until recently, the method of extracting oils was not reliant on high-temperature processes, and it is best to continue to use oils that are expeller pressed, unrefined, or cold pressed. These methods do not subject the oil to much damaging light and oxygen. It is all the better to store these oils in opaque containers in the refrigerator. Tropical oils like coconut oil tend to hold up better in high-heat cooking, such as frying or baking.

Oil has almost all yin properties, and good-quality oil, provided we digest it well, goes a long way to support good-quality yin and, therefore likely good-quality hormones. Very good-quality yin can support health in significant ways. Some oils, like those containing omega-3s, may reduce coronary incidents and total mortality. Olive oil has been linked to better cardiovascular health and a lower risk of breast cancer.[18] Conversely, poor-quality oils provide poor-quality yin. Trans fats are an excellent example of poor-quality yin. Instead of supporting cellular membrane structure, they clog passageways and create a hospitable environment for disease.

Just as progesterone balances estrogen, omega-3 fatty acids tend to balance omega-6s. Omega-3s and other high-quality oils provide super-quality yin—nourishment on a deep level, which in turn supports women's health. These oils are super yin. The brain, eyes, and heart—organs that require refined, high-quality yin to function well—have high concentrations of omega-3s. As little as 2 tablespoons of ground lignan-containing seeds such as flax or sesame (or 1½ to 2 teaspoons of their oils[19]) may help balance women's hormones and reduce bad cholesterol levels and heart attack risk.[20] Uncooked hemp oil or ground hemp seeds are said to have the ideal ratio (3 to 1) of omega-6 to omega-3 oils as well as containing GLA (gamma-linolenic acid), another beneficial substance. It is also advertised to have a high content of lipase, an enzyme that supports removal of plaque buildup from cell membranes and arteries. I am not a Western nutritionist, but I can see that this oil has wonderful-quality yin that may support a woman's hormonal balance.

These forms of yin need to be refrigerated and consumed as freshly as possible. It may be difficult to get flax oil that is fresh enough. I prefer to use oils on or in my food rather than in a capsule, so I like some hemp oil or, better yet, hemp seeds on my veggies. Cooking the oil or the seeds renders their good qualities less beneficial.

Ghee, or clarified butter, (available in many health food stores or Indian grocery stores), is very commonly used in Indian cooking and, unlike butter, may have cholesterol-lowering effects. As ghee is such a common staple in the Indian diet, it is not surprising that its effects on cholesterol have been studied there. In one study, rats that were fed both unheated and heated ghee wound up with lower cholesterol. The authors of this study concluded that including ghee in human diets may have similar results.[21]

Although omega-3s are currently in vogue, my suspicion is that we will likely get what our bodies need if we include a variety of minimally processed, high-quality, food-grade oils and fats in general in our daily diet. My favorites are olive oil, grape seed oil, coconut oil, hemp oil, ghee, and sunflower oil. I gravitate more toward certain ones for salads, others for baking, others for frying or baking, but at the end of the day (or week or month), it is easy to consume a range of oils and recipes.

CHOCOLATE

> Ayurveda requires deep spiritual insight in order to live
> in harmony with nature. Nothing in this universe is nonmedicinal;
> all substances can be used for various healing purposes.
> —*ASHTANGA HRIDAYAM SUTRASTHANAM* IX:10

While this aphorism was composed before trans fats were developed, and it would be a tough mission to find the medicinal properties of some modern-day constructs, it does easily apply to all natural substances. For example, even the prestigious *Journal of the American Medical Association* has reported the healthy effects of dark chocolate.[22] (White chocolate and even dark chocolate accompanied by milk didn't make the grade.) Its plant phenols—specifically the cocoa phenols—seem to be responsible for lowering blood pressure and delivering megadoses of antioxidants. However, Eastern medicine would caution us to remember that no one rule or food is necessarily good for everyone. Certain individuals would do well to avoid chocolate. It has been my experience that these individuals usually know who they are. These folks generally notice a very clear cause-and-effect relationship between chocolate and headaches, migraines, insomnia, or menstrual difficulties. I have had patients who would get migraines or hot flashes from even the tiniest bit of chocolate.

For the rest of us, a small amount of organic, good-quality dark chocolate may not only be good, but good for us, too. It is oily and dense and heavy, so provides yin, but also bitter and sharp, which are more yang qualities. This serves to make it a more balanced food than are some other sweets.

What to Eat in Times of Stress

The more complicated your physical, emotional, or spiritual life, the simpler your diet should be.

This is a simple rule I made up, based on Ayurvedic principles. At any given time we are either strong and need to maintain our strength and immunity, or we feel weak and need to regain it. In either case, it takes more effort to do this during the challenging times in our lives.

We can define "challenging times" as those when we are experiencing periods of high emotional, mental, or physical stress. These can be brought on by over-work, overthinking, travel, loss of a loved one, trauma, change of seasons, excessive sexual activity, and activities that we engage in beyond our natural energy level. We can tell we have excess stress when we feel weak, rundown, stressed out, or tired.

One thing about human nature is that we tend to lean on vices or "cheat" the most during the times when we can least afford to do so—that is, during the tough times in life. For example, it is most tempting to drink eight cups of coffee to get us through a night (or the day after it) when we've been up cramming for an exam, finishing a paper, nursing a baby, waiting in the hospital with a loved one, or working a night shift. It is during these very times when we need the best nutrition possible, delivered in the most easily digestible forms. We do not need to be draining our adrenal energy with caffeine when we're trying to replace what we've spent.

The idea is, we only have so much energy available to spend on physical exertion, processing emotional and spiritual experiences, and digesting our food. The more energy we allocate to physical, emotional, and spiritual experiences—including stress—the less is left for digesting our food. For example, if you are physically or mentally exhausted or "spent," the little energy you have left may be enough to fully digest a simple bowl of soup, but not complex or heavier foods, such as lasagne. The resulting poorly digested food may adversely affect the digestive system and lead to formation of the toxic sludge we call *ama*.

Supporting the digestive system is of primary importance, especially during challenging times. Following are guidelines I have often recommended for my patients. As always, you should discuss your condition with your health-care provider and immediately discontinue any behavior or remedies that result in discomfort.

When you are under a lot of stress, enjoy:

- Mostly whole, freshly cooked, nourishing food (as opposed to highly processed, canned, raw, or frozen food).
- *Kitcheri* (a rice and bean dish; see Appendix D) at least three times a week.
- Nondairy and non-tomato-based vegetable soups that are generously seasoned with turmeric, fresh ginger, and black pepper (such as the Agni Soup recipe on my Web site, www.drclaudiawelch.com).
- Rice and stir-fried vegetables with turmeric, black pepper, and fresh ginger
- Warm or room-temperature herbal teas.
- Plenty of sleep, rest, and relaxation.
- A healthy daily routine, including moderate exercise, regular meals, and meditation.
- A 10- to 20-minute self-massage daily, with warm oil appropriate to your current condition. (Skip this if you have your period, are pregnant, or are suffering from acute illness). See *abhyanga* in Chapter 26 and Appendix C.
- A daily dose of Triphala (a mixture of three herbs) is a common practice in Ayurveda, and can help maintain a healthy digestive tract, provided you have no acute illness or diarrhea, are not pregnant, do not have your period, or have other contraindicated conditions. Discuss this with your health-care practitioner. Triphala helps support a healthy gastrointestinal tract and provides a very gentle daily detox to counteract exposure to unavoidable environmental pollutants. (Triphala is available at www.banyanbotanicals.com or other places listed in Appendix A.)

Meat
TO EAT OR NOT TO EAT

I've often thought there ought to be a manual to hand to little kids . . .
called "Welcome to Earth" and one thing I would . . . tell them about is
cultural relativity . . . A first grader should understand that his or her
culture isn't a rational invention; that there are thousands of other cultures
and they all work pretty well; that all cultures function on faith rather
than truth; that there are lots of alternatives to our own society . . .
Cultural relativity is defensible, attractive. It's a source of hope.
It means we don't have to continue this way if we don't like it.
—KURT VONNEGUT JR.

We can apply this sentiment to the question of vegetarianism versus nonvegetarianism. In light of the fact that entire countries are or have been successfully peopled with both sorts of people, it's tough to argue that either is essential for maintaining health.

In my life and practice, I have seen both healthy and unhealthy omnivores as well as vegetarians. Although vegetarianism is often touted as the healthier choice, there are vegetarians who subsist on French fries, fast food, or other fare that is highly processed or otherwise difficult to digest. They may end up unhealthier than an omnivore who consumes a little meat, very little highly processed food, a lot of veggies, and whole food.

Building Blood and Strength

Many vegetarians who consult with practitioners of Chinese medicine are told they need to include meat in their diet if they want to become strong, regain strength, or "build blood." This is because meat, especially red meat, is heavy and dense. Red meat is said to increase blood, nourishing fluids, yin, and strength in the body. This it unquestionably does. *If* you can digest it. If you can't, it becomes *ama*, like anything else that is poorly digested. Meat is more difficult to digest than, say, appropriately cooked vegetables, beans, and grains. Because of this, among other reasons, traditional Ayurvedic medicine does not promote lots of meat as part of a regular daily diet. When it recommends the use of meat in the diet, it is usually in small amounts and cooked well in a stew, and in certain cases it is recommended as medicine.

Meat is not the only thing that can build blood, nourishing fluids, yin, and strength. If someone is weak, it is often due to a weak digestive system that does not digest or absorb food completely or well. Provided the amount and choice of food is appropriate and digestion is strong, then we will receive the ideal quantity and quality of yin—nourishment. If digestion is strong and there is still some deficiency of blood or nourishing fluids in the body, then it is still possible to build them with certain vegetarian foods, such as appropriately cooked seitan, beets, tofu, and many other very nourishing foods and herbs. It might take a little longer, but it is absolutely possible.

Dr. Dean Ornish, among many other experts, recommends a vegetarian diet. There are many reasons for this. One is that meat contains substances that cause an increase in homocystine levels, which in turn is associated with increased risk of heart disease. High homocystine levels irritate the linings of arteries, increasing the likelihood that they will clog, whereas the folate and vitamin B_6 found in vegetables and grains reduce homocystine levels.

Another reason to minimize the meat and maximize the veggies is that meat is a source of excessive phosphorous, which causes a loss of calcium in the body.[1]

There are some compelling arguments for keeping meat consumption to a minimum, in terms of its effect on our global environment and water and food crisis. Writing in 1971, Frances Moore Lappé in her best seller *Diet for a Small Planet*, presented startling figures on land use required for animal production versus vegetable production:

> An acre of cereals can produce five times more protein than an acre devoted to meat production; legumes (peas, beans, lentils) can produce ten times more; and leafy vegetables fifteen times more. . . . Spinach . . . can produce up to twenty-six times more protein per acre than can beef."[2]

Water, too, is inefficiently used for meat production.

A person subsisting on a vegetarian diet of 2.5 pounds of bread a day is indirectly utilizing 300 gallons of water daily. Production of food for an affluent diet of two pounds of vegetable matter and one pound of beef and animal fat a day, by contrast, requires a total of about 2,500 gallons of water daily. The 'water cost' of a pound of beef—which includes that used to produce feed as well as that drunk by the animal—is about twenty-five times that of a pound of bread."[3]

Finally, the domestication of animals for meat and the subsequent over-grazing of land is at least one factor in the creation of deserts.[4]

Belief Systems

Michael Pollan's book *In Defense of Food*[5] is a modern, concise, enlightening read on the meat issue as well as other aspects of food. Pollan is not a vegetarian and his presentation is a balanced exploration of the realities associated with meat production.

It is one thing to make our own decision about what we feel best eating, physically, philosophically, and environmentally. It is quite another to determine this for somebody else, including our family, friends, patients, or doctors. Suppose you are Jewish. You go to your doctor, who happens to be Catholic. Your doctor tells you that you will not get better unless you become Catholic. Imagine how you'd feel. It sounds ludicrous, doesn't it? But this may be the injustice committed by a health-care practitioner—or anyone else—who says someone must become either vegetarian or nonvegetarian, or else that individual will not get well. What we choose to eat (or not to eat) can be a significant component of our physical, emotional, or spiritual belief system. Offending or diverting this can adversely affect the spirit. There is a basic tenet of Traditional Chinese Medicine that says, "Blood follows qi (energy) and qi follows *shen* (spirit)." If the spirit is disturbed, energy will become disturbed and then the body will immediately or ultimately become disturbed. To injure somebody's spirit, then, can lead to disease.

I have often heard Dr. Vasant Lad, a prominent Ayurvedic physician, tell a story that relates to this very point. I am paraphrasing here. A gentleman came in to see Dr. Lad for a consultation in the days when he was a practicing physician at an Ayurvedic hospital in Pune, India. He complained to Dr. Lad that he couldn't digest anything and was getting weaker by the day. He quietly confided to Dr. Lad that he knew what his problem was. He had a gecko living in his stomach. The man knew it was there because he'd seen it in his cup of chai (spiced tea) just before he drank it. The man had been to many other doctors, both Western and Ayurvedic. Each doctor had told him that he was crazy. Such a thing was impossible and the poor fellow should consult a psychiatrist. The fellow was not inclined to see a psychiatrist because he was convinced that there was a lizard in his stomach.

So, Dr. Lad took the gentleman's pulse and told him that, yes, it was possible that he had swallowed the gecko, but fortunately there were good herbs for expelling geckos. If the gentleman would just take a decoction and spend the night, he would be given a medicated enema in the morning and would likely expel the gecko. Dr. Lad gently assured the fellow that together they would certainly be able to rid him of the gecko. Dr. Lad gave him a simple herbal decoction that evening and the next morning collected a bedpan and slipped a large and a small gecko into it before administering the enema. After the enema Dr. Lad enthusiastically explained to the patient, "I have found the most surprising thing. Not only did you have one gecko in your stomach, you had two: one big one and one little one. The one you swallowed must have been pregnant and given birth. But they are now expelled and now you should be fine."

The gentleman was ecstatic. He exclaimed, "I knew it! And you were the only person to believe me!" He was so grateful to Dr. Lad for believing him and helping him. He went home and from that moment on, was free of his digestive complaints. He would return every now and then to thank Dr. Lad for curing him.

A Western mind may be shocked by this story, but Dr. Lad was able to see how truly entrenched this man was in his belief system, and that it hadn't worked to try to change his belief. So he decided to cooperate with the man's belief system and then guide it out of trouble.

This is also a fundamental principle in the practice of aikido, a martial art. In aikido, it is essential to first blend with one's opponent's energy, flow, and direction before redirecting it. In the case of a physician, sometimes it may be appropriate to redirect a patient's beliefs, and sometimes it is beneficial to simply work within the parameters of them.

It is the responsibility of each of us to weigh the physical, environmental, and spiritual implications of our chosen diet, come to our own conclusions and proceed in a manner that we ourselves can live and feel at peace with.

Other Considerations

If you do eat meat, it may be wise to consume it in moderation and only meat that you are sure comes from low-fat, organically fed animals or fish, especially if you are pregnant, because meat delivers pesticides, insecticides, and pollutants in a much more concentrated form than do veggies and other vegetarian fare, and these pollutants are further concentrated in a mother's breast milk. Up to 90 percent of our personal exposure to dangerous pollutants in food comes mostly through meat and, less so, through dairy.[6] We will see in Chapter 25 how damaging these chemical pollutants can be. Additionally, if you eat a lot of meat, you are likely doing so in place of veggies, which, with their undisputed and well-deserved reputation for having all the right stuff, are the preferable choice.

What about the body's need for protein and calcium? Over the years I have encountered people who are very concerned about getting enough protein in their diet. Many of these folks have turned to protein drinks daily to supplement it. The problem is, I have found that protein or shake drinks, which Ayurveda describes as heavy, cold, and dense, are usually hard to digest, especially first thing in the day on a regular basis. As food that doesn't digest well ends up causing trouble, this is cause for concern. As we will see, soy (which is an essential component of many of these shakes) has an affinity with the endocrine system. If consumed in a form that is readily digestible, it will have a good effect. If not, it may have a detrimental effect. Another possible concern is that excess protein of any sort may actually hinder the body's absorption of calcium.[7]

It may be easier than we think to achieve the minimum daily requirement of calcium, even from a relatively poor diet.[8] Eastern medicine says different people have different requirements for—and respond better to—different sources of protein and calcium. For example, one person may be heavy and lead a sedentary life and will do well to get their calcium from greens (collards, for example, have high levels of calcium), whereas a skinny person who needs more dense, heavy nourishment may benefit more from dairy or small amounts of meat. This depends on each person's current requirements and what the individual is likely to digest well. In general, a thin person already has excess yang qualities and needs more nourishing food, and a heavier person will do well to eat more lightening food.

৻৶ 23 ৶৻

What Not to Eat

Ayurveda recommends we avoid any foods that hinder digestion or create *ama*, toxic sludge. Leftover, highly processed, frozen, dehydrated, reconstituted, rotten, or burned food are all considered difficult to digest, and so serve to create *ama*. Here are a few more trouble spots.

Fast or Highly Processed Food

In the hit documentary *Super Size Me*, Morgan Spurlock ate three meals daily for thirty days at McDonald's to see how it would affect his health. Over the course of the month, he gained twenty-five pounds, his liver became toxic, his cholesterol went from 165 to 230, his libido dropped, and he suffered headaches and depression. His prescription for recovering his health, according to general practitioner Dr. Daryl Isaacs, was "to stop doing what he was doing," that is, to stop eating McDonald's food. We can generally extend this warning to include most foods at any fast-food chain and many fast snacks and prepackaged prepared foods.

The problems with fast food or other foods that have been highly manipulated and processed are numerous. I'll list them here, then expand on each one.

- They are highly processed, making them difficult to digest and assimilate, and even for our bodies to recognize them as nourishment.
- They deliver poor-quality raw material to our bodies and may potentially be carcinogenic.
- They often are made with poor-quality oils or fats.
- They don't include a lot of vegetables.
- We eat them on the go, and so don't digest them as well as if we are in a calm environment.

PROCESSED FOODS

Processed foods use several substances that the body does not recognize as food. From artificial colors to artificial flavors and artificial sweeteners, these are substances designed to trick our senses. Eastern medicine relies on our senses to determine which foods are appropriate for us at any given time. Just as a carpenter couldn't pick the appropriate tool for his job if he couldn't recognize it, we cannot determine which foods will be appropriate for us if their properties are manipulated, disguised, or altered to change their colors, flavors, and properties.

For example, there is a certain way the body has learned—through the long, slow process of evolution—to identify and process the sweet taste. According to Ayurveda, sweet foods have had a generally stabilizing and nourishing effect on the body. Until recently, the majority of sources of this taste have come from such natural sweeteners as honey, maple syrup, and other unrefined sugars, and from naturally sweet foods like yams, cooked rice, or wheat. These are all foods that do indeed provide nourishment. It is only recently that sugar substitutes such as aspartame and saccharin, devoid of calories and lacking the nourishing effects of natural sweeteners, have entered the food scene. It is confusing to the body's learned intelligence to encounter the taste it has for millennia associated with certain effects (like a boost of energy and a bulk-building effect on the body) but not get those effects. For a look at the benefits and safety issues of artificial sweeteners on the market, see the Web site www .medicinenet.com/artificial_sweeteners/article.htm. The safety issues are considerable and worth a look.

Many fast foods have high levels of acrylamide, a substance the U.S. Environmental Protection Agency defines as a colorless, crystalline solid that is probably a human carcinogen. It induces gene mutations and stomach cancer in animal tests and is known to cause damage to the central and peripheral nervous system. In April 2002, researchers at Sweden's National Food Administration deemed the results of a study so important that they disclosed them to the public even before they had been published. The findings showed that many fast foods, including French fries, bread, biscuits, and potato chips, contain alarmingly high levels of acrylamide. For example, a bag of potato chips could contain five hundred times the maximum levels deemed acceptable in drinking water by the World Health Organization. Burger King and McDonald's fries contained about one hundred times the acceptable levels. Breakfast cereals made by Kellogg, Quaker Oats, and Nestlé; and Old El Paso brand tortilla chips were also included in the study, and the news about them wasn't good, either.

The raw ingredients of all foods did not have even traces of acrylamide, but once their raw food and oils were finished being processed, fried, baked, and deep-fried at high temperatures, they did.[1] Even food that is only moderately processed, such as dried or preprepared food, may not have the same health benefits as if they were fresh. For example, the *New York Times* reported on a study by researchers at the University of Connecticut School of Medicine, wherein it was demonstrated that the cardioprotective effects of fresh garlic on rats were decreased if the garlic was crushed and left two days to dry.[2] The drying process allowed volatile chemicals to dissipate, apparently diluting their potency.

When we feed ourselves substandard edibles and process them in extreme ways, we provide our guts with substandard building blocks of nutrition. Poor-quality building blocks lead to construction of poor tissues. Poor tissues construct a feeble body.

INFERIOR-QUALITY OILS

Fast and highly processed foods are generally cooked with inferior-quality oils. Some of the better oils, such as omega-3s, can't be used in processed food because they don't have a long shelf life the way trans fats do.

WILL THE REAL VEGETABLE PLEASE STAND UP?

The benefits of vegetables do not extend to French fries and onion rings—deep-fried and processed stuff that is difficult to digest. As of this writing, the Burger King Web site lists at least ten ingredients in its French fries, including sodium acid pyrophosphate, dextrose, and xanthan gum.[3] McDonald's fries compare similarly, with about ten ingredients, including "natural beef flavor" that seems to be made from products derived from wheat and dairy, and they are prepared in oil that contains hydrogenated soybean oil with tertiary butylhydroquinone (TBHQ—a preservative that may contribute to stomach tumor formation and DNA damage in lab animals, at high doses).[4] Dimethylpolysiloxane is also added as an antifoaming agent.[5] It is also an important ingredient in Silly Putty.

Aside from some pale, limp, lettuce grown with pesticides in mineral-deprived soil, the fries and rings are about the only representatives from the veggie world you'll find in fast-food places. It might be safe to say that fast-food joints are not good sources of whole foods.

FAST FOOD VS. SLOW FOOD

Besides being highly processed, fast food is, well, fast: When we cook in a rush, we eat in a rush and don't take time to digest food before moving on to another activity. When we divert our body's transformational resources from digestive to other physical or mental activities, we cannot expect to digest our food well. This leads to *ama* formation, which contributes to disease.

We all have times when we are simply unable to cook due to time pressures and responsibilities, but we all have the choice to favor more healthy fast foods. Chinese take-out mixed vegetables, tofu, and rice can be a fast easy choice, for example. So could some simple Mexican food, such as rice, beans and *calabacitas* (a veggie dish with zucchini, onions, tomatoes, and corn). These might not be made with as high a quality oil that we might use in our homes, or be quite as fresh, but consuming these foods is likely to be better than either going without eating or eating something that is highly processed.

There is a burgeoning slow food (www.slowfood.com) movement afoot these days. It began in Europe and is spreading now throughout the world, with 100,000 members in 153 countries. It is a movement that appreciates and supports fresh, local vegetables, cooked with love and consumed with friends, in a cheerful environment, in gratitude of food.

Alcohol

There are benefits and drawbacks to alcohol. Three possible benefits of alcohol consumption are its potential to increase longevity, induce relaxation—a rare commodity in the modern world, and promote heart health. The negative effects, on the other hand, are too numerous to list. They so far outweigh the positive effects that we'd do best to explore other ways to increase our longevity, achieve relaxation, and help our hearts. Let's take a closer look.

In the spring of 2008, there was a bit of a buzz about the potential of resveratrol, an ingredient found in minuscule amounts in certain wines and in grape juice, to retard the effects of aging.[6] The hypothesis was that resveratrol might mimic the effects of famine-induced activation of a protein agent called sirtuin in humans, thereby supporting tissue preservation and maintenance. Although low doses have not been directly tested, there is speculation that wine has sufficient resveratrol to be beneficial for humans. Effects have varied in different studies on mice, showing positive results from amounts that would require the human equivalent of drinking thirty-five to one hundred bottles of wine per day.[7]

If we are choosing to drink wine to enhance longevity, based on the resveratrol studies, we might consider adding a resveratrol supplement to our daily routine, thereby avoiding the negative effects of alcohol consumption.

For many women, drinking a glass of red wine in the evening is the one relaxing thing they do in their entire day. This relaxation is precious and, no doubt, good for them. However, with a bit of effort, we can learn to relax or manage stress in other ways that won't have such a big impact on our health.

We explored the benefits of alcohol on heart health in Part II. Our conclusion: Favor the better—and proven—ways to achieve cardiac benefit, because the deleterious effects of alcohol are too impressive to ignore. If you have been drinking red wine for its resveratrol, consider replacing at least some of it with grape juice, açai juice, yerba maté, more veggies in your diet, or some other food or drink that is appropriate for you. Açai berries are said to have ten times the amount of anthocyanins (antioxidant pigments) that red wine has, and yerba maté is said to contain more antioxidants than red wine. If you want to include something in your daily or weekly routine to support heart health without risking other problems relating to alcohol, these might be worth considering.[8]

If you want to review the facts about how alcohol increases the risk of breast cancer, go to the section on alcohol in Chapter 13. It might also be useful to reread the section on alcohol in Chapter 15. Overall, research has shown that alcohol is far more dangerous than useful to us, whether we are talking about longevity, relaxation, or a healthy heart.

In Chapter 13, we saw the Million Women Study found that the risk of any kind of cancer increased as alcohol consumption increased, no matter the type of alcohol. Most of the women in the study drank an average of only one drink a day, with very few drinking three or more daily. This is typical of women in high-income countries such as the United States or Great Britain. Often we justify our drinking because of reported cardiovascular benefits, but the risks outweigh the benefits; even low to moderate alcohol consumption appeared to account for almost 13 percent of the cancers of the breast, liver, and some digestive cancers. For oral, pharynx, rectal, esophageal, laryngeal, and liver cancers combined, there were about fifteen cancers per thousand women per daily drink.[9] Alcohol also increases the risk of osteoporosis.[10]

The World Health Organization (WHO) has identified the consumption of alcohol as one of the top ten risks for worldwide "burden of disease," a measure of the loss of years of healthy life through disabling disease.[11] The consequences of alcohol use include biochemical effects such as intoxication and addiction, which contribute to traumatic events as well as personal disease. The WHO states, "Overall there is a causal relationship between alcohol consumption and more than 60 types of disease and injury. Alcohol is estimated to cause about 20–30 percent worldwide of esophageal cancer, liver cancer, cirrhosis of the liver, homicide, epilepsy, and motor vehicle accidents." Worldwide, the WHO finds that alcohol annually causes 1.8 million deaths and 58.3 million years of productive life lost to premature death or disability.[12]

In an editorial that accompanied the release of the Million Women Study, Michael Lauer, MD, and Paul Sorlie, PhD, of the National Heart, Lung, and Blood Institute in Bethesda, Maryland, wrote, "From a standpoint of cancer risk, the message of this report could not be clearer. There is no level of alcohol consumption that can be considered safe."[13]

Cola

Much as the occasional cola might be enjoyable, cola as a daily indulgence may tip the scales if you are concerned about bone density. Studies done at the Jean Mayer USDA Human Nutrition Research Center on Aging at Tufts University showed a correlation between cola consumption and bone density. Hip bone mineral density (BMD) dropped as much as 5 percent in women who drank cola every day, as compared with women who drank less than one a month. These are significant differences, and results were similar for diet cola. Results were only a bit weaker for decaffeinated cola and did not apply to noncola carbonated soft drinks.

This study also demonstrated that the lower bone mineral density was not due to lower calcium or vitamin D intake. Nor was it caused by the caffeine or sugar in the soda or by the body size of the woman. The phosphoric acid in cola beverages binds to calcium in the gut and prevents it from being absorbed.[14]

While this is particularly important information for women concerned about their bones, it is also an important consideration for those who are parents. We are supposed to gain bone mass until we are about twenty-five years old, and if young people are not maximizing that potential, they may be jeopardizing their bone density.

Because we know that clean water, fruit juice, and various herbal teas have such beneficial effects, it might be wise to consider cola only as the occasional treat, not to be regularly consumed.

Foods Treated with Pesticides and Chemicals

We will consider the effects of toxic pollutants in more detail in Chapter 27, but it is important to consider the effects of pesticides and insecticides on our health and the health of our planet. From increased risk of reproductive and other cancers to decreased sperm counts in men, the risks are too great to ignore.

Fruits and veggie consumption is one of the main things we can do to support heart health and prevent cancer, so it's probably best to not have them add to our health problems by consuming with them pesticides and other chemicals that are carriers of synthetic estrogen-like chemicals, many of which are known to be carcinogenic.

Aside from the negative effects these substances have on us, they have also contributed to the industrialization of food, which has served to deplete our soils of their nutrition. Michael Pollan's *In Defense of Food* covers this issue tidily and is a good read for anybody interested in what to eat. When soil nutrition is depleted, whatever grows in that soil also is less nutritious. Over the years, the nutrients in our food have diminished to the point that we might need to eat three times the amount of food we ate less than a century ago to derive the same nutrition.[15]

It is curious to note that much of the practice of using pesticides and insecticides can be traced back to World War II. During the war, chemicals were developed for use in chemical warfare. After the war, when they could no longer be used toward such a sinister purpose, the companies were able to find a new use for the chemicals: insecticides and pesticides. This allowed them not to waste the chemicals and, instead, to find financial reward in their continued use. Using the same chemicals that were designed to cause human beings suffering, to spray on what they eat, seems odd logic.

The use of toxic insecticides and pesticides not only has an adverse effect on human beings, but also on the environment. For insight into their role in the tragic disappearance of bees, due to what is now called *colony collapse disorder*, see the enlightening documentary, *Vanishing of the Bees*, listed in Appendix A.

Sometimes we don't want to pay the extra money for organic food, but it may not be as expensive, in the long run, as paying for health care for diseases related to consuming pesticides and insecticides. Anyone who has grown even a small vegetable patch in his or her yard knows the work that goes into growing good-quality food. Considering the work involved, it is sometimes amazing to me that organic food doesn't cost more than it does. I always feel great about paying those farmers, who, by the way, never seem as if they are becoming wealthy from what they charge. Check Appendix A for how to find the current top twelve most important foods to buy organic and the top twelve foods to avoid.

But look at where we live. We are living in a world that is polluted, where organic veggies sometimes seem outside of our budget and where it is not always possible to find them. If we become so rigid in our organic fastidiousness that we won't, say, enjoy a tasty nonorganic meal made with love at a friend's home or at a restaurant, our own stress and rigidity around this issue can itself cause problems. Rigidity and stress cause qi or *prana* to stagnate and clench, robbing our organs of vitality and our spirits of joy. We can do our best to buy and cook organic food, drink organic coffee, get fresh air, and drink clean water, especially if we suffer from environmental illnesses, but if we stress about it excessively, the stress may well add insult to injury.

The Pros
and Cons of Soy

There is a lot of confusion about soy around women's health. There is a "soy is good" camp, where soy proponents tout it as a virtual cure-all, and there is a "soy is bad" camp, which tends to portray soy as dangerous. How can we make sense of whether soy and plant estrogens (of which soy is one) are good or bad? I won't claim to clear up the whole issue here, but shall present how we might approach this from an Ayurvedic perspective.

First, let's look at what we know about soy. Soy is a powerfully rich source of a group of phytoestrogens (naturally occurring compounds in plants that act like estrogen) called isoflavones.[1] Even moderate amounts of these plant-based hormones can effect biological change.[2] Over the last decade or so, consumption of soy products, both minimally processed (like tofu, tempeh, tamari, or miso) and refined, highly processed derivatives and forms of soy (like soy isolate and concentrated powder for use in shakes and baby formulas), has exploded among adults and infants alike.

The "Bad Soy" Camp

In the "soy is bad" camp, we see some studies that have shown that genistein—an estrogen-mimicking component of soy—can interfere with a rat's hormonal function and cause physical abnormalities in growth, sexual organs, and decreased fertility.[3] Although rats and humans are different creatures, there are enough similarities that scientists take the results seriously and questions have been raised about soy's effect on humans.

The concern that soy could negatively affect infants is of particular concern because an infant's developing system is so vulnerable to permanent damage. Karl

Rozman, PhD, a University of Kansas toxicologist at the National Institutes of Health, explains that human infants consume far lower doses of soy than do lab animals and only a little of the chemical makes it to the infant's bloodstream, but also admits that there have been few controlled studies and the jury is still out.[4]

There is at least some laboratory indication that soy affects breast tissue. A 1998 study reported in the *American Journal of Clinical Nutrition* followed forty-eight women who were scheduled for a breast biopsy. Half were given a high-soy diet for two weeks before the biopsy. The other half had a diet without soy. Subsequent biopsies showed that the women who had eaten the high-soy diet had more markers of breast cell proliferation than did the low-soy group.[5] There is also some indication that soy can have a negative effect on the thyroid.[6]

Another study, reported by the journal *Alternative Therapies* in 2001,[7] showed roughly equal menopausal symptoms in women who consumed soy and those who didn't. The women in the soy group were given either soy isolate powder or casein (milk-based) protein powder. This is a point that will become important in our discussion later.

Such studies would seem to dissuade us from soy. But, it is important to note that soy isolate powder is different from more whole soy foods. In fact, Walter Willett, chairman of the department of nutrition at the Harvard School of Public Health, warns that soy isoflavone supplements should be regarded as "totally untested new drugs."[8]

Thus, the effects of highly processed and concentrated forms of plant-based hormones seem to be inconclusive at best and damaging at worst. The confusion sets in when we hear from the other side, the "soy is good" camp.

The "Good Soy" Camp

It is well documented that Japanese women who consumed 35 to 60 mg of phytoestrogens a day, in easily digestible forms of soy, such as cooked tofu, soy sauce, and miso, had a lower incidence of breast cancer than did women who consumed a more typical Western diet. However, when they would move to the United States and adopt the same Western diet, their rates of cancer would increase to the "American" rates.[9] These points have been proved through enough different studies that they are accepted as true.[10]

Other studies suggest that soy protein is beneficial both for both cardiovascular disease and for osteoporosis in postmenopausal women.[11]

So, is soy good? Or bad? Let's see if we can reconcile the two camps.

Soy: Meeting in the Middle

The form in which we ingest soy may make all the difference between whether it has a good or bad effect on our endocrine system. If it is easily digestible, it may be beneficial. If it is concentrated, powdered, and highly processed, it may not.

The Japanese women who were enjoying health benefits were eating soy foods as part of their daily diet, in forms that were minimally processed. The women in the study that showed no benefits from soy were given soy isolate.[12] Why were these women given soy isolate powder instead of tofu and other real foods?

One fundamental difference in Eastern and Western medical philosophies lies in the Eastern practice of consuming raw plants for medicinal purposes as opposed to the Western approach of consuming isolated, often concentrated "active ingredients" of the raw plant. In Eastern medicine we tend to assume that Nature has a wisdom that governs which active and nonactive ingredients belong together, and we are suspicious of teasing them apart. I recall a fruit in India that is said to be toxic if eaten without its seeds, which contain an antidote to the toxin.

There may also be a Western tendency at work here. When we in the West heard about the benefits Japanese women were experiencing, we assumed that if some soy was good, more would be better. We set about pulverizing, isolating, processing, concentrating, and powdering it. Then the resulting powder is added to baby formula, or whipped into a cold shake and sucked down in bulk. Or we ingest it in an easy-to-take pill, instead of having to cook a meal. Or we consume it in other forms that are highly processed and have a bunch of unpronounceable additives; forms such as vegetarian hot dogs, sliced "meats," veggie burgers, and other fake meats that have soy isolate as a main ingredient. And then we are surprised when we don't see the same results. We are even more surprised when, instead of delivering good effects, the soy is found to be harmful for our hormonal system, especially in infants. Thus the "soy is bad" camp emerges.

Not all Western scientists agree with the "more is better" approach. Walter Willett of Harvard cautions, "In moderation, soy is fine . . . Stuffed into everything, you could get into trouble."[13] On the online medical site www.WebMD .com, Jatinder Mhatia, a pediatrician at the Medical College of Georgia, agrees. "Only in our country are we using [soy] in a free-for-all . . . [It] has a specific indication, and we tend to use and abuse in America."[14]

As I discussed earlier, an Ayurvedic perspective would indicate that the qualities of soy match closely enough with those of estrogen that it will have an affinity with the endocrine system. Soy's affinity with the endocrine system gets its foot in the door. What it does when it gets there is the question. It is possible that whether soy has a positive or negative effect on hormonal balance may be dependent on the form in which it is ingested (that is, highly refined versus whole—or at least minimally processed) and whether it is well digested.

What Does Eastern Medicine Say About Soy?

From an Eastern medicine point of view, minimally processed, cooked forms of soy are easier to digest than forms like fake meats or highly processed soy cheeses or yogurts, which are complicated, highly processed products. Concentrated, highly processed soy powders and soy isolates are, likewise, often difficult to digest. In my practice I have found that most patients who regularly consume soy shakes, for example, will show signs of weak digestive systems or that their food is not being transformed appropriately into more biologically refined nutrition. I rarely see this problem with people who include easily digestible, well-cooked, and seasoned forms of soy regularly in their diet. There is some evidence that fermented soy products, like tempeh, miso, soy sauce, tamari, and some tofus, are healthier than nonfermented ones. Ayurveda teaches that the fermentation process increases the warming energetics of the food and may render it easier to digest. Whatever is not digested well will sooner or later act as poison somewhere in the body and lead to disease. Often it acts as poison in the very areas of the body that it has affinity with. In the case of soy, that would be the endocrine system.

The most digestible way to include soy in the diet is as moderate amounts of tofu or tempeh, well cooked, preferably with fresh ginger. A small amount of miso, soy sauce, or tamari may be beneficial if it you are not trying to have a low-sodium diet. A daily cup of warm, spiced soy milk at bedtime is not only tasty but probably digestible and nourishing, provided you find an organic, non-GMO, unsweetened soy milk to which you can add your own natural sweetener. There are indications even in Western studies that support this outlook. For example, it has been found that we receive the most benefit from soy, or other foods that contain isoflavones, if we consume small amounts of them throughout the day, every day throughout our lives. [15]

Some Western studies have also shown that the bioavailability of soy is inextricably linked with healthy intestinal metabolism.[16] This may also explain why the rat studies did not show favorable effects of soy, as rats and humans have different systems of intestinal metabolism.[17]

It may be that people with stronger digestive systems derive more benefit, or at least less harm, from highly processed and concentrated forms of soy than do folks with weaker digestive systems, but I tend to just recommend the forms that are easiest to digest.

Soy is great. And soy is suspect. It simply depends on what we do to it and how we consume it that makes it beneficial or harmful to each of us.

Some Conclusions About Phytoestrogens

After wading through soy studies, seeing its effects on patients, and considering this issue from the perspective of Eastern medicine, I have come to the conclusion that it is likely that we will find negative effects associated with overconsumption of highly processed, concentrated, cold forms of soy and positive effects associated with moderate, daily consumption of digestible, minimally processed forms of soy, cooked well, with fresh ginger or other mild spices. This conclusion is supported in at least one excellent exploration of soy's risks versus benefits for humans, wherein the authors conclude that, as long as soy is consumed in the way that the Japanese women consumed it, it is unlikely to have a negative effect on the thyroid or on breast cancer or carry the negative effects associated with estrogen in general. In fact, it is likely to be beneficial for the prevention and treatment of breast cancer.[18]

If there were comprehensive studies done on whole forms of broccoli, cauliflower, and other isoflavone-rich foods versus concentrated, highly processed versions of these vegetables, I suspect we would find similar results as with soy.

According to Eastern medicine, anything that is overused or poorly metabolized can have a negative effect. After all, even too much water can kill you. When used wisely, in minimally processed forms, in daily diet and digested well, plant foods can support hormonal balance and provide excellent benefits. I think it likely that phytoestrogens, consumed in this manner would not have negative effects on estrogen-dominant conditions such as heavy bleeding or estrogen-sensitive tumors, because I trust the body would not usually transform unadulterated building blocks into material that will harm it. But because there is confusion around this, and to be on the safe side, I generally recommend that women with signs of estrogen dominance, like fibrocystic breasts or uterine fibroids, avoid plants like soy and herbs like *shatavari*—a famous Ayurvedic herb commonly used for women's complaints—that are thought to be especially rich in phytoestrogens.

25

Essential Elements of a Healthy Lifestyle

Ambition is the thief of the spirit.
—KIRPAL SINGH, TWENTIETH-CENTURY INDIAN SAINT

As we pass the life landmarks of age thirty-five and then fifty, our yin sex hormones gradually decline and, along with them, the generous buffer we had for handling ways of life that weren't working for us. Luckily, our willingness to tolerate things that don't work for us may wane as well, and our commitment to living the good life, whatever that is for each of us, grows. Diet, job, family, relationships, exercise, our environment, and a host of other factors contribute to the quality of our lives. If we pay honest attention to how each element of our lifestyle affects us, we often have the choice to eliminate or tweak those aspects that are causing trouble.

In this chapter we'll look at the aspects that make up a lifestyle and talk about how to work with them to reduce stress and improve health. In the next chapter, we'll focus on specific stress-management techniques for coping with whatever still interferes with our happiness and well-being.

Trapped on the Modern Treadmill

Before we go any further, let's look at one of the most common things I have seen in my practice: People feeling trapped in lives they don't want to be living. It seems unlikely that a woman can enjoy herself—and her own company—if she is miserable in her life. Running from the bedroom to the kitchen to the car to school to the job to extracurricular activities to events to errands, back home, to the TV, computer, and phone, she finds herself drained and unbalanced.

Unfortunately, as we do all this running around, we are modeling it for our children. Multitasking has so much become the norm for the growing generation that it is difficult to have a ten-minute conversation with teenagers without their concurrently sending, or reading text messages. They seem proud of their ability to multitask.

One of my mentors counseled his students to give their full attention to one thing at a time, to complete that thing and then move on. This allows qi or *prana* to concentrate rather than scatter. When qi scatters, we end up spending more of it quickly.

I recently had dinner with my friend Patty—a nurse—at a new restaurant in town. The food was fantastic, but it took a half hour to be seated and another half hour to get our food. While we were waiting to be seated, we noticed the proprietor didn't have a waiting list. She simply remembered which party was to be seated next. We congratulated her on her memory and she seemed understandably proud of it. Then, as we sat waiting for our food, we began to understand why the long wait. The strikingly beautiful young woman—probably in her mid to late twenties—was not only the proprietor and hostess, she assisted the two busboys, took orders, and brought them to the tables. This young woman was rushing gracefully about, juggling about three different jobs. In a pair of three-inch heels.

Patty and I felt as if we were witnessing a poignant, familiar tragedy at its inception. This girl had learned that she could do it all and have it all, but she hadn't learned yet that it would have its price. For a few quiet moments we could see her future. Neither Patty nor I are prone to repressing our thoughts, so as we were leaving we gushed about how good the food was and said we hoped the hostess could hire a little more help, as we noticed she was doing everything herself. She responded to our concern by letting us know that her main job was interior design and this was a side endeavor and she was doing fine, thanks to a little yoga and meditation and following her passions. It was a familiar story.

All this rushing stimulates the mobile, ambitious yang qualities in our life. Initially this may feel exciting, but in the long term, it depletes yin and leaves the body and spirit poorly nourished. Then, not only do we suffer ourselves, but we no longer have the reserves to be able to extend care to the other relationships in our lives.

One thing that we are tempted to do when we spend our days multitasking is to spend our nights watching TV. One thing I have noticed in my own life is a relationship between depression and the amount of TV I watch. As the latter increases, so does the former. It is odd to take a break from multitasking by watching television, as television itself is a form of multitasking, what with the shows presented in short fragments interspersed with multicommercial breaks.

Aside from the questionable effect on our spirit and mind, there is evidence that watching TV is associated with physical troubles as well. It has been shown that two hours a day of TV watching was associated with a 23 percent increase in obesity and a 14 percent increase of diabetes. Therefore, one easy prescription for a healthier lifestyle: Watch less than ten hours of TV a week.[1]

In the last century, change has advanced at a breakneck speed, and the lifestyle that has accompanied these changes has had undesirable results. We have less time for real connection with our spouses, children, and friends and are divorced from the land and protected from the realities of changing seasons and weather—including sunshine. "Having it all" apparently includes having more than we bargained for. If our quest for it all was satisfying us, maybe it would be worth it, but discontent seems to pervade our society. As James Thurber quipped, "Nowadays men lead lives of noisy desperation."

And what are these results? Despite tremendous technological, medical, and scientific advances, we see a rise of a group of distressing health concerns. We are the first generation in which our children are likely to live shorter lives than their parents.[2] Two-thirds of adults and 15 percent of children in the United States are considered obese. And we are exporting this disturbing probability. In one generation, Asians have gone from having one of the lowest rates of modern diseases to having one of the highest. Obesity, cardiovascular disease and diabetes are some of the other side effects of modern life[3] and have an effect on hormonal balance—and conditions it affects—as well. For example, postmenopausal obesity may increase a woman's risk of breast cancer.[4]

The Good News (Yes, There Is Some!)

As we look at the prevalence of these diseases it is easy to feel disheartened, but there is ample cause to take heart. Cardiovascular disease, obesity, and diabetes are "completely preventable for at least 95 percent of people just by changing diet and lifestyle,"[5] says Dr. Dean Ornish, a pioneer in the effects of lifestyle and diet on these major diseases. Using state-of-the art equipment, Dr. Ornish has demonstrated the efficacy of low-cost, simple changes in diet and lifestyle.

Engaging in a healthy lifestyle and diet can decrease obesity and benefit a woman's reproductive organs. And we're not the only ones who can benefit.

Dr. Ornish finds that prostate cancer can be preventable, even reversible. Compared with 9 percent of participants in a control group, there was regression of tumor growth in 70 percent of men who adopted positive diet and lifestyle changes.[6]

Ayurvedic medicine has been practiced for thousands of years in India. The foundation of this medical system lies in lifestyle and diet. Ayurveda is especially strong at assessing what sort of lifestyle is appropriate for which individual. Although it is beyond the scope of this book to help you determine what your constitution is and what are the most appropriate exercise routines for you, there are some universal factors.

We have already looked at the role of diet, the first pillar of health. Here we'll look at several other components of lifestyle.

Relaxing into a Routine

A lifestyle is nothing but the long-term pattern made up of our daily routine and habits. Having a daily routine, called *dinacharya* in Ayurveda, is one of the most important elements of Ayurvedic medicine and a crucial part of our health. In Ayurveda, we have a daily routine in which we do the same things at the same time every day, if possible. When the body adjusts to a daily routine and learns to count on it, the nervous system can relax.

In Ayurveda, the ideal routine is a bit morning-heavy, from waking sometime between three AM and dawn, to meditating, grooming, exercising, and bathing. Something closer to dawn may be more appropriate for many, as sleep is a precious commodity in the modern world, though if her life is already balanced, a woman may find waking earlier enriching. In any case, the idea is to fit in the really important things—meditation, self-care, yoga, physical exercise, and breathing exercises—before breakfast unless we are sure they work better for us later in the day. From breakfast on, we are left to address the rest of life's demands. Now, I don't expect anybody to immediately start waking up at dawn, but if most of the crucial elements of a healthy life are worked into a routine, we are less likely to forget them. They will become, well, routine. Starting early sets the tone for the day (much the same way early childhood sets the stage for life), and ensures that some of the most important things we can do to maintain or restore our health will not get lost over the course of the day.

Here is a detailed daily routine that incorporates many elements of a healthy lifestyle and stress management:

1. Wake early (at the same time every day).

2. Clean your face, teeth, and mouth. Brush your teeth, scrape
   gargle with some warm water. The tongue accumulates bacter
   helps diminish their numbers. While your local drugstore m
   rubber tongue scrapers, I prefer the Indian-style stainless-steel ones.
   find sources for these in Appendix A.

3. Drink a glass of warm water. This stimulates a bowel movement and cleanses
   the gastrointestinal tract.

4. Eliminate.

5. Apply cooling salve or cool water to the eyes. This refreshes the eyes.

6. Gargle with salt water and use a neti pot to irrigate the nasal cavities with salt
   water. These steps should only take about 3 minutes total. Put ¼ teaspoon of
   noniodized sea salt in the bottom of your neti pot, fill with warm water, and follow the clear directions that come with the pot. You can find where to get this
   in Appendix A. We are all exposed to a multitude of pathogens every day, especially if we work or live with a lot of other people. Being exposed to pathogens
   is not the problem. The problem is proliferation of the pathogens, which often
   occurs in the nasal passages or throat. Rinsing the nasal passages and gargling
   with salt water helps us avoid proliferation of bacteria and viruses that we are
   exposed to and prepares us nicely for doing some breathing exercises, which we
   will discuss later.

7. Meditate, engage in quiet contemplation or read inspirational material for 15 to
   60 minutes. If you don't have a meditation practice, this could be a time of prayer
   or gentle breathing exercises that you can learn from a yoga practitioner. In any
   case, the goal is to quiet the mind. This is useful for calming the spirit.

8. Apply warm oil to your body. It is ideal to massage it in for about 15 minutes,
   but even a simple application of oil, which only takes a few minutes, is beneficial.
   This encourages the nervous system to be calm for the rest of the day. It can be
   a powerful medicine for calming a threadbare nervous system and gradually
   restoring hormonal balance. (See page 291 to learn how to do this.)

9. Follow your self-massage by bathing and dressing.

10. Take a brisk half-hour walk, followed by 5 to 10 minutes of gentle yoga. This is
    useful for calming the spirit. In general, if you are very thin or weak, a slow,
    stretchy restorative yoga, tai chi, or qi gong routine will be good. If you are heavy,
    a more vigorous form of exercise, such as a strenuous, vigorous form of yoga or
    jogging could be appropriate. If you are unsure which is best for you, consult
    an Ayurvedic lifestyle counselor. Appropriate exercise encourages a calm spirit
    and smooth flow of qi and nourishing fluids. Remember: Blood follows qi and qi
    follows the spirit. If the spirit is calm, and qi and blood flow smoothly, and hor-
    mones will be more balanced. It is not a problem to exercise later in the day, if
    that works better in your life or in certain seasons, weather, or climates, but it is
    important to include exercise in your life and doing it first thing in the day en-
    sures it won't be missed.

11. Do 5 to 15 minutes of gentle alternate-nostril breathing (see page 245 to learn how) or other exercise, such as tai chi or qi gong (see page 220), that is designed to move qi or *prana* smoothly in the body. These practices can focus the mind, quietly energize the body, and calm the nervous system. If you feel your nervous system and your mind are already calm, and your hormones are balanced, you may not need to do this step, but the more anxious you are, or the more imbalanced your life or hormones, the more important this is. It really requires the full 15 minutes daily to resolve hot flashes, night sweats, and anxiety.

   As you already need to wake up, brush your teeth, and do other basic self-care, the extra things that will add time to your daily routine are the gargling, doing the neti pot, applying oil to your body, exercising, and doing some breathing exercises, if you feel the need. Adding these steps will increase your routine by about an hour. This is assuming you haven't been exercising to begin with. If you have been exercising anyway, it may not add much time at all to your routine.

12. Cook. If you won't have time to cook later in the day, cook in the morning for the rest of the day. If you will have time to cook later, then just cook breakfast.

13. Have breakfast, lunch, and dinner at the same time every day.

14. Remember to breathe deeply throughout the day.

15. Spend the evening quieting the mind and body, in preparation for bed.

16. Retire at the same time each evening.

This routine is one that would work for just about anybody, health permitting, but can be modified and tailored for each individual, according to one's special needs or considerations. If the routine feels daunting, and you start only with five minutes of meditation and a fifteen- or twenty-minute walk, you will still benefit.

Exercise

Although exercise is a huge part of health maintenance and disease prevention, in practice there is minimal emphasis on it in our Western medical system, especially, it seems, as we age. Consider a study that showed that primary care physicians provided exercise counseling to 22 percent of men aged forty-five to fifty-four, yet they counseled only 9 percent of women over age seventy-five.[7] Whether this is because we are a society more attuned and committed to the well being of younger people than we are to our elders, or whether it is a sexist issue, could be debated. Whatever the reason, generally, the older the patient, the less exercise counseling they receive. This should prompt us not to rely on our health-care practitioners to encourage and educate us about appropriate exercise, but to educate and inspire ourselves.

Exercise is essential at any age, to move qi or *prana* throughout the body, encourage sufficient blood flow, vitality, and digestive capacity. It is important at every age, but in different amounts and at different levels of intensity. No exercise or too much exercise are both problematic. Not exercising allows qi to stagnate. When qi stagnates, we suffer from irritability, depression, stiff muscles, poor digestion, poor waste disposal, and other maladies. When we exercise too much, our muscles consume our available qi and nutrition, thereby starving our organs and depleting our bones.

Strenuous exercise might be more appropriate in youth, when we have plenty of yin, whereas more gentle exercise may be more appropriate as we age, when there is less yin. In India it is sometimes said that people should focus on physical yoga for the first third of their lives, breathing exercises for the second, and meditation for the final. This also depends on whether we have too much or too little yin at any given time.

STAGNANT ENERGY, STAGNANT SUBSTANCE

According to Eastern medicine, there can be stagnation of either yin or yang, that is, of substance or of energy in the body. Stagnant energy leads to stagnant substance. To maintain health, we require continuous smooth movement of thoughts, energy, blood, and substance. Our bodies are constantly and simultaneously undergoing a process of building new cells and tissues, maintaining them, and eliminating tired, old cells to make way for fresh new ones. Our tissues carry out these processes in a healthy manner if qi is moving smoothly through them.

Eastern medicine teaches that one of the most effective ways to move energy is through breath. If breath stagnates, then energy can stagnate. Breath stagnates when we are nervous or anxious because we tend to hold our breath at those times. This can lead to various maladies. For example, you may usually have a bowel moment in the morning, within a half hour of waking. Suppose one morning you know that you need to leave for a trip shortly after you wake and, upon waking, you realize you forgot to make two important phone calls and you need to make them before you leave. Anxiety strikes. You hold your breath. It is highly likely that this will throw off your natural rhythm and you will become temporarily constipated. This is a case of stagnant breath becoming energetic stagnation and manifesting as physical stagnation.

Most forms of exercise involve breath stimulation. Just about any kind of exercise will support movement of energy. We do not have to pant to achieve this beneficial effect. All we have to do is breathe fully. Whether it's jogging, swimming, tai chi, qi gong, yoga, *pranayama*, or meditation, we are likely to breathe with less tension, more deeply and smoothly, and therefore increase energy circulation.

What is appropriate exercise?

That's the question—and the answer may be different for each of us. Whereas training for a marathon might be a good practice for one person, it may lead another to endocrine, menstrual, or nervous system disorders. Conversely, where gentle restorative yoga may be just the ticket for the woman who has too much activity and stress in her life, it may do very little to support another woman who has a sedentary life. Remember that too much exercise can be just as damaging as too little, as both can severely affect hormone balance, essential to a woman's health. It is for each of us to discover what exercise is appropriate for us. Eastern medicine offers excellent direction in this arena. In general, these guidelines usually work well:

If a woman has a lot of stress or multitasking in her daily life, or a very slender or delicate constitution or tends to fear and anxiety, she likely needs to protect her yin. Therefore, a gentler form of exercise would be most beneficial. More strenuous activity may simply consume even more yin, increase her stress, and prove detrimental. Gentler forms of exercise include:

- Brisk walks, gentle hikes, bike rides, tai chi, or qi gong for 30 minutes daily, exchanging 5 to 10 minutes of any of those exercises with a gentle form of yoga 3 to 7 times a week, to maintain flexibility. It is best to exercise outdoors, weather permitting, when it is neither too hot nor too cold.
- If you are very tired or have flu, cut out any fast movement and replace your usual exercise routine with restorative yoga or gentle *pranayama*. Most yoga studios offer classes in restorative yoga, or you can learn it from a class and then do your own version.

If a woman has a competitive personality, she may be drawn to team or competitive sports or to push herself beyond her physical limits. She may prefer to think that her body is as invincible as her mind, even if her body is calling "uncle," giving her signs that it is depleted. She may tend to ignore these signals and push herself beyond what is healthy. It would be best for her to calmly consider if her body is truly feeling as strong as her mind, and be sure to only engage in friendly exercise that doesn't wear her out. She may do well to learn to surrender to the pace of her body, something we will consider later.

When her yin is depleted, it is generally better for a woman to choose exercises that focus on building and smoothly circulating qi or *prana*, rather than to focus on strengthening her muscles. It is good for her to include at least thirty minutes of tai chi, qi gong, or gentle *pranayama* every week, so that she begins to develop a relationship with her own subtle flow of energy.

If a woman has a sedentary life, or a very sturdy, strong constitution that tends to be overweight, she may have excess yin and would do best to increase yang, by engaging in a more strenuous exercise routine. This could look like:

- A very brisk 1-hour walk, bike ride, hike, or vigorous yoga session, daily
- A 30-minute brisk walk, bike ride, or hike daily, plus an extra 2-hour hike on the weekend or an extra weightlifting class at a gym a couple times a week
- A 30-minute jog or run daily
- A 30-minute brisk walk, bike ride or hike, plus a couple of strenuous yoga classes a few times a week

YOGA

Many Western women are beginning to learn yoga, yet we have not shed the idea that a good workout is one that involves panting and sweating. All too often I am finding young women who are substituting some energetic form of yoga for other exercise and fitting it into a busy life. As one young woman recently told me, "I know this is probably backward, but I chose Bikram yoga because I could show up at the studio, sweat a lot, get in a good workout faster, and get back on the road."

This may work, short term and to a certain extent for young women, but usually is an increasingly inappropriate practice for women over age thirty-five. There are many stories of women who have healed their menopausal symptoms by enjoying a regular yoga practice,[8] but in my experience, they haven't done it by doing an intense practice that simply increases their stress or consumes their yin.

This more-is-better approach to exercise is foreign to the very roots of yoga. Ayurveda, a sister science to yoga, teaches that strong, healthy people should exercise only to half the capacity of their strength during cool weather and to stop exercising once there is the appearance of sweat on forehead, nose, armpits, or joints of the limbs, or a feeling of dryness in the mouth. During hot weather or when one is feeling weak, even milder exercise is recommended, lest the body's nourishing yin elements be depleted.

Yoga, tai chi, meditation, and qi gong have all been shown to have powerfully positive physiological effects in general and for menopausal women specifically.[9] For example, the September–October 2001 issue of *Yoga Journal* reported that yoga can help prevent breast cancer in three important ways: helping balance the hormones, supporting the immune system (mostly by stimulating lymph flow), and helping support a healthy relationship for women with their bodies and environments.[10]

Before perimenopause, the hypothalamus stimulates the pituitary gland to produce important reproductive hormones. These in turn, stimulate production of estrogen and progesterone. During perimenopause, the ovaries reduce hormone production. When the pituitary gland senses these low hormone levels, it sends continual messages to the ovaries to produce more. This struggle causes hormonal fluctuation that is somewhat stressful to the body. The resulting estrogen surges, for example, can be associated with stubborn weight gain. Gentle, restorative yoga postures can relax the nervous system and thereby improve the functioning of the endocrine system, which supports the body to adapt to hormonal fluctuations.[11] For many women, stress, fatigue, and overwork trigger hot flashes. Yoga can help balance this. It is nice to have a yoga practice established before menopause, so its good effects can already be in place.

Yoga is also a form of stretching and may have a strongly beneficial effect on heart health. We saw in Chapter 15 that increasing our physical flexibility correlates with increased flexibility of heart vessels.

Tai Chi

Tai chi, like some forms of yoga, is a gentle exercise that can have positive effects. People taking a tai chi class for forty minutes, three times per week for sixteen weeks, can have improved immunity to various viruses, better responses to vaccines, and significant improvements in their physical functioning, pain levels, vitality, and mental health.[12] Tai chi stimulates the brain's balance system. It also simultaneously requires mental focus and a meditative quality that has been proven very effective in lowering stress.[13] When my husband and I spent a month in China, we were struck by the fitness and grace we saw in the older people, hundreds of whom met in the public parks around dawn to practice tai chi together.

Walking

One of the simplest exercises is one of the most positive. Over and over, studies show that brisk walks are as beneficial as more strenuous activities. The perk with walking is that it is not likely to damage the joints as much as jogging, running, or weight lifting. And all you need is a pair of sneakers. And though a good pair is preferable, I can speak from experience that even an old pair (embarrassingly old, in my case) can serve for a very long time. Five hours of brisk walking per week can reduce the risk of heart attack by 50 percent, but even only about three hours per week (or about half that time for more rigorous exercise, such as jogging or dancing), has been shown to reduce the risk of heart disease by 35 to 40 percent.[14] If walking is your exercise of choice, the trick is brisk. At least three miles per hour—twenty minutes per mile. Strolling, window-shopping, or walking a dog that stops every few minutes to do its business just doesn't cut it.

Along with benefiting the heart, walking is a medicine for hormonal balance. Invoking the macrocosm versus microcosm law of Eastern medicine, we see that aligning with natural cycles of our external world supports internal cycles. Walking outdoors, preferably at the same time every day, aligns us with the natural rhythms of the seasons and light of the day. The function of the pineal gland is not a fully understood part of the endocrine system, but it is generally associated with biorhythms. I have had patients with irregular menstrual cycles or cycle-related acne who added a daily half-hour brisk walk outdoors to their routine and within a couple months had regular cycles and clear skin.

Walking also benefits the spirit. It has been demonstrated that by the end of a sixteen-week period, depressed patients who took a brisk thirty-minute walk or jog three times a week experienced as much relief as patients treated with standard antidepressant medications. Given that almost a third of depressed patients don't respond to medications and others cannot or will not tolerate their uncomfortable side effects, exercise is a medicine not to be ignored. It is useful to note that in this study the patients who exercised took a little longer to experience relief than the patients on drugs, but within sixteen weeks, results in both groups were comparable.[15]

If you've never exercised, it's never too late to start. Women who had previously led sedentary lives had the same reduced rates of health problems as did those who were active, once they included brisk walking into their daily routine.[16]

Whatever type of exercise is appropriate for our individual requirements, Eastern medicine emphasizes the movement of qi or *prana*. Movement of bones and muscles is secondary, because, if qi is moving in the body, blood will circulate smoothly and all the bodily tissues will receive nutrition and effective waste removal. So, whatever exercise we choose, it is of primary importance to develop an awareness of what qi feels like and what it feels like when it is circulating smoothly. Tai chi and qi gong usually offer a palpable experience of qi. Some yoga classes emphasize stretching and calisthenics over the tangible feeling of qi. While these are useful, it is best to find a teacher who experiences the smooth flow of qi themselves and can help you feel it. Once you know what smooth-flowing qi feels like, and how to move it yourself through awareness, you can apply this skill to any exercise that suits you.

Sleep

Sleep encourages yin qualities and, like any other aspect of yin, needs to be consistent and enjoyed in the right amount. Although too much can increase excessive yin and leave us sluggish and lethargic, too little is also damaging to health. There are longtime practitioners of meditation who naturally reduce their need for sleep, but if we try to reduce sleep without changing other aspects of our lives, it may cause trouble. Too little sleep contributes to diminished yin, fatigue, lightheadedness, lowered immunity, and endocrine disorders. It creates a relative excess of yang, leading to excess circulating stress hormones. We have seen the many problems this fosters. If it goes on too long, our adrenal glands get exhausted and stop being able to produce enough stress hormones to meet our demands. Cortisol levels then bottom out, leading to obesity[17] and other signs of adrenal burn out.

Sleep is one of the most natural, easy ways to support good-quality yin in the body. It is one of the most nourishing, restorative things we can do. The body knows when we need rest and it tells us. Fatigue is a basic, natural signal from our body, like hunger or thirst. If we ignore or override it, we contribute to imbalance. When we feel spacey or confused, we might just be tired. Unfortunately, we often misinterpret or ignore our body's signals. Although we may readily respond to our body's hunger by eating and drinking when we are thirsty, we often ignore fatigue.

If we feel tired, we think something is wrong. Nothing is wrong. We are just tired. We need rest. Sometimes a lot of it, if we've gone for years vetoing our body's signals.

WHAT TO DO ABOUT INSOMNIA OR INSUFFICIENT SLEEP

If you don't get enough sleep or insomnia bothers you, try the following suggestions:

- Stick to a routine of when you wake and go to bed, as much as possible. If you have too much yin in your life, try sleeping no more than six hours a night. If you don't have enough yin, sleep as long as you can until you regain balance. Then find what works best for you.
- Do not use your bedroom as a workspace, a place to read, or to watch TV. Use it only for sleeping and making love.
- If you can't sleep (and can tolerate dairy), get up, have a mug of warm milk with a pinch each of nutmeg and saffron, and then go back to bed.

- Avoid caffeine in general and especially more than one cup (or any) after noon.
- Make sure to exercise at the same time every day, and outdoors, if possible. This is helpful in aligning with nature's rhythms and may benefit the pineal gland functions, which support our natural biorhythms.
- Avoid alcohol, especially more than one glass of wine weekly. It might help get you to sleep, but it won't help you stay asleep. Even if you drink alcohol early in the day, it can affect your sleep patterns.
- Apply warm *bhringraj* oil (see Appendix A) to the soles of your feet and your scalp before bedtime. If it is cold where you sleep, wear a nightcap so that you don't get chilled. Wear socks if you don't want the oil from your feet to get on your sheets.
- Use the last couple of hours before you go to bed to allow your mind to relax and unwind. These are not good hours to get excited or worried or disturbed about your research project, your paper, your book, your relationships with others or yourself, or to have that discussion about money, the children, the amount of time you or your partner spend working, or any topic that tends to lead to discord. It is a good time to turn off the phone or only use it for pleasant conversation.
- For the worries that you do have in your head, give them to God, the Universal Divine energy, the Absolute, Whatever or Whoever you call it. As the saying goes, "God is up all night anyway." Indulging your worries by feeding them attention will only serve to strengthen your tendency to worry. Better to occupy your mind by turning your attention to anything besides what you are worried about. You could read something inspirational, focus on alternate nostril breathing for 5 to 15 minutes, or pay attention to soothing music.
- Discuss the appropriateness of Banyan Botanical's Tranquil Mind, Sound Sleep, or other Chinese or Ayurvedic herbal remedies with your Ayurvedic or TCM health-care practitioner. Dr. Christiane Northrup has many suggestions for insomnia supplements in her book *The Wisdom of Menopause*.
- If all else fails, you might try bioidentical progesterone for your insomnia. There is some indication that it can do what synthetic hormones cannot. Although Premarin may actually increase brain cell excitability and progestins in general are not calming, bioidentical progesterone may be.[18] Studies have demonstrated that progesterone has a soothing effect on the central nervous system and the brain.[19] I still consider bioidentical hormones a third-tier strategy, that is, one to be used only after lifestyle and diet change and herbal remedies have been tried. It is always best to treat the underlying cause of the hormone imbalance, even when the best choice of supplements are available for treating its symptoms.

Relationships

My spiritual teacher advised me, when I was seven or eight years old, "Keep good company. Good company makes a man great." This advice has stayed with me to this day and seems as sound now as it did in my childhood.

Over the course of life, I've reflected on what exactly "good company" is. I feel that it is the company of those who inspire me, among other things, to be a truly kinder, more honest person. "Company" includes the people we spend time with at work, as well as at home. If it's hard to find good company, I've found that it helps to spend time alone, and find inspiration through books or pastimes.

If our relationships are in disarray, it takes a toll on our emotions, stress levels, and, ultimately, physical health. Naturally, one of the most important relationships is that with a spouse or life partner. If this relationship is healthy, our nervous system relaxes, stress isn't produced, and we can knock this off the list of troublesome lifestyle factors. In fact, if our main relationship is healthy, we can expect our heart to pump better and to live longer. However, if our relationship is strained, we can expect trouble. One stressful conversation can increase stress hormones *for more than twenty-two hours*. If this is our daily fare, we may experience anything from more intestinal and gastric ulcers to more difficulty recovering from illness, surgery, and heart conditions; increased blood pressure and heart rate; certain types of joint pain and other difficulties; more cavities and gum disease; and a shorter life span. We have already looked at the long-term effects of increased stress hormones on women's health issues. And it appears that the effects of marital stress are stronger and longer lasting on women than men.[20]

So finding ways to heal our relationships becomes a priority for our health. Perhaps the most important relationship to heal is with ourselves. If I am not happy with myself, it is unlikely that I will find peace in my other relationships.

Environment

Where we live is as relevant to our health as what we do. Trying to maintain hormonal balance in an environment that is rife with hormones from external sources may be possible but is a bit of an uphill battle.

External, or exogenous, hormones are substances produced outside the body that may act like or affect hormones inside the body. They include synthetic, patentable hormones and bioidentical hormones, both of which we discussed in Chapter 6. They also include environmental and plant estrogens, which we looked at in our exploration of diet and will revisit briefly here. All of these exogenous hormones can act as hormones in the body and affect the endocrine system.

Some external estrogens that degrade quickly in the body can have quite positive effects. Beneficial results have been associated with consumption of plants like soy, cauliflower, and broccoli. Other, usually synthetic, forms of external estrogens are found in a stunning array of chemicals that can amplify the negative effects of estrogen, enhance production of "bad" estrogens (see Chapter 3 if you need to refresh your memory on the difference between good and bad estrogens), and remain in the body anywhere from hours to days or even years. Since World War II, environment-polluting chemicals, many of which are termed endocrine disruptors, have become increasingly widespread in our environment, in certain pesticides, drugs, fuels, stain-resistant clothing and furniture treatments, lawn care products, personal care items, cleansing products, and plastics, among other sources.[21] As DuPont used to say about Teflon, "It's everywhere."

And probably *in everyone*, too. In one survey of twenty-seven body burden studies (*body burden* is the term to describe the amount of environmental pollutants that are found in a person's body), every single participant was found to have PCBs and organochlorine pesticides in their bodies, even people who were born after PCBs were banned. Even unborn babies were found to have "hundreds of chemicals in their little bodies."[22] It turns out that the human body is like a sponge, soaking up whatever is permeating its environment.

PESTICIDES AND CHEMICALS

The postwar environment of the United States and Europe and widespread industrial activity in every country has produced hundreds of poisonous chemicals that are now insidiously present in our world. This environmental marinade includes a dizzying number of ubiquitous chemicals with many syllables[23] (see this endnote for a more comprehensive list). Some that are more commonly heard of are 2,4 dichlorophenoxyacetic acid (also called 2,4-D, this is a pesticide used on lawns and an active ingredient in Agent Orange)[24]; phthalates (used as plastic softeners and cosmetics, among other things); DDT (now banned); ozone-destroying CFCs (chlorofluorocarbons); bisphenol A (BPA); various chlorinated and brominated compounds such as polybrominated biphenyls (PBBs, used as fire retardants and close cousins of PCBs); phthalates; dioxin; triclosan (an ingredient in many antibacterial products) and many, many others. Some, like POPs (persistent organic pollutants) include many halogen (chlorine, bromine, fluorine, or iodine) atoms that have long half-lives (about two to ten years) in the bodies of animals and humans and in the environment. Although manufacturing processes may have improved in some areas,[25] the prevalence of these chemicals is still a concern.

An Unbroken Cycle

In the world of toxic chemicals, there is a common story: A company has a stock of a certain chemical and finds some use for it. We slowly amass data, sometimes over decades, which finally proves the chemical is toxic for humans and the environment. It is finally—and, in many cases reluctantly—banned, at least for use in the purpose it was employed. The same or another company introduces a new, not-banned use for the chemical or introduces a similar chemical that is just dissimilar enough from the banned one, to be able to avoid the ban and make its way into widespread use. So the story starts again. Here's just one as an example: When the United States began to phase out leaded gasoline in the 1960s, one of its additives—ethylene dibromide (EDB)—needed a new home. So Great Lakes Chemical Corporation, the largest supplier of EDB, began to supply it to farmers as a pesticide. When the Environmental Protection Agency abruptly suspended all agricultural uses of EDB in 1983 because of evidence that it was carcinogenic and a mutagen that was contaminating groundwater, EDB was reincarnated as a flame retardant. Back in the day, flame retardants were marketed as protection against the dangers of fire due to cigarette smoking. Flame retardants have increased in use ever since.[26] So now they're ubiquitous. They're on our clothes, furniture, car upholstery, or otherwise in contact with our bodies. EDB is not the only chemical used as a flame retardant, nor is it the only toxic one.

One or another of the chemicals I've just listed is used or released in the manufacture (or incineration) of certain plastics, packaging materials for food and drink, carpets, epoxy resins, electronics, spermicidal gels, baby bottles, lubricants, solvents, insecticides, pesticides, herbicides, lawn care products, medical equipment, toys, paints, packaging, water jugs, drugs, hormonal skin creams, cosmetics, herbicides, PVC pipes and other construction materials, cleansing products, personal care products, antibacterial soaps and products, pesticides, and flame retardants and the products saturated with them (like airline seats, furniture, pajamas, and other clothing). These chemicals can be damaging throughout their life cycles, from the way they are produced and the way they are used to the method of their disposal or their disintegration into the environment.

Often called "endocrine disruptors," some of these chemicals' molecular structures resemble natural estrogen so closely that they fit into the same receptors in the body."[27] They either bind to these receptors—so your own hormones can't—and turn genes on and off, amplify the negative aspects of estrogen, or travel to the cell nucleus, where they exert a negative effect on chromosomes or the DNA there. Once they've established themselves in these sites, they are sometimes stubborn guests. Many do not deteriorate quickly, so they may have long-lasting, sometimes even permanent, effects.

Each of us has a certain threshold of toleration. Depending on our age, how strong our constitution is, what our challenge areas are, and how much exposure we have to these endocrine disruptors, we will be more or less affected. It is possible for exposure to trigger everything from very mild symptoms to serious disorders. Possible effects include hormonal disruption; reproductive and developmental aberrations; infertility; early onset of puberty in girls; poor quality or quantity of semen; lowered sperm counts; immune system disorders; learning disabilities; cancer (especially prostate and breast cancer); insulin-resistant diabetes and other metabolic disorders; behavioral changes; damage to the skin, liver, and kidneys; neurological impairment; asthma; birth defects; and, of course, disruption of the endocrine system, among other possible problems. This does not even include the problems of direct exposure to the skin if you accidentally spill some, say, lawn pesticide on yourself. Those are more acute symptoms, like nausea, lack of coordination, difficulty breathing and other temporary problems. Recently more attention has also been given to the significant link between environmental pollutants and type 2 diabetes.[28] In addition, many of these chemicals can cause inflammation in the body. When the liver detects this inflammation in the system, it produces C-reactive protein (CRP). High levels of CRP are an indicator of increased risk for heart disease.[29] Some chemicals, like POPs, are stable (i.e., persistent), lipohilic (which means they are stored in fat tissue for long periods of time), and have the ability to act as endocrine disruptors.

Endocrine disruption caused by these chemicals can result in decreased follicle stimulating hormone (FSH), decreased natural progesterone, and blocked function of aromatase and decreased estradiol levels. We learned in Chapter 3 that if aromatase and estradiol are both affected, estradiol gets a double hit; first, because aromatase is affected so that it can't turn precursor hormones into estradiol, and second, because estradiol is directly decreased.

While exposure to these chemicals may be detrimental at any age, the most critical time is as an embryo. It is a difficult thing to study, because effects may not be revealed until thirty to thirty-five years later. An adult has mature organs and systems that are well developed and more capable of eliminating toxic substances from the body, but the developing embryo has immature organs and elimination capacity. Imprints and impressions made at this time on the child's physiology are like etchings in the child's constitutional blueprint, and carry sometimes permanent characteristics and defects forward into the child's lifetime.

Modern science knows now that, the higher an organism is on a food chain, the more concentrated these chemicals become in its body. For example, small fish exposed to chemicals in plant food and algae are eaten by bigger fish. They in turn are eaten by even bigger fish. Then a human consumes this biggest fish so that the pollutants are most highly concentrated in the human at the top of the food chain. The only organism higher in the food chain than this human being is the breastfeeding infant.

Breast milk can be a concentrated delivery system for environmental toxins. For example, in 1970, the Environmental Defense Fund found that the levels of DDT in breast milk were up to seven times greater than in cow's milk sold in stores.[30]

Bisphenol A (BPA)

When a woman is exposed to bisphenol A (BPA) during pregnancy, damage can be done simultaneously to three generations at once. The mother is affected. The unborn baby in her womb is affected, and the unborn baby's reproductive system is affected. If the unborn baby is a girl, her eggs can be affected. Current research shows that even one exposure can damage 40 percent of the eggs belonging to the unborn baby girl.[31] This is impressive, especially when we understand that BPA is not scarce. Despite the fact that the body metabolizes it within just a few hours,[32] 93 percent of Americans tested have been found to have detectable levels of BPA in their bodies.[33] Dr. Pete Myers, an expert on BPA, says, "From everything we know about this chemical, exposure in childhood increases the likelihood of kids having health problems later in life."[34] One issue here is that the metabolism of babies and children is not as mature as that of adults. Babies and children are much slower than adults to flush BPA out of their bodies.[35]

Problems don't always wait until later in life. Some problems, like prostate cancer, that used to be confined to older populations are beginning to be seen in young people, and some scientists are linking these anomalies to environmental causes.[36] For example, the results of a 2005 University of Missouri study links in utero exposure to even small amounts of some man-made chemicals, including those in oral contraceptives, to higher risk of permanent damage to cellular control systems, and fetal damage in males to prostates and urethras.[37] BPA is seen to cause prostate cancer[38] and perhaps it is due to exposure in utero as well as later in life.

Prepubescent children suffer from exposure to exogenous hormones as well. They can experience signs of hormonal imbalance, such as of premature puberty, premature growth of breasts, pubic hair, genital enlargement, or abnormally increased levels of sex hormones.

Problems resulting from endocrine—that is, hormonal—imbalance at any time in life are countless. As we've seen throughout this book, hormonal balance is central to a woman's health at any stage of life. It is key to the health of breast tissue, menstrual cycles, bone health, heart health, and most, if not all of a woman's health concerns.

In September 2009, the *New York Times* quoted Congressman Steve Israel (D-NY) on the absurdity of knowing what is in our food but not what is in the chemicals that we use to clean our house, polish our floors, and care for our automobiles, among other things: "The cleaning industry uses five billion pounds of chemicals in the United States, and we have little to no idea of what chemicals are inside these products."[39] The article was reporting on the growing pressure on chemical companies to list their ingredients. Some headway might be on the horizon, but the progress doesn't include disclosing what is meant by "fragrance" or "parfum," which are often code words for phthalates.

Pthalates

Pthalates are one of the ubiquitous classes of chemicals in our environment. They are clear and look like vegetable oil. There are no acceptable levels of phthalates. While bisphenol A is associated with hard plastics, phthalates are often used to soften plastic, making it more flexible. For example, they are present in PVC plastic, which often has a distinctive odor, as in the case of plastic shower curtains.[40] Pthalates are also used to allow lotions to penetrate into the skin and soften it, and to allow scented products to retain their fragrance longer. They can also be found in plastic packaging used as food and beverage containers, which might be used to heat food in a microwave, and in some straws. This could be problematic, as heating a medium is a common method of extracting chemicals from it. So these chemicals may leach into our lunch, our coffee, or even our organic peppermint tea.

In support of the University of Missouri study, findings from a University of Rochester study linked exposure to phthalate-related chemicals to increased risk of adverse effects on reproductive development, reproductive tissue, and other bodily tissues, including the brain. In the 134 boys that the study followed, there was a greater incidence of undescended or small testicles, small genital organs, and other abnormalities, even without exceptional levels of exposure.

Dioxin

Dioxin is perhaps one of the deadliest substances known to man. Exposure is linked to such serious ailments as cancer, heart disease, diabetes, and reproductive and developmental disorders. Its impressive ten-year half life allows it to accumulate in the environment and leach into soil, air, and water supplies, con-taminating plants, the animals that eat them, and the humans who consume the plants and animals and breathe the polluted air.

Dioxins are released through certain combustion processes. Certain situations are particularly dangerous. Hospital waste has a high concentration of certain plastics, like PVC plastics and other aromatic compounds that contain dioxin precursors. We'd almost have to expect that, right? Big building. Lots of mal-odorous plastic. Perhaps a bit less obvious is the more benign seeming practice of backyard trash burning. Burning common household trash in a drum in the backyard can release more dioxins than a plant that incinerates hundreds of tons of garbage daily but has emission controls and regulated incineration methods.[41]

This may be even more of a problem in such places as rural Japan, where open burning is a common practice and is responsible for local dioxin levels that are ten thousandfold higher than in the United States. Scientists are linking this to the significantly higher rates of endometriosis there.[42] Open burning is not con-fined to rural Japan. It is a common practice in India, for example, where I've passed by many a morning bonfire incinerating household garbage, neighbor-hood garbage, and tires. These have kept the streets clean and added some warmth to the winter mornings, but the pernicious side effects may warrant a different solution.

When we consider how harmful dioxins are, we might want to be very careful not only about what we burn purposely, but about our choices of what we fill and build our homes and offices with, in the unlikely event of their burning down. PVC is of particular concern for firefighters and others exposed to building fires, where even the fumes released by heated PVC are deadly. We have already seen that PVC products contain phthalates. PVC is a particularly nasty plastic because it also releases dioxins when it is produced or burned, [43] so it is a vehicle for toxicity throughout its life cycle.

Atrazine

The weed killer atrazine has been getting attention lately because its harmful ef-fects are also being found at lower doses than previously thought. Used on agri-cultural crops—especially corn—lawns, parks, gardens, and golf courses, atrazine is finding its way easily and generously into our water supplies. It is one of the most common contaminants of American reservoirs, and even when it's found at levels that are acceptable by federal standards, it is associated with menstrual problems, low birth weights, birth defects, and possibly increased vulnerability to cancer later in life. Low birth weights were associated with exposure to as little as 0.1 parts per billion and some impartial scientists are particularly concerned about the effects of atrazine at certain life stages, such as during the time a fetus's brain is forming.[44]

Atrazine is only one of many chemicals that make their way into water supplies. The millions of patients of pharmaceutical drugs, including synthetic hormone therapy of one kind or another, pass these chemicals out in their urine, which can eventually end up in water supplies. Waste from industrial plants, dry cleaning solvents, insecticides, discarded pharmaceutical products, pesticides, almost anything can make its way into water supplies. In an extensive article in the *New York Times*, their research uncovered more than 506,000 violations of the Clean Water Act by over twenty-three thousand companies and facilities since 2004. And these are numbers submitted by those companies themselves. The actual number is likely to be much higher.[45]

A Crucial Element

One important emerging consideration about endocrine disruptors is this: We've been thinking about them all wrong. We tend to consider that the more the exposure, the worse the effects. This premise has guided our chemical risk-assessment process and has guided our regulations. But hormones are weird. They simply don't act as many other things do. Over millennia, the body has evolved to be highly responsive to minuscule amounts of hormones and possibly respond in an opposite way than we might expect to higher doses. Consider this study, for example. Mice were fed estradiol and the synthetic hormone diethylstilbestrol (DES) to determine their effect on prostate growth. When they were fed high doses, prostate growth was blocked, whereas low doses stimulated growth dramatically. This experiment led to similar studies with BPA and the results are thought provoking, to say the least. A dose of BPA twenty-five thousand times lower than ever before tested stimulated prostate growth in exactly the same way as did low doses of estradiol. This had been missed in studies that looked at high doses of BPA, because high and low doses act differently.[46]

Although many of these chemicals exert major effects, they do so in minuscule amounts, and often our exposure to them is through mediums we can't avoid. The good news is that awareness of this issue is growing, as is awareness of the prevalence of toxic chemicals in our environment, and we are beginning to understand what we can do and what we can avoid.

Saving the Poison Maiden: How to Minimize Toxic Exposure

In India, the term *visha kanya* means "poison maiden."[47] In ancient times it is said that a young maiden would be fed successively stronger doses of poison throughout her life, starting when she was a child. Initial doses would be small enough that they wouldn't make her ill and she would develop a tolerance to the poison. She would be fed more and more, until by the time she had developed into a beautiful young maiden, she had also become an effective and deadly weapon. She would be presented to enemy kings and nobleman in an apparent gesture of goodwill. Alas. The moment the poor fellow would kiss the beauty, he would be immediately and fatally poisoned.

Although most of us are not poisoned to such a malignant degree, it is possible that we need to consider our exposure through our diet, lifestyle, and environment, so that we may avoid becoming poison maidens to any serious degree. This may be especially important when we want to become pregnant, are pregnant or breast-feeding, or are parenting young children, so that we are not unwittingly transmitting toxicity to our vulnerable, developing fetuses, babies, and children.

Whether industrial, chemical, or pharmaceutical pollutants are released in the manufacturing, disintegrating, or incinerating process, they get released into soil, water, and air. Plants then absorb them. Animals eat the contaminated plants, drink polluted water, breathe polluted air, and store the toxicity in their flesh. Humans drink polluted water, breathe polluted air, absorb chemicals through the skin, and consume polluted plants, contaminated animals, or both.[48] Animals and humans both accumulate toxins in their bodies, especially in fatty tissues. The higher up one is on the food chain, the more likely one will store large doses of toxicity. Therefore, the higher up on the food chain are the items we eat, the more concentrated doses of poison we are likely to consume. Lynn Castrodale, the Endometriosis Association's former environmental coordinator, suggests that about 90 percent of exposure to dioxins, for example, probably comes from consuming meat and dairy products.[49] Similarly, we are also exposed to high levels of mercury by consuming contaminated fish.

We are usually more directly threatened by these toxic chemicals, the more we have in our environment. This can be readily apparent near industrial plants that spew smoke into the air into local neighborhoods. It can be far less obvious in a picturesque agricultural village, but equally damaging if the industrial plant is a few hundred miles upstream and the stream is irrigating our crops. If the crops are covered with some of the nasty herbicides and pesticides, we may be in some serious trouble. It may look like paradise, but may pack an uncomfortable wallop. It is also the case that extremely remote areas are being severely affected. Many animals in the North Pole, for example, are found to have high concentrations of certain chemicals that are not being produced, used, or incinerated anywhere near them, but air and ocean current patterns have converged to deposit these chemicals there.

I am not an expert on these chemicals, the extent of their effects, and the process by which they wreak their damage, how they are manufactured, how long each one stays in the body, which are banned, which are being banned, and which are being ignored. For an expert account and a surprisingly hopeful and fun read—believe it or not—try Rick Smith's and Bruce Lourie's *Slow Death by Rubber Duck*, listed in Appendix A.

The mass of information on environmental pollutants is impressive and the number of products that contain chemicals of varying levels of toxicity are too much to fully comprehend. It is hard to remember which plastic has what chemical and which produce has the most nasty pesticides and herbicides. To cover bases as best we can and avoid too much exposure, here is a list of habits designed to minimize exposure in our daily lives.

- Try to use pots and pans and utensils that are made of stainless steel, cast iron, heat-resistant ceramic, glass, or wood, to avoid leaching out toxic chemicals into hot food and liquids.[50]
- Avoid nonstick cookware.
- Avoid using plastic "to go" cups, especially with hot liquids.
- My husband used to tell his patients that what they ate was not as important as where they shopped. He was only half joking. His advice serves well in the case of personal care products and home cleaning products. Health food stores are far less likely to carry products with harmful chemicals in them than are major supermarket chains or department stores. Check the labels and ask questions when you're not sure.
- Don't put anything on your skin that you wouldn't put in your mouth. The skin is the largest organ in the body and will absorb chemicals, as well as anything else applied to it. Try to use natural lotions or oils instead of mineral oils, petroleum products, or stuff with lots of hard-to-pronounce chemicals.
- Store food in glass, stainless-steel, or ceramic containers.
- Avoid using plastic wrap, especially on hot food.
- If you are a meat-eater, try to reduce your meat consumption and buy organic meat.
- Buy organic food and drinks when possible. As noted before, check Appendix A for how to find the current top twelve most important foods to buy organic and the top twelve to avoid.

- Avoid canned soft drinks for several reasons, one of which is that the cans are lined with BPA.[51]

- Avoid PVC products (vinyl plastics or polyvinyl chloride) or products that are associated with phthalates. PVC products are often identified with the number 3, the letter V or the letters PVC inside or underneath the universal recycling triangle. They also may have a distinct odor, like that of vinyl shower curtains. Want more information? Contact the Center for Health, Environment and Justice (www.chej.org) or Health Care Without Harm (www.noharm.com) for non-PVC medical devices. PVCs or phthalates are used in some toys, inks, hair sprays, nail polish, perfumes, plastic cling film,[52] cosmetics, medical devices, packages, and a bunch of construction materials like paint, siding, pipes, and flooring. Construction materials are considered to comprise 75 percent of PVC products.

- Try cloth shower curtains rather than PVC vinyl ones, even if they're more expensive.

- If it smells toxic, it probably is—whether it contains PVC, phthalates, or some other chemical, and therefore try to minimize smelly stuff in your building and living choices, as well as in choices related to other aspects of your environment. For example, I prefer a citrus-based wax over polyurethane to refinish cabinets, or "no VOC" (volatile organic compounds) paint over more toxic latex or oil paints, or milk paint and linseed oil over oil paint, to finish a set of drawers.

- Go green—literally: English ivy, Gerbera daisies, Madagascar dragon tree, potted mums, and variegated snake plant are just some examples of plants that are said to purify the air of at least some nasty pollutants. Place plants in any environment that needs purifying.

- Avoid organic chemicals that have "chloro" as part of their name, such as chlorophenol weed killers (e.g., 2, 4-D, which is used by some commercial lawn services).

- Have your local waste-collection agency dispose of any insecticides and herbicides you may need to get rid of.

- Don't burn household garbage.

- Avoid personal care products or household cleaning products that list "fragrance" or "parfum" as an ingredient, or call the manufacturer to be sure that the scent is not from phthalates. If you apply 126 different chemicals in twelve different products to your face, body, and hair by the time you drink your coffee in the morning, you probably aren't helping to save the poison maiden.

- Avoid room, car, or air "fresheners."

- Go to www.healthytoys.org to check out the safety of various kids' toys.

- Don't feed children sweetened candies with pretty colors. This trains them to find the taste of chemicals acceptable—even desirable—and turns them into lifelong consumers.

26

Stress Management Techniques

*The past and future take away most of our time, most of our time—
these two sprites eating into the veins of life. So forget the past,
forget the future, live in the living present. When tomorrow comes,
you'll see what will happen. When you're here,
be fully for the purpose you are here.*
—KIRPAL SINGH

Rachel was fifty-one and had been seeing me for a few years. Her periods had ended about a year earlier and she had begun experiencing hot flashes about six months before that. Thanks to acupuncture and herbs, practicing yoga, and having a daily routine, the hot flashes were much reduced since then but still irksome. One evening, when she broke into a sweat on a dinner date with her husband, he asked, "Hasn't Claudia been telling you to do that oil massage thing? Why don't you try that?" Newly inspired, Rachel began to do the daily self-massage with warm oil, called *abhyanga* that I've mentioned before. When she saw me a few weeks later, the hot flashes had disappeared.

For the next two years, she was symptom free but her relationship with her husband was straining under broken commitments and the prospect of separation, and the business she had worked for a decade to nourish was faltering. With the increased stress, her hot flashes and insomnia returned, despite her lifestyle and self-massage. She called me one afternoon. She was unwilling to take synthetic hormones or sleeping pills and hesitant to try bioidentical hormones, but felt a need for more support.

Rachel had been going to yoga classes for five years. I suggested she find a teacher well versed in *pranayama* (breathing exercises) to teach her gentle, deep alternate-nostril breathing and practice it for fifteen minutes daily. She

235

did this, and within days her hot flashes had disappeared and she was sleeping soundly. Over the next year, as her marriage ended and her business endured multiple setbacks, she found that she was symptom free as long as she practiced her fifteen minutes of alternate-nostril breathing daily. If she missed one day, her symptoms would return. As long as she was regular in her practice, she was fine. Even though this added fifteen minutes to her daily routine, Rachel liked the fact that she wasn't taking hormones, drugs, or even extra herbs. She wasn't spending an extra cent and was finding relief through her own breath.

Stress and Its Causes

We all go through times of stress, imposed by self or circumstance, avoidable or otherwise. Stress has at least three readily observable causes. The first cause is a mixture of multitasking, too much ambition and too much activity. This combination robs us of time for contemplation, relaxation, and cooking healthy food. The second cause is related to the first. It's the illusion that we are in control of everything and that if we don't keep juggling all the balls, the show will end in humiliation and disaster. This self-imposed perspective leads to an overblown sense of responsibility and tremendous fear of impending doom. A third source of stress is unavoidable external circumstances, like some illness, accidents, or the sickness or death of parents or children. Such factors also may rob us of time to devote to cooking, contemplation, and other self-nurturing practices. The fact that unavoidable events will inevitably present themselves in every woman's life means that it is even more important to resolve the first two causes of stress as consistently and well as we can, so our good habits will create a foundation that can withstand the inevitable storms to come. If we don't, we will eventually suffer exhaustion, hypersensitive nervous systems, and subsequent hormone imbalance.

Sometimes following a normal daily routine and healthy diet is not enough to counteract our levels of stress and its unbalancing effects on our bodies and minds. Incorporating stress-reducing techniques into our daily routines helps to counteract or soothe these effects. To try to establish these habits in the middle of a tidal wave of stress can be spectacularly challenging. It is better to dig the well before we become thirsty. The nervous system will be calmer in general, less likely to translate benign events as threats, and less likely to stimulate the release of cortisol and adrenaline on a continuous basis. Many of these techniques allow us quiet time to check in with ourselves daily and consider what we need to nourish the spirit as well as the body and mind.

If we have a consistent daily routine, this in itself has a stress-reducing effect. If that daily routine includes the stress-management techniques of self-massage and alternate-nostril breathing, then we have woven several especially powerful practices into our lifestyle that enable us to become calmer in general. When the nervous system is calm, cortisol and adrenaline are released far less often. Good-quality yin is then freed up to nourish our tissues, organs, and bodily systems rather than being sacrificed to meet the demands of excessive stress.

If you feel your lifestyle is great, if you don't suffer from stress or symptoms of feeling crummy and you feel fulfilled in life, then perhaps there is no need to fix what ain't broke. But if stress, the desire to self-medicate, or a lack of time (or a perceived lack of time) has led to poor eating or lifestyle habits and you find yourself feeling increasingly crummy, it might be time to reevaluate and reorganize. For example, maybe you don't have time to cook, so you eat fast food on a regular basis and you turn to antacids, laxatives, or other aids to ease the digestive troubles that result. Maybe you smoke or have a couple drinks at night to relax and you find you are getting headaches and a cough. Or maybe you watch *Sex and the City* reruns instead of taking a walk, and you are feeling depressed. If something doesn't feel right in your life and you are feeling stress and its effects on a daily, if not hourly, basis, Eastern medicine offers several techniques to address this.

First Things First

Before choosing any of these techniques, the first thing we need to do is to get rid of the poisons: alcohol, drugs, cigarettes, nonorganic coffee, any caffeine in excess of a cup or two of coffee a day, refined sugar, trans fats, highly processed foods. We can also begin to address our big stressors, such as neglected or poisonous relationships or jobs that only give us just enough to keep us from walking out the door. If we can't do this all at once, we can at least address these issues one at a time. Chances are that each of these "poisons" is actually serving a positive purpose in our delicate status quo. That is, each may be acting as part of an overall coping strategy. And coping is better than not coping. We are generally ill advised to take too much away without replacing it with something else, just as we would not wish to take away someone's crutch, even if it's too short and is throwing her back out of alignment, without giving her a cane or other healthy substitute.

In this book, we're looking at many "canes" to support a return to good health. For most of us, it would be daunting process to incorporate all of them. And all of them may not be needed. What we can do to start is pick a poison we feel we can remove and replace it with one technique or dietary recommendation that we feel we can adopt. After doing this, if life becomes healthy and balanced and happy, well and good. But if we still suffer symptoms of feeling crummy, we will need to replace or alter another poison with a healthier habit. We may need to repeat this process until the balance is tipped in favor of health and hormonal balance. How fast this happens generally depends on how many changes we need to make, how rapidly we can make them, and how long we maintain them. Ideally, we make enough changes and have the perseverance to practice them long enough that they become habitual.

Change is scary for many. We feel that if we stop running, pushing, overreaching ourselves, our lives will fall apart, something terrible will happen if we say, "No more," to what is harmful to us. But I have found, in my own life and in that of my patients, that this is not the usual outcome. On the contrary, life improves. When we make one little change and find only positive side effects, we become open to the possibility of change without disastrous consequences. With slightly less trepidation, we make another change and reap further benefits. Little by little we begin to trust that when we do the best thing for ourselves, positive effects begin to radiate to our partners, our families, and our communities.

Stress-management techniques accomplish their goal in a few ways. They serve to replace fear with faith. They adjust our perspective. They promote good-quality yang by supporting clear thinking and the ability to focus, and they promote good-quality yin by engaging in quiet, calm, still activities. Many activities may serve as stress-management techniques. How many we need to incorporate into our daily routine and how long we should practice them varies from person to person and situation to situation.

If there is minimal stress, it may be sufficient to practice a technique for only fifteen minutes. If stress is so high it's off the charts, however, we may need to devote more time to these practices. It doesn't much matter which stress-management technique we choose, as long as we choose something that works. If none of the practices I suggest appeal to or work for you, find something else. We are living in a time where choices abound and something is bound to work for each of us if we are dedicated to finding out what it is.

(Note: Be sure to read the section "What to Eat in Times of Stress" in Chapter 21.)

Spiritual Practices and Meditation

In the previous chapters, we looked at making diet and lifestyle changes. Relieving the stress that arises from our own worldview is a bit trickier. Although it is fairly straightforward to replace doughnuts for breakfast with whole-grain cereal, for example, substituting a healthy perspective on life for an unhealthy one is more involved.

Let's consider two primary causes of stress and how spiritual practices can address them. The first cause was living in overdrive to attain our desires. If having the HDTV, the SUV, and the big house represent the acme of success to us, we will probably have to work hard and long to acquire and sustain them. If reaching the pinnacle of our desires turns out to be all it's cracked up to be, well and good. But if we find we're working harder to maintain what we want than we are enjoying having it, we may suffer more stress and less health than the body and spirit are comfortable with. Our priorities may need to shift from material acquisitions to spiritual nourishment. Downsizing may play a part in this. One of my teachers, used to say, "Simplify. Simplify. Simplify." He knew that if desires are kept simple, the likelihood of fulfilling them is greater and leads to more satisfaction. And it will free up time to devote to spiritual nourishment.

Another cause of stress is the issue of control. When we believe we are in control of everything, it follows that we feel responsible for everything. "Everything" is a tall order. Our lives become an unending to-do list. This may cheat us out of what my teacher used to call each person's birthright to pursue his or her spiritual nature. He once wrote, "Perhaps more souls are lost to heaven by the sense of duty to earth than by downright sin and evil."

So how to deal with the fear that life will fall apart if we stop being in charge of everything? Through Ayurveda, I have seen that faith is the antidote to fear. It is helpful to have faith in or an actual experience of a divine presence that has our best interests at heart, but this is not essential. Even without it, we can learn that life will go on just fine without our trying to control everything.

An Easy, Use-Anywhere Meditation Technique

Dr. Vasant Lad, one of my teachers, once offered a visualization technique to address this. I don't remember his exact words, but here is a similar visualization, inspired by my memory of his work. Perhaps you could have someone read this to you until you can remember it and do the visualization on your own.

See yourself sitting quietly in a corner of your home. Watch what is happening in the room, but do not participate in it in any way. See how things go on without your participation. When you are comfortable with how that feels, see yourself floating above your home, looking in on it, without participating, and become comfortable with your lack of involvement. When you feel peace here, rise up and see the comings, goings, and activities of first your city, your state, your country, the world, and then the universe, each time becoming at peace with your lack of involvement. See how everything can and will go on without your participation.

The physiological value of this sort of meditation is that it allows us to relieve our spirits of our real or perceived obligations long enough to allow the nervous system to calm down, and to feel the experience, even fleetingly, of freedom. Whether our obligations are real or simply perceived doesn't matter to our body. It responds the same way to perceived stress as to real stress. If we can engage in a practice that suspends our sense of control and responsibility long enough, the body can catch a much-needed break. When we do this, we can notice that the world will not fall apart in the absence of our involvement. As we gain faith in this, we can increase our time in this experience, and the nervous system can begin to heal.

SOME THOUGHTS ON MEDITATION

Don't ask what the world needs. Ask what makes you come alive,
and go do it. Because what the world needs is people who have come alive.
—HOWARD THURMAN

When I was a child I knew a woman who was like a grandmother to me. She literally meditated in the woods throughout most of her life. Early on, a friend of mine, upon hearing of her, mused, "Isn't that rather selfish? She's not contributing anything to society."

I have since encountered this sentiment more than a few times. The first time it stumped me awhile. I reflected on the question over the next few years, as I watched what was going on around my meditating friend. What I noticed was, over the course of years, thousands of people—that's no exaggeration—had heard about my friend and gone to her for spiritual inspiration and counsel. I sat with her on dozens of occasions as she visited with people, and I saw each of them leave with an experience that comforted, surprised, or enlightened them on some point or another, sometimes even angered them, but always transformed them. Always inspired them. Her example of living according to her own principles usually inspired people to be better parents, spouses, teachers, students, and participants in their own lives. She never told anyone to do what she did: to move to the forest to meditate. That was *her* natural role, and I didn't see her trying to dissuade others from theirs.

I also grew up around political activists. While many of them may have achieved some good, I also saw many who frothed about inequities and appeared to me to be utterly miserable themselves. What's more, their misery seemed to spread to people around them.

These people were, as Howard Thurman put it, asking what the world needed, and they were taking a transparent and active approach to address what they perceived those needs were.

Meditation, on the other hand, made my friend come alive, and her aliveness spread like wildfire to others and changed their lives. She eventually passed away, but not before quietly affecting the lives of the thousands she came in contact with.

I am not suggesting everybody go to the forest and meditate, but I don't see that as a selfish option, either. Whether we choose that or not, including a little meditation in our lives can carry some happy side effects. Meditation could be sitting quietly, contemplating inspirational words, practicing a gentle *pranayama* technique, or following instructions from a spiritual mentor. I've included some resources in Appendix A.

It's Your Choice

Spiritual practices are distinct from religious practices in that they are not rooted in dogma. Either may involve ritual, but ritual and prescribed belief systems are not prerequisites for spiritual practices, which simply require time for us to commune with our own spirit. Whatever meditation technique or spiritual practice you choose, the result should be greater calm and a buoyancy of spirit.

It is the responsibility of each of us to be true to ourselves, to consider carefully which spiritual aid we use, applying our discrimination to the process and honestly evaluating if it is of benefit to us. We live in a time that is ripe with techniques, traditions, advice, and books from saints, seekers, and charlatans alike. In Appendix A I have listed some books that my patients or I have found inspirational.

Aside from spiritual inspiration, there are some stress-reducing techniques that can calm the nervous system and balance the mind, regardless of belief system. The practices of *abhyanga* and *pranayama* are two of the most powerful techniques I have ever witnessed.

Abhyanga: **Warm Oil Self-Massage**

The body of one who uses oil massage regularly does not become affected much even if subjected to accidental injuries, or strenuous work. By using oil massage daily, a person is endowed with pleasant touch, trimmed body parts, and becomes strong, charming and least affected by old age.[1]
—FROM *CHARAKA SAMHITA*, AN ANCIENT CLASSICAL AYURVEDIC TEXT

While acupuncture and herbs and even diet can be helpful to counteract stress and its resulting hormonal imbalance, often there is no medicine—except *pranayama*—that affects the nervous system quite as rapidly as the regular practice of *abhyanga*. One of the unique aspects of Ayurvedic medicine is its therapeutic use of oil. *Abhyanga* is the Sanskrit word for a warm oil massage. This can be self-administered or given by a practitioner and can last fifteen minutes to over an hour. In this book, I usually refer to it as "self-massage" as it's unlikely we can find a practitioner who will administer it to us every morning!

In *abhyanga,* a generous amount of warm oil, often medicated with herbs and usually warm, is gently massaged into the entire body before steaming or bathing. Although not considered a part of a daily routine or lifestyle in modern society, self-massage has a long and illustrious history in Ayurvedic medicine. It is one of the surest ways to nourish yin and support hormonal balance. It's hard to believe that such a delicious habit can be so healing. But it is.

For thousands of years, people in India have used *abhyanga* to maintain health, benefit sleep patterns, and increase longevity. The Sanskrit word *sneha* can be translated as both "oil" and "love." It is understood that the physiological effects of the application of oil on the body are similar to those received when one is saturated with love. Both experiences impart a feeling of stability, warmth and comfort.

The skin is the largest organ in the body. We feel sensations on our skin because of the nerves that enervate it. When we cover the skin with warm oil, it calms the nervous system, making it less hypervigilant and oversensitized. When the nervous system is less jumpy, it is less likely to trigger the release of stress hormones, which we have seen over and over again to be the cause of hormonal imbalance. With the release of fewer stress hormones, our endocrine system may, little by little, be able to regain a healthy balance. This may lead to the resolution of various maladies that have their roots in hormonal imbalance.

It is best not to put any oil on your skin that you wouldn't put in your mouth. It should be edible. The skin absorbs what is applied to it. Chemicals and poison can be absorbed through the skin as fast as can things that are good for it. So Ayurveda recommends we avoid mineral oils and oils with chemical perfumes or other synthetic ingredients. I generally avoid any oil that has any ingredients other than vegetable oils and herbs. And I prefer organic oils.

It is important to use oil that is appropriate for your current condition. An oil that appeals to one person may be distasteful or even cause nausea in another. If you're not sure where to start, most people can tolerate a half-and-half mix of sunflower oil and untoasted sesame oil. This can be just fine, but I've come to prefer herbal oil that is appropriate for the season and my current requirements. The Web site www.banyanbotanicals.com has some online questionnaires to help you determine which oils are best for your current condition or constitution, if you don't have access to a personal Ayurvedic consultant.

Untoasted sesame oil, herbal massage oils, and herbal powders for removing the oil from your body are available from Ayurvedic product suppliers. There is a list of suppliers in Appendix A. For a detailed description of how to practice *abhyanga*, including when not to use it, see Appendix C.

I can't tell you how many times I have had students or patients come to me and tell me that *abhyanga* has changed their lives. Literally. "Doing this has changed my life." Of all the single changes someone can make to change their life for the better, this one is right at the top of the list. It might be hard to imagine that such a pleasant practice can lead to a truly changed state of health or make a significant difference, but it is remarkable to see its transformative effect over and over. As was the case in Rachel's story at the beginning of this chapter, the regular practice of *abhyanga* can sometimes trump diet, acupuncture, and herbs in calming the nervous system, thereby having a balancing effect on hormonal balance.

Pranayama and Alternate-Nostril Breathing

Influenced by my studies of the various health-related texts of India and my experience with myself and my patients, I have come to believe that *pranayama* (breathing exercises) constitutes the most powerful and direct technique of affecting the mind that is available to most of us.

Because breathing exercises are so powerful, a little can go a long way. Certain simple exercises can at once promote good-quality yin and yang as they simultaneously relax and focus the mind. In Ayurveda it is believed that the mind affects the body. When the mind is relaxed and focused—representing a mental balance of yin and yang—the effects trickle down to the body, calming the nervous system and irrigating our tissues and organs with qi or *prana*.

Not all breathing exercises are good for everybody. Some are too stimulating for an already overstimulated life, but some are almost universally beneficial. These exercises are not complicated, but they are not always easy. Many of us have learned to hold our breath. We take shallow, short breaths, and breathe only into the upper parts of our bodies. *Pranayama* teaches us to direct *prana*, or the vehicle of the breath, into all parts of the body. At first it may feel foreign to do this and we may need some coaching to learn how. It is an important skill to apply to most breathing practices. If we don't learn this skill and, instead, just try to learn various other techniques, we run the risk of simply strengthening a poor breathing habit.

Basic Deep Breathing

To help learn how to direct *prana* and breathe a full, therapeutic breath, I often lead students and patients in the following exercise, which is best done when the stomach is empty and there is fresh air in the room.

1. Lie on your back with a pillow under your knees. Place your hands over your lower abdomen. Breathe through your nose throughout this entire exercise. Close your eyes. Imagine that your torso is like a vase. Just as when you fill a vase with water, the water fills the bottom of the vase first and gradually and fills the middle and then upper portions of the vase, feel your breath filling first your lower abdomen, then middle, then upper body.

2. Breath will follow *prana* and *prana* will follow your focus. They are as inseparable as a shadow from a tree. As breath fills your lower abdomen, *prana* irrigates the organs of elimination and reproduction. As it fills the middle portion of your torso, *prana* irrigates the digestive organs. As it fills your upper torso, it irrigates the lower, middle, and upper lobes of the lungs and the heart.

3. As you inhale, then, your breath very slowly fills first the lower, then the middle, then the upper portions of your torso and finally rises to about 8–10 inches above your head. Keep the attention here a few seconds and then allow your exhale (still breathing only through your nose) to very slowly surrender your breath back down the path it took on its way up. *Prana* will follow the breath back down through the upper, then middle portions of your torso and return to the lower abdomen.

4. Continue breathing like this for about 5 minutes. Keep your hands on your lower torso. You should feel your lower abdomen rise as you begin your inhale. As your breath fills your middle torso, it will rise, too. When it fills your upper torso, your entire torso should feel expanded. Likewise, each section should relax as you exhale your *prana* down through each section.

5. If you feel any tight areas in your body as you are breathing, you can try "breathing into" those areas until they feel free and easy. If you don't experience the feeling of "breathing into" an area, place your hand over that tight area and imagine

there is a straw that reaches into the area from outside your body. Imagine that you are not breathing through your nose but through that straw, directly into the tight area. As the breath enters the tight area, the area quickly releases and becomes free. Engage in this releasing process for about 5 minutes. Then go back to breathing fully through the entire torso. If emotions come up, continue to focus on the breath, rather than on the emotions.

6. Allow your breath to return to normal. Bring your attention back to the room you are in and slowly open your eyes.

Breathing deeply like this helps *prana* to circulate and move smoothly throughout the body, with all its tissues and organs, and the mind. It also supports digestion of emotional memories and experiences. Breathing like this is *a medicine* in and of itself. Try breathing like this at least five minutes morning and evening.

ALTERNATE-NOSTRIL BREATHING

Once you feel comfortable with this deep-breathing exercise, it may be useful to learn another breathing technique. While there are many, my favorite is alternate-nostril breathing (*nadi shodhana*). Alternate-nostril breathing is the most powerful quick technique I know for balancing hormones. I have heard that it is best to check with your doctor before engaging in breathing exercises if you have heart or respiratory disorders, but I have personally never come across anyone who has had a poor reaction to it. Occasionally people feel some heat in the body during the practice, but this quickly resolves and does not necessarily mean that the exercise is creating heat in the body. The heat does not stay after the exercise is over.

This is an exercise wherein the practitioner exhales and inhales through one nostril first and then the other, with the aid of certain finger arrangements. It is practiced in many yoga classes. Luckily, it is not difficult these days to find a yoga teacher familiar enough with *pranayama* to be able to teach this basic practice. One of my teachers, Kirpal Singh, describes a very basic form of this exercise as follows. He also recommended imagining one is absorbing qualities like mercy, compassion, love, peace and joy on the inhale, and releasing qualities like anger, lust, greed, attachment, selfishness, and pride on the exhale. It is preferable to do *pranayama* in a quiet room with fresh air. If the air in your room isn't fresh, you might consider putting a bunch of houseplants in the room in which you do *pranayama*, to help oxygenate and purify the air.

- Sitting in *padam* or *sukh asana* (a simple cross-legged position), one should close the right nostril with the thumb of the right hand and exhale the air slowly and rhythmically in one long and unbroken expiration through the left nostril.

- Now the left nostril is also to be closed with the little or ring finger of the right hand.
- The *bahya kumbhaka* (the pause at the end of the exhale) be maintained as long as possible without the least discomfort.
- Then the breath is to be inhaled, very, very, slowly, through the right nostril after removing the thumb. Follow this with *antar kumbhaka* (the pause at the end of the inhale).
- Then the order is reversed.
- All these eight processes constitute one *pranayama*. One ought to commence with five to ten *pranayamas* in the morning and in the evening, on an empty stomach, and gradually increase to twenty, together with increased *kumbhaka* (retention) without causing any inconvenience.[2]

As Rachel's story illustrated, doing alternate-nostril breathing for fifteen minutes a day can eliminate menopausal symptoms when nothing else can. Its calming effect on the nervous system and balancing effect on the hormones is quick and, usually, its only side effect is greater mental and emotional equilibrium.

Laughter

Not every stress management technique requires new skills, time, or warm oil. You can always try the time-honored healer: laughter.

While not all comedians enjoy the longevity achieved by centenarians like George Burns or Bob Hope, laughter has been shown to have positive physiologic effects that range from supporting the immune system to enhancing the quality of breast milk. This is one of those things that is . . . er . . . funny to cite studies on, as it is such an intuitive no-brainer. But studies have been done, and they show that laughter's immune-enhancing effects include lowering the level of cortisol in the blood, increasing the number of activated T lymphocytes (which fight infected and malignant cells), and supporting the quality and quantity of natural killer cells.[3]

Finding an antidote to stress seems crucial, considering that stress and depression can almost triple the risk of a heart attack[4] and affect us in all the other ways we've seen. If meditation, spiritual communion, *abhyanga*, and *pranayama* are too daunting to embrace immediately, at least we can laugh about it in the meantime.

Changing Lifestyles, Changing Lives

If all you can do is crawl, start crawling.
If you have a hundred cynical fantasies about God, make it ninety-nine.
If you can't pray a real prayer, pray hypocritically, full of doubt, and dry-mouthed.
God accepts counterfeit money as though it were real.
—RUMI

Living a stressful life serves up a double whammy. We feel miserable while we are living it and miserable again when we experience its uncomfortable results.

If we know we need to slow life down, find balance, and eat well, but we don't know where to begin, or if we fear life will fall apart if we slow down, we can start simply. Begin with one area of life. Increase the nourishing aspects, or slow down and cut out fast food. See what the effects are. After getting comfortable with this, we can make adjustments in other areas.

Little by little we may find that life becomes sweeter.

Hope

If we care for living a nice, honorable and honest life in the living present . . .
there should be little to worry for the past and nothing to become
anxious for in the future.
—KIRPAL SINGH

Forget your perfect offering. There is a crack in everything.
That's how the light gets in.
—LEONARD COHEN

A hydrangea grows outside my family's living room window. Throughout the winter, the plant looks to be a group of dead, hollow plant skeletons. In April, after a bit of sun and rain, small bright green leaves grow out of these barren-looking stalks. By summer the leaves are big and lush, and the bush sports large, almost gaudy blue and purple clumps of blossoms. The first spring I witnessed this resurrection of dry stalks, tears came to my eyes. My father had been fighting cancer and I felt particularly close to the cycles of life. It was a miracle of renewal.

Suppose we've lost touch with the joy of a slower-paced life that moves according to the needs of time and nature. It is easy to feel that we have wasted—or, worse, ruined—our lives. We wonder if it is too late to change.

Sometimes we do the best we can with lifestyle, diet, and meditation, and still we develop a serious disease. For many it is not possible to avoid all illness. I have often felt that there is no such thing as perfect health. There is only becoming aware of our challenge areas and learning how best to manage them. Even then, conditions and challenging times arise in spite of our best efforts. Although it is sometimes tempting, these are not the times to give up the good habits we have developed. Those very habits may see us through the trying times and ensure that there are pieces to pick up at the other end. It is human nature to want to lean on our vices when we can least afford to do so, but it is also the human prerogative to rise to meet challenges.

It is *never* too late to start eating well, to start learning how to release stress, to stop running ourselves ragged, and to start to take steps toward living the life we want to be living. As long as we can make changes, there is hope.

Dr. Dean Ornish has become well known in his success with reversing heart disease with lifestyle and diet changes. Even one change can produce dramatic results. Consider that a previously sedentary woman can reduce her likelihood of getting heart disease just by including walking in her daily routine.[1]

The heart is not the only resilient organ in the body. Scientists once thought brain damage was irreversible and that memory loss and mental atrophy were an inevitable side effect of aging. In recent years, however, breakthroughs in the field of neuroplasticity have revealed the brain's ability to form new nerve connections to compensate for disease or injury, to rewire, repattern, and adapt to new or changed environments.

This applies to the brain's ability to bounce back from highly stressful situations. In the summer of 2009, the journal *Science* included an intriguing report by Nuno Sousa and his colleagues at the Life and Health Sciences Research Institute at the University of Minho in Portugal. They described experiments that mapped the brain's response to stress and its resiliency. The results are striking in both areas. When experimenters subjected rats to a monthlong course of intense stress, it withered the regions of the brain that relate to executive decision-making and goal-directed behavior and stimulated regions associated with habitual activity. Stressed, the rats would then begin to engage in ineffectual behaviors and then persist in them.

The good news? After only a month's relief from the stressors, the brains of these rats—and their behavior—returned to normal. This is heady stuff. Consider it. The actual physical tissues and connections in the brain shift in response to stress or release from stress.[2]

Although a month's vacation from stress was sufficient to remedy a month of stress, it may be insufficient to counteract years of stress. That may require a bit more time, but the brain's extraordinary capacity for resilience provides solid ground for hope. The results of this study also suggest that if life is stressful, we either need to change that life or at least take a regular hiatus. Our brains are constantly forming new pathways, reinforcing those we've established, or allowing unused ones to atrophy or dissolve. The brain, like the body, consistently reflects what we expose it to. The more focus and intent we employ in the process, the quicker the results. The more focus we apply to establishing healthy patterns, the quicker the brain, as well as the body, may be able to replace their stressed-out patterns.

It often takes something drastic—being faced with the prospect of heart surgery or some other extreme proposition—for us to find the motivation necessary to change patterns that need changing. In these cases, the disease or disorder leads to better health than we could have imagined and is therefore a great gift.

Judy was fifty-two and had been having bloody stools and intestinal pain since her midforties. Things had become progressively worse over the years and she was now told that surgery was her best treatment option. When she came to see me, she was scheduled to have surgery in three weeks to remove part of her colon. I recommended she consult with her gastroenterologist to see if she could safely postpone her surgery and to give herself about three months to address her health with Eastern medicine. We developed a daily routine for Judy that included fifteen minutes of silent meditation, fifteen minutes of gentle yoga, a twenty-minute walk outdoors, and five minutes of gentle alternate-nostril breathing. She also did a couple castor oil packs every week to calm her digestive area, took some herbs, and changed her diet so it suited both her constitution and her current condition. Within a month her symptoms were only a minor annoyance. A pleasant side effect of the treatment was that the hot flashes she'd been having for the past three years were gone.

It has been six years and Judy still hasn't had the surgery. Her stools are normal and she rarely has pain. When she begins to have mild discomfort, she now knows which foods to avoid and which to favor. She has addressed some underlying anxiety and anger issues, and learned how to respond with lifestyle and dietary alterations to her body's signs of stress.[3]

Judy's story may seem miraculous, but it is not. It demonstrates the natural result of educated change.

Most of us are more comfortable with gradual, less drastic change. There is no problem with this approach, provided we aren't in dire circumstances. Making gradual change might even be easier on the body and mind. If we can't immediately change a stressful course, we can at least retreat for one weekend a month, a few weeks a year, or fifteen minutes a day. One way or another, we need to give our brain some regular, stress-free time so it can morph back into a healthy state.

Above all, we need to avoid stressing out about how quickly we change. Expecting instant gratification or making too many changes at once defeats at least part of the purpose, because stress hormones released by stressing out undo some of the good we aim for.

Frank Woodruff Buckles, born February 1, 1901, is the last verified living American veteran of World War I. The secret of his long life? He jokes, "When you start to die . . . don't." But seriously? He says, "Hope," and he adds that he "never got in a hurry."[4]

So, if gradual change is our strategy, let's consider what the first step should be.

Take Away Everything That Isn't Horse

My father once recalled—erroneously as it turned out—a sculptor's response to a question about how he sculpted such beautiful horses: "Take away everything that isn't horse." The actual quote is by Elbert Hubbard, who said, "The sculptor produces the beautiful statue by chipping away such parts of the marble block that are not needed—it is a process of elimination." I am fond of Dad's version.

In our context, the horse is your well-being. The first thing we want to do is take away everything that isn't contributing to it. Start by taking away the poison. Poison includes exposure to pollution, consumption of excess caffeine, sugar, alcohol and recreational drugs. Pharmaceutical drugs are also toxic, but it is not always possible to eliminate them without causing more damage than they are inflicting. Relationships and experiences can also be poisonous. If a certain social situation or relationship *feels* toxic, it may well be. And if we uncomfortable with or despise ourselves, our relationships with ourselves may, too, be toxic.

It is beyond the scope of this book to address the best ways of healing addictions—whether to substances or toxic relationships—but it is imperative to do so. This generally means quitting what we are addicted to or changing its nature. If we are in a toxic relationship, for example, it may or may not be ideal to get out of it. It may be better to change its nature from the inside. These days we are surrounded by support for self- and relationship improvement. We can begin individual or couples counseling, attend twelve-step meetings, find advice in the self-help section of the bookstore, or find some other way to change. It doesn't matter how we do it, as long as things improve.

If we consume poison on a daily basis, it is almost impossible to build, restore, or maintain health. Pursuing an addiction while being treated for overall health by a practitioner of Eastern medicine will prolong the healing process indefinitely. All your efforts will mostly serve to help counter the effects of the addiction rather than to improve your health.

If you have been on pharmaceutical drugs for any condition, and you are considering getting off them and trying to address your health issues through lifestyle, dietary, or herbal means, it is essential that you consult with your prescribing doctor before making a change. There can be disastrous effects from coming off medications the wrong way. If your doctor is willing to work with you, you can work out a plan together. If your doctor is unwilling, you have a couple of options. You can look for another doctor who is willing to help; or you can remain on the drugs while you allow your dietary, lifestyle, and herbal changes time to work, and then share the results with your physician. It could be that you may need to be on drugs for the rest of your life. There is a time for everything, even drugs, but bettering your lifestyle or diet can improve your tolerance of them, as well as your overall health.

Sacrifice Ambition at the Altar of Reality

In his thought provoking book *Blink*, Malcolm Gladwell describes a study in which people were given two decks of cards, one red and one blue. They were asked to turn over a card from either pile, one by one. Each card delivered either a reward or a penalty. What the participants didn't know—and didn't begin to suspect consciously until they had turned over fifty cards—is that the red pile delivered bigger rewards . . . and bigger penalties. In the long run, the slow, steady diet of small rewards and smaller penalties delivered by the blue deck would pay off. Participants figured this out by the time they'd turned over eighty cards. The remarkable thing is that by the tenth card they had already stopped choosing as many red cards *without being aware of it*. They had also started perspiring a bit on their palms and showing other signs of stress when they pulled cards from the red deck. This suggests that the body is quicker to recognize land mines than is the conscious brain. If we could just learn to listen more closely to the wisdom of our bodies, perhaps we could recognize better what is and isn't working in our lives, and we could begin to jettison the activities that don't pass our bodies' tests.

Some of my mentors are fond of saying, "It is wise to live with reality, otherwise reality will certainly come to live with you." If we are constantly trying to change what *is*, constantly pushing for things to be different, we can injure ourselves. Many of us are in the habit of chasing our ambitions, for example, even beyond the point where the body has reached its limits. We push and push and begin to get headaches; we take painkillers and push on. We begin to get constipated; we take some laxatives and keep on. We get anxious; we try Prozac or St. John's wort, and press on. We ignore the body's SOS signals to stop whatever it is we are doing to damage it. Renaissance physician Paracelsus said, "Man is ill because he is never still." Some of us need to hit the wall—have some significant crisis or illness—before we respond. Even when we finally turn our attention toward healing body and spirit, we may do so reluctantly.

Surrender to the Pace of Your Body

When we do listen to the body, we often discover it is telling us is to slow down, kick back, and chill out. Were we to surrender to the pace of the body, we might find that it is only asking us to live as we really want to live. How ironic that it takes courage to live the lives we want to live.

Kirpal Singh said, "Perhaps more souls are lost to heaven by the sense of duty to earth than by downright sin and evil." We are commonly driven to ignore our true calling by the perceived demands of our responsibilities, often until our very life comes to a close. One of my mentors, Dr. Vasant Lad, teaches his students of Ayurveda that knowing we are confused is the dawn of clarity. If we sort out what we truly need to be doing from what we are in the habit of doing, and begin to take little steps in the direction our soul is calling us to walk, we may actually get where we want to go.

Once we know what the root of the problem is, we can begin to change. Often, when we listen to the body and respond accordingly, little step by little step, life's path becomes clearer. More simple.

The following is a true story, written to me by a highly qualified woman surgeon about her journey, deep into Western medicine and concurrently into personal imbalance, then further into the root causes of health, and ultimately into her own return to health. This is her story, almost entirely in her words, and printed here with her permission. It is the story of a life that reflects everything we've discussed in this book: How ambition, while leading to some positive accomplishments, can also lead to stress, which ensures high levels of cortisol circulating in the body. How this weakens the immune and endocrine systems, and causes qi to stagnate. How these disorders begin to reveal themselves increasingly after age thirty-five, as we have progressively decreasing yin sex hormones to buffer the yang stress hormones. How beginning to slow down and eat whole foods can help restore health. How, just as it is helpful to have an doctor set a bone, it is helpful to have a qualified practitioner of Eastern medicine to help us tailor a dietary, exercise, and herbal regimen appropriate to our individual needs. How, ultimately, when we find life difficult, the most important thing to do to change it is to change how we are living it.

> *Dear Dr. Welch,*
>
> *I was recently a participant at your "Women's Transitions" seminar and benefited greatly from your wisdom. I am a Western physician—a surgeon—by training and have worked in that field for twenty years (including residency training and practice). I want to tell you a little about my history because it pertains directly to what you spoke of almost the entire course! I felt like I was a living witness to all you described.*
>
> *You are probably familiar with the workload of a Western surgical training program and I won't need to elaborate on that other than to mention I was spared every other night call after my surgical internship, graduating to every third night call for the remainder of the five years. I finished my surgical residency at age thirty-one and joined the faculty at Harvard Medical School then, teaching, doing research and doing clinical work. For the next five years I routinely worked twelve- to fourteen-hour days and often did rounds on weekends. Because I operated on people with advanced cancers, my operative days were long and grueling, many times involving operative cases that took longer than eight hours. Just before turning thirty-six, I had my first child after a long and strenuous labor necessitating an emergency C-section. I nursed him until he was nine months old. I took three months at home with him, returned working three and a half days a week, thus cutting my schedule back to forty to forty-five hours a week, and pumped milk for*

him at work and froze it. I remember having a dictation headset on my head while I dictated patient evaluations, eating lunch and pumping breast milk all the same time. Two years and one transcontinental move later, I had my second child and, four months later started my new job.

I nursed my second child for eleven months. The night I stopped nursing him I had my first glass of wine in over twenty months. (I have never drunk much, no more than maybe a glass or two of wine a month at most.) I woke in the middle of the night with severe epigastric pain and vomited blood (coffee-ground, upper GI bleed-type) several times. The next day, lab work showed that I had a fairly low white blood cell count, anemia, elevated bilirubin, and elevated cholesterol (about 225). I was started on a Prilosec (proton pump inhibitor) and sucralfate. Endoscopy two days later revealed I had gastritis and esophagitis on biopsy. I was told by my GI colleagues I would be on the medications indefinitely. I had pretty regular heartburn, sometimes waking me at night. I had very low libido. The red, itchy patches of eczema that started before I had my first child came back in full force, often in body folds. Also, my allergies started up (I had mild allergies as a child), and I was particularly bothered in the spring and fall.

I attributed this to the move, to a new climate and started on antihistamines, nasal steroids and sometimes Sudafed when the nasal congestion was particularly bothersome. I could monitor what my nasal tissue and throat tissue looked like by doing a nasal endoscopy and the tissue was chronically pale, edematous, and boggy. I also started to develop vaginal itching and yeast infections, which became chronic and were barely treated before another one started. I would use a combination of Monistat vaginally, douches, and Nystatin which stopped working and I graduated to the more powerful Diflucan (the "one time" pill), having to take that sometimes an entire week to knock off a yeast infection. I had a thyroid nodule that developed in my thyroid gland which was biopsied and found to be colloid goiter.

I was forty years old and my mother was in the terminal stages of ovarian cancer. She died that summer at age fifty-nine of ovarian cancer she had developed at age forty-five. I had been traveling across the country to see her every six weeks for the last year of her life while she was bedridden at home. I was exhausted, demoralized, and grieving. Four days after she died, my father and I had just honored her with a little ceremony and were driving on the Interstate when he fell asleep at the wheel. The car flew off the highway above a ravine, and the car roof crushed on my head as the car rolled. I remember seeing treetops move in circles and then having what is described as Lhermitte's spinal electric shocks traveling down up and down my spinal cord to my fingers and toes. There was that split millisecond in the air where I felt my whole life reeling quickly before me and I had the chance to choose to live on. It was really quite a powerful experience. My father was okay other than bruises and I was transported via ambulance strapped to a C-spine board to a hospital. I found that I had a T4 compression fracture and mostly "soft tissue" injury from my mid-thoracic spine to the nape of my neck. I returned home several days later and my youngest child, who was now barely walking, ran up to me at the airport. Because I could not lift my arms and was in great pain, I couldn't catch him and he bounced his head off the cement and had a concussion and mild seizure, for which we had to rush him to the hospital for a head CT scan (fortunately, he did not have any bleeding).

Needless to say here, I was at the very end of my rope, and I was in great physical and emotional pain and didn't think I could take much more. I started on a four-month course of antidepressants (refusing to take any narcotic pain meds) which I discontinued because I developed headaches and bruxism [teeth grinding] at night with this. I took a leave of absence from work for three months and sought the treatments of both a chiropractor and an acupuncturist when the orthopedic surgeon at the Back Institute told me, because I could still touch my toes, that I was fine and needed no therapy.

After three months I returned to work, taking weekly massages and still visiting the chiropractor. I developed a bronchitis that fall that took several months to go away. When a child patient with an infection inadvertently spit in my eye, I developed a 4+ conjunctivitis with complete closure of my right eyelid for one week and blurred vision. My internist at the time retested me for allergies and I had some marked responses (skin and RAST testing) to molds, tree, weed, grass pollens. I wasn't seeing progress, or getting to the bottom of this, and my doctors kept plying me with medications (proton-pump inhibitors, antifungals, antibiotics, antihistamines, topical steroids, decongestants, eye drops, and, now, antidepressants).

I decided I'd had it and there had to be another way. I started with a yoga therapist who helped me with some poses I could do and I developed a daily practice very slowly . . . I still had a "dowager's hump," a huge lump of swollen soft tissue from my skull base to my bra line but was now able to raise my arms above ninety degrees! I cut back on surgical cases, only doing those that would be less than two hours. I also tested myself with ALCAT (a nonstandard test that looks at white cell clumping in response to a variety of antigens) and I had a 4+ response to Candida, which, at this time was no surprise to me. It also explained to me why my white blood cell count might be so low! At times, my absolute lymphocyte and absolute neutrophil counts were well below the normal range.

I didn't know who to trust and I realized the reductionist and completely fractionated approach of Western medicine wasn't working for me and that I just *needed to listen to my body and let it tell me what it needed. In the fall of 2000, after some research, I started on my first "elimination" diet . . . that is, pretty much eating rice, vegetables, beans and a little animal protein—all organic, no processed foods, no sugars of any kind, nothing fermented, etc. for three months. (I was already off caffeine for ten years). I went through a pretty severe withdrawal, especially for sugar, the first couple of weeks, and developed some significant skin rashes.*

I started to feel somewhat better and I was continuing with the yoga practice. But I also realized I needed to work with the stress and my response to stressors in my life. So, I decided to completely stop working in September 2001 (uncanny that my first day "off" was 9/11) and devote time to healing myself. (I returned in early 2003 at one day a week.) I continued to do "research outside the box." I realized that the problems with cholesterol and recurrence of the fibrocysts in my breast were likely related to weakness in my liver and the liver probably had been somewhat trashed by all the antifungals I was taking. I also realized that my chronic low white cell count (when I checked back even to med school days, I was already developing a low white count then), sugar cravings, fatigue, etc. were probably due to adrenal fatigue to some degree. I had our backyard pool switched to saltwater, put in water filters and dechlorinators inside, made sure we ate as much organic as possible, and pretty much removed most animal protein except occasional fish and chicken from my diet.

As I read more, I decided I would do well to have my hormone levels checked as well as a daily cortisone profile . . . as I said I was beginning to think I might have some adrenal fatigue. So, I found a naturopath and asked to have progesterone, estrogen, DHEA, and cortisol levels checked (salivary). I started on some bioidentical progesterone cream the second half of my cycle as first-line therapy because my adrenals were doing overtime but not quite yet in adrenal fatigue. I was on this for three years or so to start turning things around. The high cortisol profile (and overstimulated immune system) also explained to me why I was having increasing allergic symptoms, chronic yeast infections, and low white blood cell count, at least in part. My immune system was on chronic alert and responding to everything.

I asked my yoga therapist if she knew anything about cleansing and where I might go and she had several suggestions. After more research, I decided that I might like to try the Ayurvedic Institute in Albuquerque and went for my first panchakarma in spring 2002. With the dietary changes I had made, I was feeling quite a bit better but still had a low white blood cell count, gastric reflux, etc. and occasional yeast infections and still elevated cholesterol, especially LDL. With the first panchakarma treatment, I felt exhausted and developed a brilliant red rash on every crease in my body as well as a rip-roaring vaginal yeast infection. I finished out the panchakarma and these temporary symptoms resolved by the time I left.

After I returned home, I stayed on the prescribed diet for two weeks and felt better than I had felt in twenty years! I have continued to do panchakarma once a year since then and have incorporated an Ayurvedic diet prescribed for my constitution.

So, as I head into menopause, I have gradually incorporated all of this along with daily meditation over the past two years and finally, lastly, pranayama practice along with the daily gentle yoga practice of one hour. I bike a few times a week, garden, and walk the dogs every day. I work one day a week teaching residents in the operating room and I am slowly, very slowly, studying a couple distance learning courses for Ayurveda. I write poetry and paint now as stress relievers. In my mind, the largest part in all this is the mind part, and how I responded to stressors, essentially, my coping techniques. I have explored the roots of how I learned to cope with stress and have learned some new ways that better serve me.

I also see an acupuncturist/herbalist here who does acupuncture on me once or twice a month and has given me some Traditional Chinese Medicine herbal medicines for sleep. I don't as yet know of an Ayurvedic practitioner locally. I get massage a couple times a month as well and started daily abhyanga, especially in the fall and winter starting a year ago.

As you mentioned in your seminar, I had always "bulldozed my way" through things and that just wasn't working anymore. (By the way, I see that some of my women medical colleagues my age who continue to bulldoze are now developing their autoimmune diseases from cortisol burnout: myasthenia gravis, Hashimoto's thyroiditis, Grave's disease, chronic alopecia [hair loss], to name a few.)

So, at this time, I still will develop a little eczematous rash in what I call my indicator areas, as well as fatigue right before and during my period, especially if I've had a stressful month or if I've eaten any chocolate or wheat. And when I say chocolate, I mean a chocolate-covered strawberry or two, not a bar of chocolate.

My white blood cell count is now normal, my LDL ("bad") cholesterol has dropped 40 to 50 points and my HDL ("good") cholesterol is now 86! I have a very low C-reactive protein, and no thyroid autoantibodies and normal thyroid levels. I might get one cold every year or so which is quite mild and goes away quickly . . . I used to get five or six a year and they hung on for quite a while.

I believe my mother's death and my rollover car accident were incredible gifts to me . . . to shake me up and help me listen to my body as it had so much to teach me! On the other hand, listening to my own body helped me understand a great *deal I didn't understand as a Western practitioner . . . [such as] cases of severe adult-onset allergies and chronic sinusitis, pediatric yeast infections, patients with chronic fatigue and multiple chemical sensitivities, and the list goes on, including the rise in autoimmune diseases, especially in women. I am not castigating Western medicine . . . and I would be the first to have a bone reset or a spleen removed if I had internal injuries from a motor vehicle accident. However, I have learned its limitations and reductionism can be crippling, too. Thank you for indulging me to listen to my story.*

I am in awe of this doctor's story. Her persistence and commitment to finding what worked to improve her health and her life, is an inspiration.

The latest scientific studies show that the body has a remarkable capacity to begin healing—and much more quickly than we once knew—if we address the lifestyle factors that often cause these chronic diseases. These studies, like the doctor's story, show that integrative medicine can make a powerful difference in our health and well-being, and testify to how quickly these changes may occur and how dynamic their mechanisms can be.

Breakthroughs in medicine are not always new drugs, complicated machines, or medical procedures. Today, we are on the verge of a breakthrough that involves simple changes in diet, lifestyle, and behavior, based on informed choices.

Making Choices

Sometimes choices are better made by the body than by the mind. The body often gives us signals if we are choosing a path that is not in our highest good. If you are not sure how to listen to your body—that is, you can't tell when your shoulders tighten up, you start breathing more shallowly, you begin to perspire, or you have some other sensation that is indicating that you are heading in an uncomfortable direction—you might try the following activity. It might help you make life choices, big or small, and discover the true inclination of your spirit.

Consider a choice that you need to make. This could be anything from, "Should I go back to school?" to "Should I accept Marjorie's invitation to dinner?"

Put it in the form of a question and write it down. Under this create two columns. Label one "Fears" and the other "Seductions." In the Fears column, write down any fears preventing you from making the choice. This might be anything from, "I'm afraid I can't afford school" to "I'm afraid Marjorie won't like me if I decline her invitation." From the sublime to the ridiculous, write down every fear associated with the question at hand. Then, in the Seductions column, list the things that are luring you into making the choice. "If I go back to school, I will be able to make more money." "Marjorie is friends with my boss. If she likes me, I might receive more favor from my boss." "If we eat at that new restaurant I might see that guy I have a crush on." What makes this exercise work at all is to look completely honestly at the fantasies—fearful or attractive—that are secretly motivating your response to the choice at hand.

Usually money, prestige, and the feeling that we might miss out on something are powerful motivators behind our fears and seductions: I'll be able to afford to buy a new car . . . Through association with someone more powerful or famous, I might get ahead . . . What will people think of me? . . . I'll miss out on something . . . Someone else will snap it up . . . I won't be able to make ends meet . . . Someone will think I'm dumb, slow, arrogant . . .

Once you have completed your evaluation, look at what you've written and tell yourself, "None of this is real." Rip up the paper and throw it away. What is left? A yes or a no. From the little voice of your heart. The thing is either right for you or it is wrong for you. The voice of your heart is ignorant of your likes and dislikes, your reasons and excuses. That's why you can trust it. Go back to school? Yes or no. Go out to dinner? Yes or no. The answer, underneath the fears and seductions, generally reflects reality. We may have twenty-three reasons why our reality is wrong, but that misses the point. The point is to live with reality. (Otherwise reality will definitely come to live with us.) Most of us have come to believe our fears and seductions are real. It might be surprising to think that they're not. We may even refuse to believe this.

If there is not a clear yes or no, I tend to defer to this advice from one of my teachers: When in doubt, do nothing. Eventually something becomes clear.

This is not to say that there are never obstacles between what is right for us to do and doing it. But the obstacle is not really a fear or a seduction. It may be a situation. Maybe there is no money (right now). This is not to say that can't change. Money shows up sometimes. There are ways to make it. Not having enough money is not always an insurmountable obstruction. Knowing what is right for us gives us a handle on our emotional reality. Looking at the feasibility of cooperating with that gives us a handle on another aspect of reality. Then we can come to terms with it and adjust our desires or circumstances accordingly, or we can simply digest reality (that is, breathe through it and ensure that our qi or *prana* is not getting stuck anywhere when we think about it) and see what changes. Change is a constant. We can be sure that what is so today will be different tomorrow, even if only slightly.

Remember that what we believe has a strong physiological effect. A striking example: In clinical trials involving the hair-growth stimulating drug Rogaine, a full 20 percent of the men using a placebo lotion grew "minimal to dense hair."[5] The power of positive thinking can change your reality.

By the way, if one of your reasons not to do something that is right for you is that other people might think you are crazy, consider a book title my husband remembers seeing one day called *What Other People Think of You Is None of Your Business*. We never read the book. We never had to. The title said it all—and we regularly remind ourselves of its message.

Self-Blame vs. Self-Responsibility

Sometimes we find ourselves in a situation we know is detrimental to our health and we know what we need to do, not do, eat, not eat, and so on, yet for one reason or another, we find it untenable to change the situation. It can be a source of guilt or resentment when we can't do what needs to be done. Other times it is tempting to duck out of our own responsibility by blaming our inaction or problematic actions on an external circumstance.

If life needs changing, we can't expect someone to come in and do it for us. We can begin by being honest with ourselves. Is there something we can do that we are not doing? Do we know this and continue to ignore it? If we are ignoring change that needs to be made, there are often two possible reasons for this. The first falls in the category of what Ayurveda calls *prajnaparadh* ("a crime against wisdom"). Suppose I get home after a long day at work. I'm tired. I know that I should cook myself a nourishing, easily digestible meal and take a walk, but I choose instead to microwave some mac and cheese, eat a doughnut, and watch *South Park*. I know the food choices are highly processed, poor choices of nutrition and that *South Park* is equally vapid. But I make these choices anyway. It is understandable because life is hard sometimes and we just need to chill out. But if this becomes a way of life, I will only cause myself more suffering. In this case, my actions lie within the bounds of free will, and I need to find a way to change my behavior.

The second reason we might ignore changes we need to make is due to ethical obligation or forces outside one's control. This is a poignant reality of life. Take the same example, where I arrive home, tired after a long day and know what I should do to revive and nourish myself: the home-cooked meal, the walk, maybe a bath, *abhyanga*, and a hot cup of milk. Otherwise I might even get sick, because

I'm feeling just on the verge. But when I arrive home, I find my eighty-two-year-old neighbor has fallen and broken his hip. Do I leave him there, prioritizing my own well-being? Of course not.

Or, suppose I never make it home that evening to take care of myself in the first place. A tornado has swept through the area and when I arrive where my home should be, there is only rubble. Some things are clearly beyond our control.

Nature Throws Us Curve Balls

Because nature throws us curve balls—things outside of our ability to choose, like the timing of our eighty-two-year-old neighbor's accident, our child's illness or an ailing parent—it is important not to indulge too much in laziness or procrastination when it comes to making the healthy changes that are within our control. We need to educate ourselves so we understand how diet, lifestyle, and environment affect us, and make choices that encourage balance. If we are educated, we make those choices not out of allegiance to dogma but out of appreciation of health. We need to be honest with ourselves and have the courage to do what brings us closer to balance. Once we have experienced balance and health, we will not want to sacrifice them again. The joy, clarity, and vitality that we nurture and experience can help us through those times when we are thrown the inevitable curve ball.

How Long Does It Take to See Change?

If you are able to eliminate poisons and change your lifestyle and diet, there is no question that you will see change. If your initial imbalances are minor, you can expect change fairly quickly. A month can be enough time. If you are starting out with major imbalance, you can usually expect it will take longer to turn around. There is no set rule, of course. Serious conditions can change surprisingly quickly and mild issues are sometimes very stubborn. I regularly see people with long laundry lists of issues they've suffered for decades, issues that all but fully resolve within three to six months of simple changes in diet and lifestyle. It is so common that I have ceased to be shocked, though I continue to be amazed by the healing power of nature and the simple changes that allow us access to those powers. In general, though, you can expect that the more serious your imbalance and the longer you've had it, the stricter you will need to be about your changes and the longer they will take to achieve.

The Three-Tier Treatment Strategy Revisited

At the beginning of Part II, I outlined the three-tier treatment strategy I recommend. Now that we've been through all the details of a healthy diet, lifestyle, and stress management, I'd like to revisit these principles. Here they are:

1. Make appropriate diet, lifestyle, and stress-reduction changes first.
2. Use natural herbs and remedies when extra support is needed.
3. Use surgery or pharmaceutical drugs, including bioidentical hormones, in an emergency; as a stopgap measure when physical, mental, or emotional symptoms are unbearable; or to manage such symptoms when first-tier and second-tier strategies are insufficient.

THE FIRST TIER

Within the first tier, there are things that you can do on your own and things for which you will want to enlist an Ayurvedic lifestyle and diet counselor. The things that you can do, you will need to include in a daily routine that you adhere to as much as possible. By now you have probably started taking some of the "baby steps" I recommended in Chapter 8. The emphasis there was to start with what's doable. Here I want to give you an assessment of which dietary changes are probably the most important to implement first.

1. Eat mostly organic, whole, minimally refined, and freshly cooked foods. Include a lot of vegetables, grains, beans, some high-quality fats, and dairy (if you can tolerate it). Eat organic and very minimal meat, if you eat it, well cooked in small amounts.
2. Avoid highly processed, refined foods like packaged, prepared foods; white sugar; white flour products like bread, pastries, cookies, cakes, and too much pasta. And all trans fats.
3. Avoid very spicy food.
4. Avoid cold drinks with meals.
5. Eat at the same times every day, when you are hungry and calm.

The next crucial step is to establish a daily routine that includes meals, exercise, spiritual practice, and self-care. This is the hardest step you will have to take. Taking herbs, pills, or bioidentical hormones is easy compared to changing your life, and changing your daily routine amounts to changing your life. Nobody can do this step for you. I find that the best way to gain inspiration to continue to form and practice healthy habits is to continue to educate myself. Ayurveda offers a most elegant approach to individual lifestyle and dietary coaching. You can learn the basics for yourself, using the educational resources listed in Appendix A. You can also consult with an Ayurvedic lifestyle and diet counselor.

After you've practiced your ideal daily routine for a few months, you may find that many of your initial complaints have dissipated and that you have less stress and depression and more energy. If you still have stress in your life, you may need to consult with an Ayurvedic or Traditional Chinese Medicine practitioner, or try therapy, twelve-step programs, meditation retreats, or other supports, but your life will better be able to support those changes. Whatever you do to address stress, it should make you feel more balanced, not less. Minimizing the release of stress hormones prevents them from dominating your hormonal landscape. This is the first crucial element to restore hormonal balance.

If you have an addiction to sugar, alcohol, or tobacco, or habitually use other recreational or pharmaceutical drugs, you may wish to address that only after having practiced your daily routine for a few months. You may find that you are in a more balanced state of physical and mental health at that time and are better able to support these important changes.

If you have uncomfortable symptoms that do not abate, you may need to employ the second-tier treatment strategy while you are learning your routine or even after it has become habitual.

THE SECOND TIER

This strategy calls for the use of herbs and natural remedies. Relying on herbs to provide what we are not able to provide through our lifestyle and diet is okay in moderation and as an intermediate measure until our tier-one measures are able to restore balance. To rely on herbs without making those appropriate changes is not sustainable. Not for us and not for our planet. These days it is not uncommon to find a busy woman ignoring her lifestyle and diet and leaning on supplementation from herbs. Meanwhile, agricultural space the world over is dwindling and suffering from contamination by various pollutants. While Ayurvedic and Chinese herbs are truly boons for an ailing humanity, we cannot expect either India or China to produce remedies for the entire world. They will not be able to supply a growing demand forever. We may eventually need to grow our own herbs and prepare our own medicines locally, in the same way that we are beginning to understand the need for eating locally.

Having said this, there are certainly times that we need these supplements in addition to the first-tier strategy. It often takes a little time to figure out how to reduce the stress in life or to learn appropriate dietary and lifestyle changes to make. Depending on the symptom or condition that you are experiencing, you may experience wonderful results from consulting with a qualified practitioner of Ayurveda or Traditional Chinese Medicine and receiving an herbal prescription. I have listed some remedies in Appendix A; however, it is far preferable to any reference material, to see a practitioner who can consider your individual needs.

Ideally, herbal remedies would be a stopgap measure until your life has been balanced long enough to have regained hormonal balance. I admit this is easier said than done. Sometimes herbs are used for a long time or indefinitely if a woman's history of imbalance is severe, long-standing, or both, and her symptoms have progressed beyond the ability of lifestyle and diet alone to manage.

THE THIRD TIER

Sometimes, someone is working on getting a daily routine in place and has been taking herbs for some time (say, three to six months), yet still experiences significant discomfort related to hormonal imbalance, whether before, during, or after menopause. It is in this sort of situation that the third-tier strategy, bioidentical hormone supplementation, can really do the trick. I still think of this as a stopgap measure that I would lean on only as long as necessary and with the lowest effective dose. If and when diet, lifestyle, and herbs are sufficient to restore and maintain balance, then it will be time to consider gradually removing bioidentical hormone supplements from the mix.

You can contact a local compounding pharmacy and inquire as to who they recommend to work with as an expert to prescribe the ideal combination of bioidentical hormones for you. Often there are at least a few nurse practitioners who specialize in bioidentical hormones. I also recommend reading Dr. John Lee's *What Your Doctor May Not Tell You About Menopause*. This is especially helpful if you are in an area or country where bioidentical hormones are not readily available and you may have to find a source and learn how to effectively use them yourself.

Sometimes this third-tier strategy involves taking another pharmaceutical drug, for either temporary or long-term support. This is between you and your health-care providers to consider, discuss, and decide.

Take-Home Messages from Part III

In this part of the book, we have looked at many, many changes that support hormonal balance and health. We may not be able to incorporate all of them, but we can do what we can. Let's look at a compilation of all the points.

TAKE-HOME MESSAGES ABOUT DIET

Here are the things that you can do to give your body the nourishment it needs.

- Eat meals at regular times every day.
- Eat in a calm, clean environment. If you are upset or distracted, you could eat perfect foods yet not digest them well.
- Eat only when you are hungry. If you never have a true appetite, increase your exercise, especially in the early morning, and take the following remedy a half hour before meals: Thoroughly chew a thin slice of fresh ginger with a pinch of rock salt and a spray of lime juice.
- Eat the right quantity of food. My teacher used to say it is best is to eat one-third the capacity of your stomach, drink one third, and leave one third empty. He also used to say that you should stop eating just one bite before you are really satiated. I've heard that the size of the stomach changes with how much we habitually eat. Rather than get too literal with this advice and try to calculate the actual capacity of the stomach, I like to take the spirit of it. I find it best to eat almost to the point of satisfaction so the digestive fire is never overly taxed.
- Chew your food thoroughly. Take a deep breath and a moment of quiet after swallowing your last bite and before going on to your next activity.
- Eat most foods warm. Cold food is more difficult to digest. If you are going to eat raw or cold food or drinks, it is best to consume them at midday or in hot weather, when the warmth of the atmosphere can support your digestive fire.
- Enjoy drinks at room temperature, warm, or hot. Cold drinks hinder digestive capacity.
- Consume organic foods and drinks whenever possible.
- Eat simple food when life is complicated. The more complicated your physical or emotional life, the more simple your food should be.
- Enjoy mostly whole, freshly cooked foods including cooked grains, beans, vegetables, and some fruit. If you are too thin, favor more nourishing, heavy, dense foods like yams, squashes, stews, some beans, dairy—if you can tolerate it, and whole grains. If you are too heavy, favor more lightening motivating foods like greens, light soups, some spices, some beans, and less grains.
- Enjoy beans, which are about equally nourishing and motivating. They are often difficult to digest if not prepared well. To make them more digestible, soak them in cool water overnight and then cook them until they are mushy, preferably with a piece of kombu and with spices like cumin, coriander or ginger, and a pinch of asafetida (also called *hing*), which aids digestion. When the beans are finished cooking, you can discard the seaweed if you don't like its taste or texture.
- In general, when you eat heavy foods like grains, beans, dairy, or mashed potatoes or squashes, consider adding some turmeric, black pepper, and ginger to them in the cooking process. Cumin, coriander, and fennel are also suitable for most people. Considering that, as you may well be eating grains, legumes, or dairy on a regular basis, you will also be reaping the benefits of these amazing spices.

- Eat a moderate daily amount of organic, non-genetically-engineered soy foods in forms that are easy to digest, like tofu, tempeh, or miso cooked with fresh ginger, or warm, spiced soy milk, provided you're not allergic to soy.
- Be a vegetarian or eat a small amount of organic meat. Be sure it is organic, as any meat concentrates environmental pollutants more than dairy and much more than vegetables and fruits. If you choose to eat meat, consume it in a form that is easily digestible, like a couple of ounces chopped and cooked in a soup.
- Eat lots of veggies.
- Veggie sprouts, especially broccoli sprouts, are packed with vitality. Have two to three tablespoons of broccoli sprouts, daily, if you have access to them and can digest them. If you can't digest them well raw, you can add them to stir-fried veggies, steamed veggies and soups, when they are finished cooking (For kits and supplies to grow your own sprouts, see The Daily Gardener in Appendix A.)
- Eat some dark chocolate daily, if you know you can tolerate it. Having a small square or a piece the size of a truffle, except when you are sick or have poor digestion, probably can't hurt and might be beneficial. Skip it if it gives you migraines, menstrual pain, or any other uncomfortable symptom.
- Drink unrefined or "cloudy" varieties of fruit juice at least three times a week.
- Use extra-virgin olive oil and other cold-pressed, high-quality oils.
- Have somewhere between a couple of teaspoons and a couple of tablespoons of fresh, ground hemp seeds, sesame seeds, or flaxseeds or oil daily. Check with your health-care practitioner to determine the best dosage for you and try to use this fresh on your food, instead of in a capsule. Remember to refrigerate these omega-3 oils and keep them in opaque bottles. Do not heat or cook with these oils.
- Use pots, pans, and utensils made of stainless steel, cast iron, heat-resistant ceramic, glass, and/or wood to avoid toxic chemicals leaching into hot food and liquids.[6]
- Store your food in glass, ceramic, or stainless-steel containers instead of plastic, to avoid estrogenic chemicals leaching into your food.

Here is a list of diet-related things to avoid.

- Foods that cause you to have uncomfortable digestive symptoms. If you have gas, bloating, heartburn, intestinal noise, diarrhea, or constipation, you are not digesting well. You will need to change either what or how you are eating.
- Frozen, canned, or leftover food. It is considered old and harder to digest than freshly cooked foods.
- Refined sugar. There is nothing inherently wrong with the sweet taste. It is nourishing for the body, provided it is associated with naturally sweet foods like apples, yams, grains, or natural sweeteners like raw honey, maple syrup or barley malt, and it is taken in moderation. But refined sugar is highly processed and, like other highly processed foods, comes with nasty side effects. For example, over the past twenty years, the U.S. per capita consumption of sugar has in-

creased from 26 to 135 pounds a year.[7] Not surprisingly, diabetes has increased 70 percent in the past decade alone.[8]

- Cold food. It's harder to digest than warm foods. Some cold food, like ice cream or salad, is okay in the middle of the day or in warm weather, when environmental heat supports your internal digestive fire. This is why we tend to enjoy salads and ice cream more in the summer, and hot chocolate and soups in the winter.
- Cold or carbonated drinks, because they tend to hinder digestive capability
- Raw food (fruits, veggies, salads), especially in the morning and evening. They are okay to have in the middle of the day or in summer.
- Highly processed or fast foods, and products made with refined white flour such as pasta, white bread, cakes, pastries, cookies, and breakfast cereals
- Highly processed or cold forms of soy, like soy isolate powder (especially if it is consumed cold), soy shakes, soy-based fake meats, or soy ice cream. Especially avoid these in the morning, evening, or cold weather, when there is no environmental heat to support the capacity of your digestive fire, as they are difficult to digest. Also avoid them if you have symptoms of estrogen dominance, like uterine fibroids or fibrocystic breasts. If you are not sure, check with your healthcare practitioner.
- Saturated fat and trans fat. Avoid deep-fried food. It is heavy to digest.
- Caffeine, especially in coffee. If you do drink coffee, be sure it is organic. Nonorganic coffee is grown with chemicals that can disturb hormonal balance.
- Alcohol. It interferes with calcium metabolism, healthy breasts, and sound sleep. It is also associated with increased risk of many cancers, including breast cancer.
- Phosphates. They decrease calcium absorption. Foods that contain phosphates include cola, root beer, alcohol, coffee, and meats.
- Nonorganic meat, fish, and dairy. Meat contains the highest concentration of estrogen-like chemicals. The higher on the food chain, the more true this is. Dairy contains lower concentrations than meat, but more than fruits and vegetables.
- Nonorganic food in general, especially if you are pregnant or nursing. The estrogen-like chemicals that go into its production cause hormone-sensitive disorder in the body, and fetuses and infants are especially vulnerable to their damaging effects.
- Freaking out if you have to eat nonorganic food sometimes. The stress of being rigid and fearful may well outweigh the negative effect of a little nonorganic food.
- Eating while anxious, upset, emotional, bored, or distracted. It disturbs digestion.
- Eating on the go. It also disturbs digestion.
- Excessively spicy foods, unless you are positive that you are someone for whom this is a healthy practice
- Heating, eating, or storing food or drink—especially if they are hot—in plastic or Styrofoam containers or plastic "to go" cups, because estrogenic chemicals

may leach into your food and drink. If you have to use plastic containers or lids, be sure your food is at room temperature before covering or storing it.

- Using plastic wrap on your food, especially hot food, for the same reason.

TAKE-HOME MESSAGES ABOUT LIFESTYLE

- Emphasize overall health over symptom management. If you suffer from one of the conditions we explored in Part II, refer to those sections for specific recommendations.
- Have a daily routine. This allows the nervous system to relax. Your routine should incorporate all the important elements of your life. Try to include the most important ones early in the day, before other events of life obstruct your efforts.
- Have an exercise routine that is appropriate for your current condition. Start by learning how to feel qi or *prana*. Then choose a 20-minute daily exercise routine that is good for you. In general, if you are too thin, a gentle stretchy form of yoga, tai chi, qi gong, or other gentle routine is best. If you are too heavy, more vigorous forms of exercise, like strenuous forms of yoga or jogging, are more appropriate. In any case, look to improve or maintain your flexibility so that, at a minimum, if you are sitting on the floor with your legs straight in front of you, you can bend from your hips and touch your toes. In addition to your regular exercise routine, add a brisk 20- to 30-minute outdoor walk outdoors at the same time every day. Outdoor exercise is beneficial to support your internal natural rhythms.
- Include at least a little meditation or quiet contemplation in your daily routine. This allows a minimum of a few minutes a day when you feel free of responsibility. It also affords a sense of communion with yourself and the Divine.
- Do *abhyanga* (warm oil self-massage). This is one of the best ways to calm the nervous system. Calming the nervous system means fewer stress hormones in the bloodstream. Fewer stress hormones mean less demand on yang, which means less draining of yin and, ultimately, better-balanced hormones.
- If you are extra stressed, and have no contraindications, practice some gentle *pranayama* (breathing exercises) daily. Like *abhyanga*, it has a quieting effect on the nervous system, and a balancing effect on the mind and hormones.
- Learn how and when it is okay to cheat on your diet or in your lifestyle habits. As a general rule, cheat only a little and only when you feel healthy and rested. We can least afford to lean on vices when we most want to. In times of stress, we need to eat and live as well as possible.
- Use discipline to achieve balance and then employ awareness to keep it there. Don't trust your cravings until you are balanced and healthy. You may need to consult with an Ayurvedic diet and lifestyle consultant to support you initially, until you are clear about which foods are best for you.
- Educate yourself on your current condition and the appropriate lifestyle and dietary choices for you. I find Ayurveda offers a most elegant approach to learning

these things. I have listed some educational resources in Appendix A. You can also find an Eastern health-care practitioner to guide you with diet and lifestyle choices. Ayurveda and Traditional Chinese Medicine both have excellent diagnostic and therapeutic aspects, but in the United States it is easier to find an experienced TCM practitioner than an experienced Ayurvedic practitioner to address specific maladies. See Appendix A for how to find a practitioner of either TCM or Ayurveda.

- Digest emotions as you do food. Buried, denied, or unprocessed emotions become mental *ama* (toxic sludge) in the same way that undigested food becomes physical *ama*.

- End or improve any toxic or strained relationships, including the relationship with yourself. Do whatever it takes: individual or couples counseling, twelve-step programs, support groups, whatever.

- Eliminate any poisons in your life, to the extent possible. If this means pharmaceutical drugs, first improve your diet and lifestyle, then work with a practitioner of Eastern medicine to address the malady for which you are taking the medications. When you are ready, talk with your prescribing physician to determine if, when, and how you can get off them. If your poisons come from recreational drugs or sugar, look in Appendix A for resources to help heal these addictions. Traditional Chinese Medicine has some very useful tools.

- Respect your body's natural urges. When you are truly hungry, eat. When you are truly thirsty, drink. When you are truly tired, rest. Surrender to the pace and needs of your body.

- Laugh.

- Engage in mentally stimulating but not stressful activities.

- Do less multitasking and give more full attention to one thing at a time.

- Watch less than ten hours of television a week.

- Avoid environmental pollutants like PVC products, BPA, phthalates, and dioxins.

- Avoid organic chemicals that have "chloro" as part of their name, such as chlorophenol weed killers (e.g., 2, 4-D, which is used by some commercial lawn services).

- Have your local waste-collection agency dispose of any insecticides and herbicides you may need to get rid of.

- Don't burn household garbage.

- If you have to be exposed to environmental pollutants, surround yourself or your environment with houseplants like English ivy, gerbera daisies, Madagascar dragon trees, pot chrysanthemums, and variegated snake plants.

- Only put on your skin what you would consider putting in your mouth. Avoid chemical-packed lotions from major department stores.

- Only use cleaning and personal care products that you are sure do not include toxic chemicals in their ingredient lists.

APPENDIX A
RESOURCES

Balanced Life Retreats

Balanced Life retreats are designed to support women throughout the world to practice what is written about in this book, and to learn further about women's health; diet; what smooth, free, easy flow of *prana* feels like; and other selected topics. These retreats include vegetarian meals, good yoga, tai chi, or qi gong, and prime education from world-class instructors, including Dr. Welch. They also include time off, in beautiful, natural settings. See Dr. Claudia Welch's Web site for details (www.drclaudiawelch.com).

Several excellent books, correspondence courses, online beginning courses, and increasingly more Ayurvedic lifestyle and diet consultants are now available to help educate people on their constitutions, how to identify their current conditions, and which exercises and diets will be ideal for them. If you already practice the basics of a healthy lifestyle and diet, then you can refine your choices and programs with further education. This is especially important if you are facing a specific health challenge.

ONLINE INFORMATION ON AYURVEDA AND DR. CLAUDIA WELCH

- Dr. Welch's Web site, www.drclaudiawelch.com, includes Dr. Welch's speaking and Balanced Life retreat schedules, introductory information on Ayurveda, a beginning online course on Ayurveda, recipes, and links to other useful information and resources.
- Banyan Botanicals in the United States, www.banyanbotanicals.com, has online tests to determine your *prakruti* (constitution) and *vikruti* (current condition) along with information on these written by Dr. Welch.

COURSES

Ayurveda

- An in-depth beginning Ayurveda online course by Dr. Claudia Welch is offered through www.drclaudiawelch.com and hosted by www.bigshakti.com. This course covers the fundamental principles of Ayurveda and is an excellent avenue for study if you are not able to dedicate years to in-person programs and want to either add Ayurveda to your existing yoga or health-care practice, or to incorporate it more deeply into your life. It covers the five elements, 20 *gunas*, three *doshas*, six tastes, the doshic subtypes, *agni*, *ama*, Prakriti, Vikriti, and other fundamental Ayurvedic principles.

- A correspondence course on Ayurveda with Dr. Robert Svoboda is available at the Ayurvedic Institute, www.ayurveda.com or 505-291-9698.
- Professional training in Ayurveda is offered at several excellent institutions in the United States, including:

  - American University of Complementary Medicine, Beverly Hills, CA, www.aucm.org/program.asp?ProgId=16.
  - The Ayurvedic Institute, Albuquerque, NM, www.ayurveda.com.
  - California College of Ayurveda, campuses in Northern and Southern California, www.ayurvedacollege.com.
  - Kripalu School of Ayurveda, Lenox, MA, www.kripalu.org/article/351/.
  - Mount Madonna Institute, Watsonville, CA, www.mountmadonna institute.org/ayurveda.

For the most up-to-date information, check the schools and training directory at the National Ayurvedic Medical Association Web site, www.ayurveda-nama.org.

- Professional training in Ayurveda is offered in Great Britain as well. Contact the Ayurvedic Practitioners Association, 23 Green Ridge, Brighton, BN1 5LT, 01273 500 492, www.apa.uk.com, info@apa.uk.com.
- For professional training in Amsterdam, contact the Academy of Ayurvedic Studies, W. G. Plein, 255 1054 SE Amsterdam, 020-840 1887, www.ayurvedicstudies .nl, info@ayurvedicstudies.nl.
- For information on Ayurveda in the Czech Republic, contact Dr. Frej-Ecce Vita, V Luhu 709/7, 14000 Praha 4-Nusle, the Czech Republic, (+420) 272765131, mobile (+420) 603221522, fax (+420) 272760985, www.ayurveda.cz, info @ayurveda.cz.
- For information on Ayurveda in Germany, contact 0049 2652 527756, info@ euroved.com.
- For authentic Ayurvedic education in India, contact:

  - The Ayurvedic Institute. If students complete the first year program in the United States, they can go on to study with Dr. Vasant Lad in India.
  - Jiva Ayurveda, near New Delhi: www.ayurvedic.org.
  - Punarnava. Students of Ayurveda may well find what they are looking for among this group of resources: www.punarnava-ayurveda.com.
- For information on Ayurveda courses in New Zealand, visit http://ayurlab .ayurlab.com.

Traditional Chinese Medicine

- The Accreditation Commission for Acupuncture and Oriental Medicine has a list of accredited schools in the United States; contact www.acaom.org.

- If you are a licensed health-care practitioner, such as an MD, DC, nurse, PT, and so on, and you want to add TCM to your toolbox, you can learn a surprising amount from a 100- to 150-hour program. My husband, Dr. James Ventresca, founded Acupractice Seminars, which trains in the most practical aspects of TCM and has developed a reputation for excellent instructors and friendly schedules. Weekend programs are taught in various locations in the United States. Visit www.acupracticeseminars.com.

PRODUCTS

Ayurvedic Herbal Remedies and Oils

- In the United States:

  - The Ayurvedic Institute (in the United States): 505-291-9698 or www.ayurveda.com. They also have tongue scrapers.
  - Banyan Botanicals: 888-829-5722, www.banyanbotanicals.com. For *bhringraj* oil, general massage oils, online assistance determining your constitution and current condition (*prakruti* and *vikruti*), tongue scrapers, neti pots (also called nasal rinse cups), triphala, and other remedies. Banyan Botanicals is committed to supplying products that are organic and sustainably harvested.
  - Floracopeia, Inc.: 206 Sacramento Street, Ste. 304, Nevada City, CA 95959, www.floracopeia.com. Floracopeia offers high-quality essential oils and promotes sustainable harvesting practices.
  - Organic India: 888-550-8332 or www.organicindiausa.com. This is the company that puts out all those wonderful tulsi teas you see everywhere nowadays. Also committed to organic and sustainably harvested herbs.
  - Sarada Ayurvedic Remedies: 877-541-5836 or www.saradausa.com. For rich, authentic, constitution-appropriate oils.
  - The Vitamin Trader: 800-334-9310 or www.vitamintrader.com. A good source for high-quality, low-cost supplements, including many Ayurvedic and Chinese medicinal formulas.

- In Great Britain: Pukka Herbs: www.pukkaherbs.com. Pukka, like Banyan, is also dedicated to organic and sustainably harvested herbs.

Traditional Chinese Herbs and Remedies

- Traditional Chinese Medicine suppliers often sell their remedies only to licensed practitioners of TCM, but some are available at health food stores or online sources such as Blue Dragon Herbs (www.bluedragonchineseherbs.com), which carries organically grown TCM herbal formulas.

Western Herbal Brands and Products

Look for these products at health food stores or online.

- Lakshmi's Garden, the Natural Place to Cultivate Health. A. Terrel Broussard has a background in Ayurveda, as well as Western herbology. He and his wife, Kim, make these and other products, in small batches, with love:

  - Milk Thistle Tincture. This Western herbal formula can help support liver function, if you've been exposed to environmental toxins and pollutants. Supporting liver function can also support hormonal balance. 413-329-5440 or www.wholebeingtherapy.com.
  - Relax and Recover. A calming formula to help the system counteract the effects of modern stressors.

- The Vitamin Trader: 800-334-9310 or www.vitamintrader.com. Along with many Ayurvedic and Chinese medicinal formulas, the Vitamin Trader also carries Western herbal formulas.

Growing Your Own Greens, Year-Round

- The Daily Gardener, www.thedailygardener.com, will get you started growing your own veggie sprouts at home. Use them in salads, steamed veggies, stir-fried veggies, soups, and more. A total of 10 minutes a day, usually much less, yields affordable, local greens year round, even when feet of snow are covering the ground.

PRACTITIONERS AND COUNSELORS

How to Choose and Use Practitioners of Ayurveda and Traditional Chinese Medicine

There is no legally recognized certification or licensure for Ayurvedic practitioners in the United States. In India, it takes a five- to six-year full-time program to become an entry-level Ayurvedic physician. Although we don't have this in the United States, we do have one- to two-year programs that give an adequate basis of education for their graduating students to help clients understand dietary and lifestyle considerations quite elegantly. Sometimes students of these programs find a way to further their studies beyond these one or two years. They may travel to India to study or find a mentor with whom to continue to develop their skills. Depending on how motivated and dedicated the graduating students are, they may either move on with their life and forget much of what they have learned, or they can apply it regularly and develop further experience.

It is important to ask a prospective Ayurvedic counselor about his or her education, background, and experience. If the counselor's only education is a few seminars, you might want to look for someone with at least a year of in-depth study at one of the schools listed in this section or something comparable. Because you will be coming up with a life and diet plan together, it is also important to feel a good personal connection with the counselor you choose. No matter who you are, what your problem is, or how serious it is, I feel it is of inestimable benefit to address your lifestyle and diet, and I don't know of a better way to do this than with Ayurveda. To address concerns with herbal remedies, look for a practitioner who has studied them beyond a one-year program, either with an extended program or a mentor.

A well-trained practitioner of Traditional Chinese Medicine is equipped to address chronic and acute pain and internal medicine issues. These practitioners mostly use acupuncture, herbs, cupping, *gua sha*, and *moxa* (a heat therapy) as therapies. Having been trained both in Ayurveda and TCM, I find Ayurveda to more elegantly address issues of lifestyle and diet, but TCM to be extremely effective with its main tools of treatment. I have also found that students of TCM usually have more clinical education. In the United States, there are many accredited four-year schools devoted to TCM, and it is a licensed, certified profession in most states, so most of these schools are able to offer significant clinical training to their students. For these reasons, it is usually easier to find a clinically well-trained practitioner of TCM than it is to find a good Ayurvedic counselor. It is wise to make sure your practitioner graduated from an accredited school of TCM, and it is probably best to consider how long the individual has been in practice and whether that practice is thriving.

I feel the ideal situation is to have an Ayurvedic counselor for education about appropriate lifestyle and diet for one's specific constitution and current health concerns, and to also have a relationship with a TCM practitioner. If your Ayurvedic counselor does not have considerable herbal education, I would look to a TCM practitioner for herbal solutions and its other therapies for acute or chronic conditions. If the TCM counselor's dietary and lifestyle advice differs from what your Ayurvedic counselor is telling you, you might need to experiment a bit and find out which works better for you.

How to Find an Ayurvedic
Counselor in the United States

- Ask around. Word-of-mouth recommendations are the best way to find someone good.

- Go to the professional membership listing of the National Ayurvedic Medical Association Web site (www.ayurveda-nama.org) to find someone in your area.

- Call the Ayurvedic school(s) closest to you to see if there is someone in your area. They often have a list of their graduating students and where they practice or know of them.

How to Find an Ayurvedic Counselor Outside the United States

- For Ayurvedic consultations in Great Britain, please contact:

  - Sharon Jackson, Ayurveda Lifestyle, The Barn, High Street, Misterton DN10 4BU, 01427 890833, fax 01427 890977, ayurvedalifestyle.co.uk, sharon@ayurvedalifestyle.co.uk.
  - Rebecca and Sascha Kriese, Ayuseva, 23 Green Ridge, Brighton, BN1 5LT, 01273 500 492, www.ayuseva.com, health@ayuseva.com.
  - Sebastian Pole, MAPA, MRCHM, MURHP, Traditional Herbal Medicine, Ayurveda, Chinese, and Western herbalism, 01225 466944, www.sebastian pole.com, sebastian@pukkaherbs.com.
  - Dr. L. Eduardo Cardona Sanclemente, MSc, Ayurveda (London), PhD, DSc Basic Medical Sciences (France), 128 Camberwell New Road, London SE5 0RS, 44 207 564 4020 or 44 7764 951076.

- For information on Ayurveda in the Czech Republic, contact Dr. Frej-Ecce Vita, V Luhu 709/7, 14000 Praha 4-Nusle, The Czech Republic, (+420) 272765131, mobile (+420) 603221522, fax (+420) 272760985, www.ayurveda.cz, info@ ayurveda.cz.
- For information on Ayurveda in Germany, contact 0049 2652 527756 or info@euroved.com.
- For authentic Ayurvedic treatment in India, contact:

  - www.punarnava-ayurveda.com. Students and seekers of Ayurvedic care at any level may well find what they are looking for among this group of resources.
  - Jiva Ayurveda, near New Delhi, www.ayurvedic.org.

- For information on Ayurveda in New Zealand, visit http://ayurlab.ayurlab.com.

How to Find a Traditional Chinese Medicine Practitioner

- As with Ayurvedic counselors, word-of-mouth is always the best way to find somebody good. Ask around.
- Check the "Find a Practitioner" page on the National Certification Commission for Acupuncture and Oriental Medicine Web site (www.nccaom.org).

Places for Panchakarma *in the United States*

I referred to the practice of *panchakarma* in several chapters of this book, including in Chapter 12. It involves the internal consumption and external application of herbal oils, administration of sweating therapies, specific diets and herbs, and routines in a very careful order, designed to draw out *ama* (toxic material) from deeper tissues and eliminate them from the body. It is a practice that generally requires the patient to undergo treatments for one to four weeks.

If you choose to do *panchakarma,* it is important to find a practitioner very experienced and specifically trained in *panchakarma* techniques and theory. An Ayurvedic lifestyle and diet counselor may be very qualified to counsel on these things but not to provide *panchakarma.* A couple Ayurvedic doctors and I are part of a trust—Satya Ayurveda Trust—that is in the process of creating a Web site, http://satyaayurveda.org, which will list spas that are certified in authentic, safe Ayurvedic treatments. You can check that site or my Web site, www.drclaudiawelch.com, for updated information, though if there is nothing there, you can contact the following sources.

- The Ayurvedic Institute in New Mexico: 505-291-9698 or www.ayurveda.com.
- The Ayurvedic Center of Vermont: 802-872-8898 or www.ayurvedavermont.com.
- Dr. John Douillard's LifeSpa in Colorado: 866-227-9843 or www.lifespa.com.
- Laksmi's Garden in Western Massachusetts, at www.lakshmisgarden.com.

Places for Panchakarma in India

- Kare: www.karehealth.com.
- Poonthottam: www.poonthottam.org.
- Punarnava: www.punarnava-ayurveda.com.
- Other places: http://satyaayurveda.org.

Help in Healing Addictions

- Twelve-step programs. These are programs for all kinds of addictions and situations. It might take a little experimenting to find which resonates most with your nature and needs.
- Radiant Recovery, founded by Dr. Kathleen DesMaisons: www.radiantrecovery.com.
- Eastern practitioners. Ask your Ayurvedic or Traditional Chinese Medicine practitioner to see if they work with addictions. That may be a good place to start. If that is not sufficient, then twelve-step programs and other programs that specialize in addictions may be necessary. If you find you are putting off kicking

whatever it is that you are addicted to for more than three to six months, it is probably time to get extra help.

RECOMMENDED READING

Ayurveda or Yoga

I find that it is possible to read TCM books cover to cover without getting a practical handle on the best way to eat and live, while effort put into learning Ayurveda tends to be amply rewarded. These books and sources are easy read and navigate.

- Nicolai Bachman, *The Language of Ayurveda*. This is a good reference book if you really get into the study of Ayurveda and want to actually pronounce stuff correctly, plus it has a good glossary of Sanskrit terms used in Ayurveda. Contact www.sanskritsounds.com.
- Dr. John Douillard's books, including *Perfect Health for Kids*, North Atlantic Books, 2003, and *Body, Mind and Sport*, Three Rivers Press, 2001.
- Books by Dr. Vasant Lad, including *Ayurveda: The Science of Self-Healing*, Lotus Press, 1984, and *The Complete Book of Ayurvedic Home Remedies*, Three Rivers Press, 1998.
- Timothy McCall, MD, *Yoga As Medicine: The Yogic Prescription for Health and Healing: A Yoga Journal Book*, Bantam Books, 2007.
- Judith H. Morrison, *The Book of Ayurveda: A Holistic Approach to Health and Longevity*, Simon & Schuster, 1995.
- Big Shakti: A source for authentic information on Ayurveda, Tantra and yoga: www.bigshakti.com. Big Shakti currently hosts Dr. Welch's beginning online Ayurveda course.
- Books by Dr. Robert Svoboda, including *Prakriti: Your Ayurvedic Constitution*, Lotus Press, 1998.
- *Ayurveda Today*, a quarterly journal on Ayurveda associated with the Ayurvedic Institute and featuring an article by Dr. Vasant Lad each month: www.ayurveda.com.
- *Light on Ayurveda Journal*, a peer-reviewed journal featuring articles by many current authors: www.loaj.com.

Hormones or Menopause

Educating ourselves about our health concerns, hormones, and changes that menopause brings is beneficial, no matter what age we are, as we will all go through it if we haven't already. Read, talk to your doctors, your complementary health-care providers, local herbalists, and friends who've been where you are or where you are headed. Relating to menopause, I recommend Dr. John Lee's *What Your Doctor May Not Tell You About Menopause* and Dr. Christiane Northrup's

The Wisdom of Menopause, whether or not you are in it, heading imminently toward it, or have it behind you. Understanding this change helps us understand any stage of life we happen to be in. Here are all my recommendations for reading on hormones and/or menopause.

- Natalie Angier, *Woman: An Intimate Geography*, Anchor Books, 2000.
- John R. Lee, MD, with Virginia Hopkins, *What Your Doctor May Not Tell You About Menopause: The Breakthrough Book on Natural Progesterone*, Warner Books, 1996.
- Susan M. Love, MD, with Karen Lindsey, *Dr. Susan Love's Menopause and Hormone Book: Making Informed Choices*, Three Rivers Press, 2003.
- Christiane Northrup, MD, *The Wisdom of Menopause: Creating Physical and Emotional Health and Healing During the Change*, Bantam Books, 2001.

Birth Control Options

- Jane Bennett and Alexandra Pope, *The Pill: Are You Sure It's for You?* Allen & Unwin, 2008.
- Francesca Naish and Jane Bennett's Natural Fertility Management Web site: www.nfmcontraception.com.
- Toni Weschler, MPH, *Taking Charge of Your Fertility: The Definitive Guide to Natural Birth Control, Pregnancy Achievement, and Reproductive Health*, Quill, an imprint of Harper Collins, 2006.

Puberty, for Adolescents

- Shushann Movsessian, *Puberty Girl*, Allen & Unwin, 2004.

Diet and Lifestyle from Contemporary Thinkers and Filmmakers

- Kathleen DesMaisons, *Potatoes Not Prozac*, Simon & Schuster, 2009.
- Michael Pollan, *In Defense of Food*, Penguin, 2008.
- *Vanishing of the Bees*, a full-length documentary, explores the reasons behind the "mysterious" collapse of hives called "colony collapse disorder" and the impact of our food and lifestyle choices on the health of bees. Honeybees are a predominately female society and the film also touches briefly upon the bees and their connection to the feminine aspect of the divine. Covering the global scope of this story in America, Europe, Australia, and Asia, this documentary examines the alarming disappearance of honeybees and the greater meaning it holds about the relationship between mankind and Mother Earth. To learn where you can view this remarkable movie or to host a viewing, go to www.vanishingbees.com.
- Top ten foods to buy organic: Any meat, any dairy, celery, peaches, strawberries, apples, blueberries, spinach, kale, and potatoes. (The Environmental Working Group [EWG] regularly updates their "dirty dozen" list of fruits and veggies with the most pesticide residue, at www.foodnews.org/sneak/EWG-shoppers-guide.pdf.)

Cookbooks and Recipes

- Mollie Katzen, *The New Moosewood Cookbook*, Ten Speed Press, 2004.
- Usha Lad and Dr. Vasant Lad, *Ayurvedic Cooking For Self-Healing*, Ayurvedic Press, 1994.
- Amadea Morningstar with Urmila Desai, *The Ayurvedic Cookbook*, Lotus Light Publications, 1990.
- Check out Anna Sapritsky's recipes at www.ayurvediclight.com. I have personally sampled her cooking and can attest that it is super.
- Check out the "recipes" page on Dr. Welch's Web site, www.drclaudiawelch.com/articlesnpubs/art_recipes.html.

Inspiration for the Spirit and Meditation

- Anything written by any saint.
- Brother Lawrence, *The Practice of the Presence of God*, available from many publishers.
- Books by Pema Chodron.
- Carol L. Flinders, *Enduring Grace, Living Portraits of Seven Women Mystics*.
- *A Short Course in Kindness: A Little Book on the Importance of Love and the Relative Unimportance of Just About Everything Else* by Margot Silk Forrest (who is also the brilliant editor of this book you are holding): www.ashortcourseinkindness.com.
- *Namarupa: Categories of Indian Thought*, a beautiful offering of photography and topics by people grounded in various Indian traditions, available at www.namarupa.org.
- Books by Eckart Tolle.
- The Web sites www.banyanbotanicals.com and www.bigshakti.com both offer relaxation and meditative *pranayama* CDs.

More Information on Environmental Toxins

PVCs or phthalates are used in some toys, inks, hair sprays, nail polish, perfumes, plastic cling film,[1] cosmetics, medical devices, packages, and construction materials such as paints, siding, pipes, and flooring. Construction materials are considered to comprise 75 percent of PVC products. PVC products are often identified with the number 3, the letter V, or the letters PVC inside or underneath the universal recycling triangle. They may also have a distinct odor, as do vinyl shower curtains. For more information:

- The Center for Health, Environment and Justice for general information: www.chej.org.
- Health Care Without Harm, for non-PVC medical devices: www.noharm.org.

- Healthytoys.org, for information on which toys are safer and which are more toxic.
- Visit www.safecosmetics.org.
- Rick Smith and Bruce Lourie, *Slow Death by Rubber Duck*, Alfred A. Knopf, 2009. An informative, well-researched, and—believe it or not—funny and hopeful book on the toxic pollutants in our environment, how they get into us, and what we can do about it. The authors offer a helpful slogan for remembering which plastics are okay and which are dangerous: "4, 5, 1 and 2. All the rest are bad for you."
- Sources for BPA-free baby bottles are listed at www.toxicnation.ca/node/161.

APPENDIX B
AN INTRODUCTION TO AYURVEDA AND TRADITIONAL CHINESE MEDICINE (TCM)

THE HISTORY AND MODERN PRACTICE OF AYURVEDA AND TCM

Ayurveda is to India what TCM is to China. They are both medicinal paradigms complete with the study of anatomy, physiology, diagnostic, and treatment theories, tools, and practice. How old each system is, and which is older, depends on who you ask, but both are thousands of years old. Originally they were oral traditions and, as paper became available and then widespread, they have become sciences that can be studied on one's own or in universities. The entry-level degree for either TCM or Ayurveda, in China or India respectively, is a five- or six-year full-time course.

Today in the United States, many full-time, four-year courses in TCM are offered at accredited colleges, and many states grant licenses to practice it. In New Mexico, for example, the licensee is a doctor of Oriental medicine (DOM), and DOMs are recognized as primary care providers.

Ayurveda has yet to be a licensed profession in the United States, but programs providing an education in this discipline are increasing in number, quality, and hours, and it is not difficult to find graduates of these programs—often called practitioners, consultants, or counselors—that are well qualified at least to counsel people on a diet and lifestyle appropriate for their constitution or current conditions.

WHAT TO EXPECT FROM AN AYURVEDIC OR TCM CONSULTATION

If you were to get a consultation by a practitioner of either TCM or Ayurveda, you could expect a scenario something like this: The practitioner might

- Ask you questions about your main complaint
- Ask you questions about your life, weather, or diet preferences; your habits; your emotional state; and whether you are happy in your life. Some questions might seem unrelated to your main complaint, but your answers will give insight into your constitution, current imbalances, and requirements. This is important because the same complaint can have many possible causes, and treating the cause can have a better long-term result than simply treating a symptom.
- Take your pulse and look at your tongue. These are diagnostic tools that both systems use to ascertain the state of the elemental influences on your constitution,

your organs, systems and even mental or emotional states. These are not essential tools of the trades. Not everyone uses them, but they are very valuable, either as the sole basis of diagnosis, or as adjunct tools.

- If it is within their scope of practice, the practitioner may palpate your abdomen or other parts of your body. Abdominal palpation is a very common practice especially in TCM, to help determine the condition of the elements or organs, depending on the perspective of the individual practitioner.

- When it comes to treatment, most U.S. Ayurvedic practitioners are confined to educating their clients on appropriate lifestyle and diet. This is not an unfortunate limitation, as lifestyle and diet considerations are arguably the two most important factors in health. Some Ayurvedic practitioners have increased scope of practices because they hold licenses in allied fields of health, such as massage therapy, Western medicine, or TCM. Depending on his or her scope of practice, a practitioner of Ayurveda will likely either prescribe, or educate you about, lifestyle and diet changes, including mediation, yoga, *pranayama* (breathing exercises), herbal or other natural remedies, sweating therapies (*swedana*), the internal and external use of oil (*snehana*), or stimulation of acupressure points—called *marma* points in Ayurveda. It is also possible that the practitioner will recommend *panchakarma*, a detoxification program that is beyond the level of training of most Western practitioners but a common practice in India, where the practitioners usually have more extensive training in this process. (I've listed resources for *panchakarma* in Appendix A.)

- A TCM practitioner will likely treat with, recommend, or prescribe acupuncture; moxibustion (heat treatments using *moxa*, a dried herb [*Artemisia chinensis, A. indica*, or, more rarely, *A. vulgaris*] that is molded into many different forms and burned over, or in some cases, directly on, the skin); herbal therapies; or tai chi or qi gong practices. Ayurvedic practitioners often rely more heavily on lifestyle and diet changes than do TCM practitioners, who usually prescribe acupuncture and herbal remedies.

- In either case, don't be surprised if you're given homework such as, "Don't eat spicy foods" or "Eat less processed foods." Your homework could be surprising, such as, "Exercise less." At their best, both systems recognize that imbalance usually arises from inappropriate lifestyle and diet habits and that is where changes need to happen for permanent relief.

Although both systems have similar visions of how the body is organized and functions, it is uncommon to find two practitioners who practice in exactly the same way. This is because it is possible to diagnose and treat individuals using any one of the fundamental principles as a lens through which to view the patient's health. Every lens is valid, but some are more practical for certain purposes.

Here are some of the underlying principles that guide each system.

THE FIVE ELEMENTS

Both Ayurveda and TCM describe the human body as being a microcosm of the macrocosm of the universe. Both describe the building blocks of the universe as five elements. These elements are not like the ones you find in chemistry's table of the elements. Rather, they are five archetypal groups of qualities that have resonance with each other.

In Ayurveda, the five elements are Earth, Water, Fire, Air, and Ether. In TCM they are Earth, Metal, Water, Wood, and Fire. Metal and Wood are not analogous to Air and Ether. Despite each system's five elements being different, however, both systems describe ways those elements interact and form the universe as well as the human body. Although I don't refer to most of these elements directly in this book, there is one exception. We looked at the role of *agni*—the fire element, as it is understood in Ayurveda. It is described as hot, dry, sharp, and light and will have those qualitative effects on the universe or the body.

In the external world, the sun is an example of the expression of *agni*. In the body, *agni* manifests as warmth and the digestive fire that transforms food and drink into a more refined substance that is biologically useful to the body. As we saw in Part III, when *agni* is weak, food is poorly digested and becomes *ama*, or somewhat toxic, biologically useless material in the body that only serves to cause obstruction and create an environment that fosters disease.

While the elements comprise the universe, they also comprise the body. The body organizes them so that they manifest as various tissues, organs, systems, and proclivities. In fact, each human being has his or her own unique proportions of the elements. One person may have more fire element than another, for example, and therefore would tend to be hotter and drier and weigh less than would someone with less fire and more earth. The idea that each individual has a unique constitution allows for more refined diagnostic and treatment strategies than would universal dicta.

In TCM, each element is associated with certain organs and functions in the body. For example, the Lungs are associated with Metal, Kidneys with Water, Liver with Wood, Heart with Fire, and Spleen with Earth. A TCM practitioner, using five-element theory as the primary lens through which he or she views a disorder, might focus on the health of your organs or how your symptoms are related to the elements. When TCM talks about organs, it is not looking at them in the same way that Western medicine does, even when it uses the same names for the organs. Whereas Western medicine will focus on the placement and physical functions of an organ, TCM will look at the associated physical and emotional considerations and will not necessarily limit an organ's placement to its location in the body. It will also consider an energetic pathway related to that organ to be part of it.

Both Ayurveda and TCM associate tastes with elements. They both recognize the sweet, salty, sour, pungent (spicy), and bitter tastes, and Ayurveda considers astringency to be a sixth taste. Both systems have different ways of describing the associations, but use them as a basis upon which to prescribe herbs and constitution-appropriate diets. We talked about tastes, especially the pungent one, a little in Part III.

THE THREE *DOSHAS*, CONSTITUTIONAL TYPES, AND CURRENT IMBALANCES

In Ayurveda, the five elements are associated with three forces or *doshas*: Vata, Pitta, and Kapha. Vata modifies the Air and Ether elements, Pitta the Fire and Water elements and Kapha the Earth and Water elements. The concept of *doshas* is unique to Ayurveda and is often used to describe an individual's unique constitution, called *prakruti*.

For example, a person with a Vata predominant *prakruti* tends to be thin, tall, imaginative; and prefers warm weather. Someone with Pitta predominant *prakruti* tends to have moderate weight; be highly ambitious and bright; and functions better in cool than in hot weather. A Kapha individual tends to be a bit round, loving, solid, and consistent; and prefers dry weather.

Doshic theory is also frequently used to describe someone's current *doshic* condition, called *vikruti*. For example, someone with high Vata would tend to have insomnia, worry, anxiety, and restlessness. High Pitta would exhibit frustration and signs of heat in the body, such as peptic ulcers, migraines, or irritability. Someone with increased Kapha might feel depressed, lethargic, or overweight.

These are just a few possible expressions of the *doshas*, but it would be unwise to jump to conclusions about which type you might be, or what might be out of balance, without quite a bit more investigation. For help determining your natural constitution and which *dosha* might be out of balance, seeing a practitioner in person is the best choice, but you can go to "Don't Know Your Dosha" on the home page, or "Determining Imbalances" under the Ayurveda page, at www .banyanbotanicals.com, at least for initial guidance.

Doshic theory is one lens through which it is possible to understand health and disease, and one that is very popular in Ayurveda today. *Doshic* theory and the idea of individual constitutions are valuable tools for diagnosing, treating, and self-awareness. See Appendix A if you are interested in learning more about them. We do not use the concepts of *doshas* in this book, as the lens of duality was more practical for our purposes.

PRANA OR QI: THE LIFE FORCE

The life force permeates every living thing and every living cell. It enters and enlivens the body at the time of conception and leaves the body at the time of death. It is carried on the breath but is not synonymous with breath. It is called *prana* in Ayurveda and *qi* in TCM, and the two terms are used interchangeably in this book.

We can nourish qi or *prana* with air, food, and drink and can nourish, cultivate, or manipulate it through various breathing techniques or exercises such as qi gong, tai chi, or yoga.

When there is sufficient qi or *prana* in the body, and it circulates smoothly, we are healthy. When there is insufficient qi, it is moving in the wrong direction, or it is constrained or blocked somewhere, then health is compromised. It is very common for a practitioner of either TCM or Ayurveda to consider how best to maintain, replenish, or support a patient's qi or *prana*.

MERIDIANS, CHANNELS, AND POINTS

While each cell in the body requires qi or *prana* to function, TCM theory teaches that there are certain pathways—called meridians—wherein the flow of qi is concentrated, and there are certain points on those pathways where qi naturally tends to gather even more. These pathways are the meridians described in TCM, and their points are called acupuncture points. Twelve of these pathways are related to organs in the body and eight to patterns that were formed in the fetus even before the organs are formed. When qi flows smoothly through the meridians, the associated organs and tissues tend to be healthy. When the flow of qi is diminished or obstructed, ill health is fostered.

Ayurveda also understands *prana* as enlivening every cell, and flowing through channels, called *srotamsi*. These channels incorporate tissues, organs, or systems, and *prana* needs to move smoothly through them to maintain optimal health. One difference between TCM meridians and Ayurvedic channels is that the channels in Ayurveda lay within the body, whereas the meridians of TCM include pathways along the surface of the body. However, Ayurveda does describe points that lay on the surface of the body—called *marma* points—where *prana* collects.

Both acupuncture and *marma* points can be stimulated to affect associated meridians, organs, or channels. TCM uses pressure, needles, magnets, tools, heat therapies, or oils to stimulate acupuncture points. Ayurveda usually uses pressure, heat therapies, or oils.

To learn the meridian, channel, and point theories requires in-depth study. Eastern medicine considers the smooth flow of qi or *prana* through pathways in the body to be of paramount importance in health, and that diminished or obstructed flow contributes to disease.

GUNAS (QUALITIES): LIKE INCREASES LIKE AND YOU CAN TREAT WITH OPPOSITES

Ayurveda explains the elements and *doshas* by their *gunas*, or qualities. We can say for example, that Fire is light, hot, and sharp; Water is cool and heavy; Air is light, dry, and mobile; or that Kapha is stable, heavy, and cool.

"Like increases like" is a fundamental tenet of Ayurveda. Whatever qualities we are exposed to though diet, lifestyle, and environment increase those same qualities in our body and mind. When any quality is unduly increased, it fosters some kind of discomfort.

Treating with opposite qualities means that we can usually treat the increased quality by employing its opposite quality. For example, chills may be an indication of too much cold quality in the body and we would usually treat it by heating up the body with warming herbs, drinks, foods, or environments.

Hot and cold are important qualities that apply not only to the physical temperature of substances such as foods, drinks, or medicines. Hot and cold also describe the inherent nature of a substance and its effect on the body. For example, chile peppers are heating and watermelon is cooling, no matter what their physical temperature. In this book, we call these inherent warming or cooling effects *energetics*.

Ayurveda uses twenty main *gunas* or qualities to describe substances in the universe. These are categorized as ten pairs of opposite qualities that serve to describe the relationship of duality that exists inside and outside of our bodies.

THE RELATIONSHIP OF DUALITY: YIN AND YANG

Ayurveda describes the relationship of duality as ten pairs of *gunas* that represent the relationship between *brmhana* or *santarpana*, which means "building" or "nourishing," and *langhana* or *apatarpana*, which means "reducing," or "lightening." In TCM it is the same relationship, but different language: yin and yang, respectively. For a more in depth look at these relationships, please read Chap-

ter 2, page 13. When we consider disease from the point of view of the five elements or three *doshas*, things can get complicated. Consider how many various
combinations are possible when there are five, or even three factors that interact
in complicated ways. The theory that describes the relationship of duality is a
simpler one we can use to view and understand the world and its affairs.

DIAGNOSIS AND TREATMENT

TCM and Ayurveda both regularly employ any one or more of the various tools
and strategies just detailed, to diagnose or treat their patients or clients. Treatment
is based on diagnosis. We can consider an individual's *prakruti*, *vikruti*, the current
condition of their elements, organs, *doshas*, *prana*, *qi*, meridians, channels, or
qualities. These are all perspectives that require a lot of education to attain pro-
ficiency, and it is worthwhile to either seek further education yourself, or seek
the counsel of health-care practitioners for diagnosing and treating according to
those theories.

In addition to these perspectives, we could also focus on someone's current
conditions and requirements from the point of view of duality, which we explore
in this book.

Whereas TCM practitioners rely heavily on yin and yang theories to guide diagnosis and treatment, the modern practitioner of Ayurveda often favors *doshic*
theory. Different principles work better to describe different phenomenon.
Whereas five element theories may best explain one malady, *doshic* theory may
more elegantly explain another. In this book, we don't talk about five elements
or three *doshas* because we emphasize the role of hormones in women's health
and, when it comes to hormones, no theory is more applicable than the theory
of duality.

APPENDIX C
ABHYANGA,
OR
AYURVEDIC
WARM-OIL MASSAGE

Abhyanga is the anointing of the body with oil. A voluminous amount of oil, often medicated with herbs and usually warm, is massaged into the entire body before bathing. The benefits of *abhyanga*, according to the ancient, classic texts of Ayurveda, are many:

- Imparts softness, strength and color to the body
- Decreases the effects of aging
- Bestows good vision
- Nourishes the body
- Increases longevity
- Regulates sleep patterns
- Benefits skin
- Strengthens the body's tolerance
- Imparts a firmness to the limbs
- Gives tone and vigor to the tissues of the body
- Stimulates the internal organs of the body, including circulation
- Pacifies Vata and Pitta and harmonizes Kapha (the three major constitutions in Ayurveda—see Appendix B)

HOW TO PERFORM *ABHYANGA*

1. Put about ½ cup of oil in an 8-ounce squeeze bottle or heat-resistant glass measuring cup, and place in a pan of hot water until the oil is pleasantly warm. The best kind of oil is one that suits your current condition. For help determining this, you can go to "Determining Imbalances" on the "Ayurveda" page at www.banyanbotanicals.com.
2. Sit or stand comfortably in a warm room on a towel that you don't mind ruining over time with oil accumulation.
3. Use a towel to sit on while you are applying your oil. Use the same towel for this every day. It will get saturated with oil more quickly than will the towel you use to dry off. Make sure you're protected from any wind.
4. Apply all the oil to your entire body.

5. Massage the oil into your entire body, beginning at the extremities and working toward the middle of your body. Use long strokes on your limbs and circular strokes on your joints. Massage your abdomen and chest in broad, clockwise, circular motions. On your abdomen, follow the path of the large intestine; moving up on the right side of the abdomen, then across, then down on the left side. Massage your body for 5 to 20 minutes, with love and patience. The closer you can get to 20 minutes, the better.

6. At least once a week, give a little extra time and attention to massaging the oil into your scalp and feet. Apply oil to the crown of your head and work slowly out from there in circular strokes. Oil applied to the head should be warm but not hot. When you massage your feet, be sure to wash them first when you get in the shower, so you don't slip.

7. Enjoy a warm bath or shower. Don't soap off the oil. Rather, just rinse with water. Special herbal powders, some even as simple as chickpea flour, can be used to remove excess oil from the skin and circumvent the dryness that often accompanies the use of soap.

8. When you get out of the bath, towel dry. Keep a special towel for drying off after *abhyanga* because it will eventually get ruined due to the accumulation of oil.

9. Put on a pair of cotton socks to protect your carpet or flooring from the residual oil on your feet.

10. Enjoy!

WHEN OR HOW NOT TO DO *ABHYANGA*

- Over swollen, painful areas or masses on the body, without the knowledge and consent of your health-care practitioner
- Over infected or broken skin
- When there is high *ama* (toxicity, often indicated by a thick, white coating on the tongue), great physical discomfort, or acute illness. It is best to check with your health-care practitioner to see if you have any contraindications, before practicing *abhyanga*.
- When you have acute fever, chills, or flu
- When you have acute indigestion, or directly after taking emetics or purgatives
- When you have a medical condition, unless your health-care practitioner says it is okay to do *abhyanga*.
- During the menstrual cycle. Some women don't like to stop *abhyanga* during their cycle. If you chose to do it during your cycle, it is best to only apply the oil gently and for only about 5 minutes.
- During pregnancy

LAUNDRY, CLEANING, AND PLUMBING TIPS

Some people eventually stop doing *abhyanga* because they report that their towels or sheets are getting rancid and ruined, their plumbing is getting clogged up, and

their bathtub floor is getting sticky with oil accumulation. Others
to find a way around these problems. One of my patients reported
were getting ruined. I asked her if she'd stopped doing *abhyanga*
She laughed and said, "Hey—ruin my towels or ruin my life? It's

If you'd rather not do either, try these tips:

- Keep one towel for sitting on when you apply the oil and one that you use only
  for drying off after your shower. The first will get ruined the quickest. The second
  will, too, eventually, even with the best laundry techniques.

- I asked Susan, a massage therapist friend, what she does to keep her sheets clean.
  She adds a few tablespoons each of vinegar and baking soda to the hot water,
  once it has filled the washbasin. She told me that this can be a volatile mixture
  when combined and can eat right through the pipes, as well as the oil. When
  added to laundry water, though, the corrosive mixture will have stopped its de-
  structive fizzing action by the time the washer drains. There are also some commercial products that Susan tried, which she read about in *Massage Magazine*.
  They worked, but she didn't care for the smell. If you can't get all the oil out,
  you might plan to replace your sheets or towels about twice a year.

- Although it is ideal to practice *abhyanga* in the morning, some people don't have
  time then and prefer to do it in the evening before bed to calm themselves down.
  If you turn out to be one of these people, wear a "special" set of natural-fiber
  nightclothes for at least an hour after your shower, after your *abhyanga*. They
  will absorb most of the remaining oil on your skin. And, if you got oil in your
  hair, put a towel over your pillow, to protect it.

- Keep a bottle of dish detergent in your shower or tub. When you are done washing, squirt some on the tub or shower floor and spread it around with your feet,
  sort of mopping up the floor. Let the shower flow over it and wash everything
  down the drain. Doing this every time you wash after *abhyanga* prevents an accumulation of oil. If your balance is poor, the shower floor is slippery, or you
  fear you might slip, make sure that you hold on tight to something stable while
  you do this. Or get somebody else to do it or find another way to keep the floor
  clean. Please don't slip and hurt yourself. That would defeat the purpose.

- When you launder oily towels and linens, there is a risk of their catching fire if
  they are too oily or too hot. If a towel is very oily, it's better to throw it away.
  If you dry these fabrics in a dryer, it's better to use low heat. Do not to leave oily
  towels in a hot car. I actually know someone who was laundering a lot of oily
  sheets and towels for a spa, left the hot linens in the hot sun in his car with the
  windows up, and the linens spontaneously combusted, causing fire damage to
  the inside of his car.

- Pour a little environmentally friendly drain cleanser down your drain once a
  month. I have been told that cold water, used with soap that can dissolve in cold
  water, causes the oil to bead up and wash along the drain better than does hot
  water, which makes it stay liquefied and stick to the plumbing. I have not tried
  this, but it is worth investigation.

APPENDIX D
HOW TO MAKE *KITCHERI* AND GHEE

KITCHERI

In Ayurveda, the things that we ingest are divided into three categories: poison, neutral, and medicine. *Poison* is defined as anything that hinders digestion. *Neutral* is anything we ingest that gives support and nourishment without either aiding or hindering the digestive process. *Medicine* is anything we ingest that aids the digestive process.

Kitcheri, a dish of moderately spiced beans and rice, is a unique food because it fits both the neutral and medicinal categories. It not only provides nourishment for the body but, due to its spice combination, it also benefits digestion. This makes *kitcheri* a food of choice for times of stress on the body, such as during a change of seasons, periods of overwork, or illness. It is a particularly good choice of food for a monodiet—a fast on a single food. For example, if you feel like cleansing or giving your digestive system a little break from its usual workout, it can be helpful to take one day a week to eat just *kitcheri* provided you are not engaging in strenuous physical activity and you decide with your health-care practitioners that a monodiet fast is advisable for you.

There are variations to the basic *kitcheri* recipe. The following recipe is a basic and easy one to start with and is usually balancing for everyone.

**INGREDIENTS (USUALLY AVAILABLE AT
HEALTH FOOD STORES OR EAST INDIAN GROCERIES)**

2 TO 3 TABLESPOONS GHEE (RECIPE FOLLOWS)
$\frac{1}{2}$ TEASPOON BLACK MUSTARD SEEDS
$\frac{1}{2}$ TEASPOON CUMIN SEEDS
$\frac{1}{2}$ CUP SPLIT YELLOW MUNG DAL BEANS, RINSED WELL,
    SOAKED OVERNIGHT, AND DRAINED (SEE NOTE)
1 SMALL PINCH OF ASAFETIDA POWDER
1 TEASPOON TURMERIC
1 TEASPOON ROCK SALT
1 CUP ORGANIC WHITE BASMATI RICE, RINSED WELL
    AND DRAINED.
4$\frac{1}{2}$ CUPS WATER IF USING A PRESSURE COOKER, OR
    ABOUT 6 CUPS IF USING A REGULAR POT
1 TEASPOON GROUND CUMIN
1 TEASPOON GROUND CORIANDER
4 TO 5 THIN SLICES FRESH GINGER

Using either a pressure cooker (much faster) or a heavy-bottomed pot, heat the ghee over
    medium heat. Ghee burns easily, so be careful. Sauté the mustard and cumin seeds in the
    ghee until the seeds pop. Add the drained mung dal, asafetida, turmeric, and salt. Stir until
    the mixture starts to stick to the bottom of the pan. Add the rice, water, cumin, coriander,
    and ginger. Stir well, making sure nothing is sticking to the bottom.
If you are using a pressure cooker, fasten the lid and turn the heat to high, letting full pressure
    build up. Once the pressure has built up, turn the heat to low and let cook for 5 minutes.
    Then take the cooker off the heat and let sit until there is no more pressure and you
    can safely open the lid.
If you're using a regular pot, cover and bring it to a boil over high heat, then turn the heat
    down and let it simmer until both the rice and dal are mushy, about 30 minutes.
You may have to experiment with how much water you use to find a consistency you like.
    Clearly, the more water, the thinner the consistency. A thinner consistency is preferable
    if your digestion is weak. You will notice that *kitcheri* will thicken quite a lot when it cools
    and you may need more water than you think.
Serve *kitcheri* hot. Garnish with fresh cilantro, coconut, and lime.
To provide the best quality of energy to your body, *kitcheri* should be made the day that you
    plan to eat it.

NOTE: IT IS BEST TO USE MUNG DAL WITH THE HULLS STILL ON IF YOU TEND TOWARD CONSTIPATION.

Serves 6

GHEE

Heat one pound of unsalted organic butter over low heat in a heavy-bottomed pot. Do not
    stir the butter at all during this whole process. The butter will begin to simmer and will
    make a little crackling noise. After 15 to 20 minutes, there will be a thin covering on the
    top and a thicker, curdlike sediment stuck to the bottom of the pot. At this point you
    need to watch the ghee very carefully so it doesn't burn. When the crackling sound has
    almost entirely stopped, the butter is a completely clear, beautiful golden color through
    to the bottom, and there are only a few air bubbles on the surface, the ghee is done. Let
    it cool for an hour and strain it carefully while it is still liquid into a clean glass container.
    Be sure that the sediment at the bottom of the pan remains there; it contains the impu-
    rities from the butter and can be discarded. The foamy layer on top of the ghee is fine.
    Ghee can be kept at room temperature or refrigerated for a long time, even months.
    Just smell it if you're not sure if it's still good. If it smells rancid, it should not be eaten.

If you don't feel like making ghee, you can buy it at most health food stores
or East Indian grocery stores. I recommend avoiding vegan products that are designed to have a butter or gheelike consistency. They do not carry the same benefits and may be more difficult to digest and assimilate.

APPENDIX E
CASTOR OIL PACKS
FOR UTERINE HEALTH

I have found this to be a wonderful remedy for moving stagnant energy and blood in the uterus and helping to restore normal periods, if done according to these guidelines and under the supervision of a health-care practitioner.

GENERAL DIRECTIONS

Purchase the castor oil and wool flannel castor "pack" from the Ayurvedic Institute (505-291-9698), online or from a health food store.

Fold the flannel into a shape that is good for the area you will be using it on. For menstrual-related disorders, this is the area between the belly button and the pubic bone and five to six inches to each side of the belly button. Warm the castor oil. Massage some into the area the pack will be covering. Pour some on one side of the flannel pack. It does not need to be dripping with oil, just moistened. Place the pack, oil side down, on the whole area. Put a plastic bag large enough to cover it over the pack, to protect your towels and clothes from the oil. Put a hot water bottle on the pack, to keep it warm. Place a folded towel over this. Leave the pack on for 90 minutes.

HOW OFTEN TO USE IT

Check with your health-care practitioner. For patients with severe pain and stagnation in the uterus, I would often prescribe castor packs daily for thirty to sixty days, except during a woman's period—or any time when she is bleeding—to bring maximum benefit. If the situation was a little less severe, I would recommend three days a week, except during the period, for thirty days.

In either case, after the thirty to ninety days, reduce the frequency of the packs to one to three time a week for one to three months, depending on how stubborn the symptoms remain or how much they improve. Then reduce the frequency again, to once a week for one to three months, and then to twice a month as needed.

WARNING AND IMPORTANT NOTE

Do not use castor oil packs during your period, an acute illness, or if you are pregnant.

After beginning to use castor oil packs, it is *very* common for the first menstrual cycle—or possibly two—to be quite a bit heavier and/or more painful. Subsequent cycles should be more regular and far less painful than before beginning the castor packs. Eastern medicine explains this as stagnation clearing from the uterus.

APPENDIX F
FOOD GLOSSARY

Asafetida (also called by its Hindi name, *hing*): A strong-smelling, heating, pungent spice common in Indian cooking. Usually only a pinch is used, but is said to support easier digestion of beans.

Hing: See *Asafetida*.

Honey: A natural sweetener made by bees. Golden honeys tend to have a warming energetic and the whiter varieties (more rare in the United States) tend to have a more neutral or even cooling energetic. Ayurveda teaches not to cook or bake with honey, so maple syrup or organic cane sugar might be better choices for those purposes. There is honey made from local bees and honey processed by large industrial plants. Local bees generally get treated better, and are less likely to suffer from disease and hive collapse (see the excellent documentary, *The Vanishing of the Bees*, to understand the story. Go to www.vanishingbees.com.) As an added benefit, people with allergies often find some relief using local honey or taking a small amount of local bee pollen.

Kombu: A seaweed that comes in strips. It is not pleasant to eat plain, but is used to support healthy digestion of beans, or to add trace minerals to soups, stews, or casseroles. Generally one or two sticks are cooked with the beans or other foods and then are pulled out and discarded after the food is finished cooking.

Maple syrup: A natural sweetener that comes from boiling down the sap from maple trees. It is considered to have a slightly cooling energetic.

Miso: A fermented soybean paste used primarily as a kind of a soup stock. It is best to add it instead of salt, to taste, after the soup has been made. Do not boil miso, as that destroys some of its beneficial qualities.

Mung dal: A type of bean that is commonly used in Indian cooking, said to be easier to digest than most beans. It comes split or whole and with or without the husk. In general, if you lean toward constipation, it is better to use mung dal that still has its hull. Split mung dal cooks faster.

Natural sweeteners: Raw honey, organic cane sugar, sucanat, date sugar, gur (an unrefined sugar from sugar cane that is common in India), coconut sugar, maple syrup that has no added corn syrup or other ingredients (look for pure maple syrup). I tend to avoid agave syrup and stevia, as they are more processed, or, as in the case of stevia, it packs more of the sweet taste into a very small amount, than our bodies may have evolved to deal with efficiently.

Seitan: This is wheat gluten. It is made by washing dough until all the starch is left and then the remaining gluten is usually cooked with spices. It is considered nourishing and yin-building. It may be difficult to tolerate if you have difficulty digesting wheat or gluten.

Soy sauce: A salty liquid condiment made from fermented soy beans and sometimes with the addition of other grains as well. It can be used in place of salt. I use it interchangeably with tamari (see below).

Spices: Common spices for savory food include turmeric (which gives curry its classic yellow color), cumin, coriander, paprika, and black pepper. Common spices for dessert foods: cinnamon, cloves, cardamom, mace, nutmeg, and saffron.

Tahini: A paste made from ground sesame seeds. It can be made from the roasted seeds, which give it a nuttier taste, or from raw seeds, which makes the final product a little thinner.

Tamari: A salty liquid condiment made from fermented soy beans and sometimes with the addition of other grains as well (if you cannot tolerate wheat or gluten, read the ingredients label carefully). It can be used in place of salt. I use it interchangeably with soy sauce (see above).

Tempeh: A dense patty made of fermented soybeans. Can be sliced and fried for sandwiches, added to soups, fried or baked, and eaten as the protein in a meal.

Tofu: Made from soy milk made from soybeans, tofu usually comes in cakes. It can be made in a process that involves fermentation or not. It is used widely in savory as well as sweet dishes.

Whole grains: These are entire or cracked grains that are not polished or processed beyond taking the hulls off them. Some common examples: any variety of brown rice, quinoa, millet, buckwheat, barley, bulgur.

ACKNOWLEDGMENTS

My spiritual father, grandfather, and great-grandfather.

My husband, Dr. Jim Ventresca, for letting me write (often instead of banging nails), for believing I would eventually finish this book and it would be good, for his infallible support and tremendous heart, for his trusting, constant, and fun partnership and incredible love. I am a deeply fortunate woman.

Dr. Kathleen DesMaisons, for encouragement and direction when I first mentioned this book to her about a decade before completing it, for her comments on the various stages of the book, and for helping bring it to fruition through connecting me to Margot Silk Forrest.

Margot Silk Forrest, for her incredibly skillful, familiar, and heartfelt editing. There were more than a few times when I had tears of gratitude for her. I truly get why everybody acknowledges their editors so effusively. She threw me lifelines. When I felt writing to be a forced march, she marched next to me and pointed out charming distractions along the way. Incredible talent. And such kindness.

Merloyd Lawrence, who took time for an unknown author.

Renée Sedliar, executive editor at Da Capo for her enthusiastic advocacy of this book, her skilled editing suggestions, and her kindness. (Does kindness run in editors, or did I just majorly luck out?)

For everyone at Da Capo for betting on the new kid.

For Dr. Robert Svoboda, beloved mentor, champion, friend.

For my other dear mentors, family and friends, all who have demonstrated to me that there is more than one way to live a life. Millie P., Russell P., Judith P., Amy S., Nina G., Dr. Vasant Lad, Hart De Fouw, Om Prakash Sharma.

For the incredible insight of the many practitioners and writers dedicated to women's health, including Dr. Christiane Northrup, Natalie Angier, Gina Kolata, Toni Weschler, MPH, Dr. John Lee, and others, all of whose shoulders must be sore from the rest of us standing on them.

For our chat fests around health and for contributing to the heart health information: cardiologist, Dr. Jane Schauer.

For fact checking or commenting on various parts of the book: Dr. Premal Patel, Dr. Ranjan Shah, Dr. Eric Bachman. For Dr. David Williams, for helping me get my mind around numbers in general and in the NIH/WHI study specifically and being available for other questions along the way.

For their transcription skills, lessons, encouragement, or support along the way: Joyce DeForge, Pat Pritchett (may he rest in joyful, productive peace), Professor Robert E. Gussner (Swami Anand Jina), Dr. Larry Dossey, Virendra Singh and his beautiful family, Ramu Pandit, and Vagish Shastri. Patty McKinnon (from whom I stole many meals, and the term "take-home messages"), Wynn Werner, Catherine and Scott Cote, Usha Lad, Joseph Goldfedder, LAc, Aparna and Manjit Kailey, Dr. Pranav and Yesu Lad, Kevin Casey, Tammy Van Eycke, Ellie and Ron Hadsall, Sue Galaviz, Laura Humphreys, the staff at the Ayurvedic Institute, Dr. Sharon and Simon Jackson, Anna Sapritsky, Easter Bonnifield, Traci Olsen, Denise Baron, Nick Lawrence, Zia O'Hara, Jim and Nancy Grundy, Kristen Rae Stevens, Brian McDonald, Virginia Shilson, Professor Fred Smith, Sharon Scaltrito, Judith Morrison, Bea Doyle, Dr. Susan Sandage, Aletha De Fouw, Dr. Ramkumar Kutty, Sarada Vonn Sonn, Rose Baudin, Leela, Dr. Scott and Chandra Blossom, Thomas and Bianca Hughes, John Baudoux, Kent Bicknell, Don and Charlotte Macken, Dr. Swami Shankardev Saraswati, Jayne Stevenson, Dr. Bryan and Katie Flamm, Dr. Tansy Briggs, Joanne Marie, Shamaz and Dominique, Zhander and Emma, Deepak Singh, Jon and Ann Sairs, Swami Shivananda, Robert Moses, Eddie Stern, Hilary Garivaltis, Prashanti de Jager, Dr. Drea Brown, Bette Timm, Nicolai Bachman, Dr. Joseph Goldfedder, Sensei Dr. James Cornfield, Dr. Eduardo Cardona-Sanclamente, Rebecca and Sascha Kriese, Sebastian Pole, Dr. Cate and Eric Chason, Beecher Grogan, Ben Hewitt, Les and Lil Griffiths, Elia Davis, Dr. Peter Wong, Dr. Will Peplinski, Dr. Renee Rossi, Cecilia Biglieri, Purvi Bhatt, Melissa Di Rito, Kim Giunta, Lexie Neonakis, Melissa Camacho, Carmon Maron, Parul Thakkar, Sneha Shah, Sneha Raichada, the other Bharatiya Behens, Kathleen O'Connor, Coen Van Der Kroon, Rolf Jost, Alessandra Franceschetto, Lynn Weinberger, Russell Weinberger, Loretta Barrett, Nick Mullendore, Annie Lenth, Iris Bass, Neville Bedford, Dr. Timothy McCall, Alexandra Pope, Jane Bennet, Duncan Hulin, Dr. Martina Ziskova and Monika, Dr. John Douillard, Dr. David Frej, and the students of the Ayurvedic Institute and Kripalu School of Ayurveda. And for Kumar Batra, may he rest in sweet peace.

For my patients, who have taught me so much and have shared their hearts and lives with me.

I like to write in cafés, especially when I get stuck. A few cafés, and their staff, were especially hospitable and didn't charge me rent: Coffee at Dawn in Tijeras, New Mexico, and the Shipwreck Café in Naufrage, Prince Edward Island.

For my family. My father and Gail, for their love, helping me get this book edited, and for their invaluable support throughout my life. My mother, for her love, feeding me whole foods, and having spiritual books and visitors from various traditions around the house when I was a child. My mother-in-law, Mildred Ventresca, for welcoming me into her heart as a daughter and friend, and being the loving matriarch of a beautiful family. Charlie Ventresca, for bestowing kindness on everyone around him, and instilling this kindness in his children. For Anne Lynn, Peter and Debbie Burke, Greg and Suzue Worth, Catherine Lowther, Bruce Lowther, Sarah Lowther. For my beautiful, talented, heartfelt, and wholehearted (if not full-blooded) siblings: Paula, Jenny M., Samantha, Elanor, Greta, Brodie, Michael, Casey, Aviva, Zia, Jenny B, Jody, Maria, Chris, Sean, Troy, Mark, Trevor, Dave, and Jacob. For Graham, Yasha, Ben, Gus, Charan Jyot, Emerson, Aidan, Eli, and Angus. For my siblings-in-law and their kids, all of whom have given me such joy and the fantastic experience of being part of a loving, good-natured, Italian family: Bob, Nick, Shelly, Patti, Paul, Dr. Chuck, Janice, Frankie, David, Jason, and Danny. The girls, too, to whom this book is dedicated.

NOTES

CHAPTER 1   THE STRESS EPIDEMIC

1. Alessandra Stanley, "The New Modern Woman, Ambitious and Feeble," *New York Times*, May 5, 2007.

2. Jason Lazarou, MSc; Bruce H. Pomeranz, MD, PhD; and Paul N. Corey, PhD, "Incidence of Adverse Drug Reactions in Hospitalized Patients: A Meta-analysis of Prospective Studies," *Journal of the American Medical Association* 279 (1998): 1200–1205.

3. In Ayurvedic medicine, the terms *santarpana* and *brmhana* mean "nourishing" or "building" and correlate with yin. *Apatarpana* and *langhana* mean "reducing" or "lightening" and correlate with yang.

4. Deepak Chopra, Dean Ornish, Rustum Roy, and Andrew Weil, "'Alternative' Medicine Is Mainstream: The Evidence Is Mounting That Diet and Lifestyle Are the Best Cures for Our Worst Afflictions," Opinion, *Wall Street Journal*, January 9, 2009.

CHAPTER 2   HORMONES: AMBASSADORS OF YIN AND YANG

1. Denise Gellene, "Is That a Hot Cup of Coffee or Are You Just Glad to See Me?" *Los Angeles Times*, October 24, 2008.

CHAPTER 3   SEX HORMONES: THE AMBASSADORS OF YIN

1. A. V. Sluijmer, M. J. Heineman, F. H. De Jong, and J. L. Evers, "Endocrine Activity of the Postmenopausal Ovary: The Effects of Pituitary Down-Regulation and Oophorectomy," *Journal of Clinical Endocrinology and Metabolism* 80 (1995): 2163–67.

2. Natalie Angier, *Woman: An Intimate Geography* (New York: Anchor Books, 2000), 204.

3. Jane Bennett and Alexandra Pope, *The Pill: Are You Sure It's for You?* (Crows Nest, NSW: Allen and Unwin. 2008), 121.

4. Ibid., 63.

5. John R. Lee, MD, with Virginia Hopkins, *What Your Doctor May Not Tell You About Menopause: The Breakthrough Book on Natural Progesterone* (New York: Warner Books, 1996), 155.

6. Ibid., 40–41, 68.

7. Ibid., 34.

CHAPTER 4   STRESS HORMONES: THE AMBASSADORS OF YANG

1. Christiane Northrup, MD, *The Wisdom of Menopause: Creating Physical and Emotional Health and Healing During the Change*.(New York: Bantam Books, 2001), 62.

2. C. M. E., Abdurrahman Altindag, MD; Ozlem Altindag, MD; Mehmet Asoglu, MD; et al., "Major Depression (Stress) a Risk Factor for Osteopenia in Premenopausal Women: Relation of Cortisol Levels and Bone Mineral Density Among Premenopausal Women with Major Depression," *International Journal of Clinical Practice* 61, no. 3 (2007): 416–20.

3. Ibid.

4. *The John R. Lee, M.D. Medical Letter*, March 2003, 3.

5. I. Michael Borkin, NMD, "Women's Hormones 101," *Alternative Medicine*, September 2000, 72.

6. *The John R. Lee, M.D. Medical Letter*, 5.

7. Ibid., 6.

8. Ibid., 3.

9. Ibid., 6.

10. Gale Berkowitz, "UCLA Study on Friendship Among Women: An Alternative to Fight or Flight" (2002). *Current Psychiatry Report* 4, no. 6 (December 2002): 441-48.

11. A. Frasch, T. Zetzsche, A. Steiger, and G. F. Jirikowski, "Reduction of Plasma Oxytocin Levels in Patients Suffering from Major Depression," *Advances in Experimental Medicine and Biology* 395 (1995): 257–58.

12. L. Torner, N. Toschi, G. Nava, et al., "Increased Hy-Pothalamic Expression of Prolactin in Lactation: Involvement in Behavioural and Neuroendocrine Stress Responses," *European Journal of Neuroscience* 15 (2002): 1381–89.

CHAPTER 5   UNDERSTANDING HOW YIN AND YANG HORMONES INTERACT

1. R. E. Nisbett, K. Peng, I. Choi, and A. Norenzayan, "Culture and Systems of Thought: Holistic versus Analytic Cognition," *Psychological Review* (2001): 291–310.

2. I. Michael Borkin, NMD, "Women's Hormones 101," *Alternative Medicine* (September 2000): 70.

3. Ibid., 77.

4. Ibid., 67.

CHAPTER 6   WHY NOT JUST TAKE HRT/SYNTHETIC OR BIOIDENTICAL HORMONES?

1. Gina Kolata, "Menopause Without Pills: Rethinking Hot Flashes," *New York Times*, November 10, 2002.

2. Jane Bennett and Alexandra Pope, *The Pill: Are You Sure It's for You?* (Crows Nest, NSW: Allen and Unwin, 2008), 52–53.

3. A woman needs to take the pill exactly according to its instructions, or it is not as effective as most assume it is, and there are plenty of women who stray from exact compliance.

4. Carolyn J. Crandall, MD, MS; Aaron K. Aragaki, MS; Rowan T. Chlebowski, MD, PhD; et al., "New-Onset Breast Tenderness After Initiation of Estrogen Plus Progestin Therapy and Breast Cancer Risk," *Archives of Internal Medicine* 169, no. 18 (2009): 1684–91.

CHAPTER 9   MENSTRUATION

1. Natalie Angier, "Radical New View of Role of Menstruation," *New York Times*, September 21, 1993.

2. Ibid.

3. Ibid.

4. Joanna Colwell, "Re-Examining Breast Health," *Yoga Journal*, September–October 2001.

5. Devra Lee Davis and H. Leon Bradlow, "Can Environmental Estrogens Cause Breast Cancer?" *Scientific American*, October 1995, 167.

6. Malcolm Gladwell, "John Rock's Error," *New Yorker*, March 13, 2000.

7. Dr. Stephen T. Chang, *The Complete System of Self Healing: Internal Exercises* (London: Tao Publishing, 1986), 94.

CHAPTER 10   MENSTRUAL DIFFICULTIES

1. Dan Lewerenz, "Diet May Disrupt Menstrual Cycle," Compuserve News service, March 3, 2002.

2. Ibid.

3. Ronald A. Chez, MD, "Etiology and Treatment of Uterine Fibroids" *Alternative Therapies* 8, no. 2 (March–April 2002).

4. Amy Zintl, "New Treatments for Fibroids," *Ladies' Home Journal*, November 2001.

5. Ibid.

6. I. Michael Borkin, NMD, "Women's Hormones 101" *Alternative Medicine*, September 2000, 67–79.

7. *The John R. Lee, M.D. Medical Letter*, March 2000, 7.

8. Vicki Hufnagel, MD, with Susan Golant, *No More Hysterectomies*, rev. ed. (New York: Plume Books, 1989).

9. Zintl, "New Treatments."

10. Natalie Angier, "Finally, the Spleen Gets Some Respect," *New York Times*, August 3, 2009.

11. Sharon Begley, "The Estrogen Complex," *Newsweek*, March 21, 1994, 77.

12. Nina Martin, "Fertility?" *Organic Style*, May–June 2003.

13. Chez, "Etiology."

14. http://findarticles.com/p/articles/mi_m0ISW/is_259-260/ai_n10299307/.

CHAPTER 11   BIRTH CONTROL

1. Gail Collins, "What Every Girl Should Know About Birth Control," *New York Times*, May 7, 2010.

2. www.toronto.net/directory/0XD9.html.

3. Associated Press, "Hormone-Taking Is Linked to Dementia," May 2003; *Journal of the American Medical Association*, http://jama.ama-assn.org; Women's Health Initiative, www.whi.org.

4. Nancy Gibbs, "Love, Sex, Freedom and the Paradox of the Pill," *Time*, May 3, 2010, 42.

5. W. D. Mosher, G. M. Martinez, A. Chandra, et al., "Use of Contraception and Use of Family Planning Services in the United States, 1982–2002," advance data from Vital and Health Statistics, no. 350, National Center for Health Statistics (2004).

6. Gina Kolata, "Menopause Without Pills: Rethinking Hot Flashes," *New York Times*, November 10, 2002.

7. *The John R. Lee, M.D. Medical Letter*, May 2000, 7.

8. Jane Bennett and Alexandra Pope, *The Pill: Are You Sure It's for You?* (Crows Nest, NSW: Allen and Unwin, 2008), 45.

9. Ibid., 52–53.

10. *The Lancet* 347 (June 22, 1996): 1713–27.

11. Bennett and Pope, *The Pill*, 52–53.

12. Jane E. Brody, "Hunt for Heart Disease Tracks a New Suspect," *New York Times*, January 6, 2004.

13. Daniel Q. Haney, "Inflammation Triggers Heart Attacks," *Wisconsin State Journal*, August 04, 2002.

14. *The John R. Lee, M.D. Medical Letter*, December 2001.

15. *The John R. Lee, M.D. Medical Letter*, September–October 2001, 4; *American Journal of Obstetrics and Gynecology* 185 (2001): 380–85; *Medicine and Science in Sports and Exercise* 33 (2001): 873–80.

16. Ernst Rietzschel and Jennifer Mieres, "Oral Contraceptive Use: More Carotid and Femoral Atheroschlerosis Later in Life," November 6, 2007, news briefing at American Heart Association Scientific Sessions, Orlando, Florida, as reported in *New England Journal of Medicine* (2007): 357.

17. Bennett and Pope, *The Pill*, 11.

18. Natalie Angier, "Radical New View of Role of Menstruation," *New York Times*, September 21, 1993.

19. Bennett and Pope, *The Pill*, 281; Sherrill Sellman, *Mothers, Prevent Your Daughters from Getting Breast Cancer* (Tulsa, OK: Get Well, 2003).

20. BBC News, http://news.bbc.co.uk/go/pr/fr/-/1/hi/health/3414021.stm, published January 20, 2004.

CHAPTER 12   FERTILITY AND CONCEPTION: THE FOUR CRUCIAL ELEMENTS

1. Stephen S. Hall, "The Good Egg: Determining When Life Begins Is Complicated by a Process That Unfolds Months Before a Sperm Meets an Egg," *Discover*, May 2004, 30–36.

2. Ibid., 37.

3. Jane Bennett and Alexandra Pope, *The Pill: Are You Sure It's for You?* (Crows Nest, NSW: Allen and Unwin, 2008), 45.

4. Sherrill Sellman, *Mothers Prevent Your Daughters from Getting Breast Cancer* (Tulsa, OK: GetWell International, 2003), 141.

5. Claudia Kalb, "Should You Have Your Baby Now?" *Newsweek*, August 13, 2001.

6. Ann Pappert, "What Price Pregnancy? A Special Report on the Fertility Industry," *Ms.*, June–July 2000.

7. Ibid.

8. Hall, "The Good Egg," 38.

9. Ibid., 39.

10. Rebecca Mead, "Eggs For Sale: Wanted: Highly Accomplished Young Women Willing to Undergo Risky, Painful Medical Procedure for Very Large Sums," *New Yorker*, August 9, 1999.

11. Ibid.

12. Ibid.

13. Todd Dvorak, "Doctors Marvel at Tiny Transplant Survivor," Associated Press, April 15, 2004.

14. Pappert, "What Price Pregnancy?"

15. Ibid.

16. BBC News, "Smoking 'Cuts IVF Success Rate,'" April 7, 2005.

17. BBC News, "Chemicals May Damage Male Babies," May 27, 2005.

18. BBC News, "Concerns over 'Female Chemicals,'" May 3, 2005.

19. Ibid.

20. Sharon Begley, "The Estrogen Complex," *Newsweek*, March 21, 1994, 76.

21. Ibid.

22. Associated Press, "Pollution Alters DNA in Mice, Study Finds," *New York Times*, May 18, 2004.

23. Ibid.

24. BBC News, "Passive Smoke Link to Miscarriage," May 12, 2004.

25. Sandra Blakeslee, "Serious Riders, Your Bicycle Seat May Affect Your Love Life," *New York Times*, October 4, 2005.

26. Jorge E. Chavarro, MD; Walter C. Willett, MD; and Patrick J. Skerrett, "Fat, Carbs, and the Science of Conception," *Newsweek*, December 10, 2007.

27. Ibid.

28. Ibid.

29. Emma M. Frans, Sven Sandin, Abraham Reichenberg, et al. "Advancing Paternal Age and Bipolar Disorder," *Archives of General Psychiatry* 65, no. 9 (September 2008): 1034–1040.

30. Nicholas Bakalar, "Bipolar Disorder Tied to Age of Fathers," *New York Times*, September 8, 2008.

31. Mariko Thompson "Pregnant Pauses: More Women Are Trying Special Treatments to Boost Biology," Comcast online news service, August 5, 2002.

32. Claudia Kalb, "Should You Have Your Baby Now?" *Newsweek*, August 13, 2001.

33. Thompson, "Pregnant Pauses."

34. BBC News, "Smoking 'Cuts IVF Success Rate.'"

35. Judith Hanson Lasater, "When You Want to Have a Baby . . . but Can't," *Yoga Journal*, November 2001.

36. Ibid.

37. Ibid.

38. Ibid.

39. Ibid.

CHAPTER 13   BREAST HEALTH

1. Coral A. Lamartiniere, "Protection Against Breast Cancer with Genistein: A Component of Soy," *American Journal of Clinical Nutrition* 71, no. 6 (June 2000): 1705S–7s.

2. Sherrill Sellman, "Breast Cancer: Detection or Deception?" *Nexus*, May–June 2001, 39.

3. Joanna Colwell, "Re-Examining Breast Health," *Yoga Journal*, September–October 2001.

4. Devra Lee Davis and H. Leon Bradlow, "Can Environmental Estrogens Cause Breast Cancer?" *Scientific American*, October 1995, 166.

5. Colwell, "Re-Examining Breast Health."

6. Lamartiniere, "Protection Against Breast Cancer."

7. Ibid.

8. Davis and Bradlow, "Can Environmental Estrogens."

9. Sharon Begley, "The Estrogen Complex," *Newsweek*, March 21, 1994, 77.

10. Davis and Bradlow, "Can Environmental Estrogens."

11. Ibid.

12. J. W. Fahey, P. J. Ourisson, and F. H. Degnan, "Pathogen Detection, Testing, and Control in Fresh Broccoli Sprouts," *Nutrition Journal* 5, no. 1 (April 21, 2006): 13 [e-pub ahead of print]; L. Tang, Y. Zhang, H. E. Jobson, et al., "Potent Activation of Mitochondria-Mediated Apoptosis and Arrest in S and M Phases of Cancer Cells by a Broccoli Sprout Extract," *Molecular Cancer Therapeutics* 5, no. 4 (2006): 935–44; M. W. Farnham, K. K. Stephenson, and J. W. Fahey, "Glucoraphanin Level in Broccoli Seed Is Largely Determined by Genotype," *HortScience* 40, no. 1 (2005): 50–53; J. W. Fahey, K. K. Stephenson, A. T. Dinkova-Kostova, et al., "Chlorophyll, Chlorophyllin and Related Tetrapyrroles Are Significant Inducers of Mammalian Phase 2 Cytoprotective Genes," *Carcinogenesis* 26 (2005): 1247–55; X. Haristoy, J. W. Fahey, I. Scholtus, and A. Lozniewski, "Evaluation of Antimicrobial Effect of Several Isothiocyanates on *Helicobacter pylori*," *Planta Medica* 71 (2005): 326–30.

13. Maggie Fox, "Trans Fats Linked to Breast Cancer Risk in Study," ed. Xavier Briand, Reuters, April 14, 2008.

14. Jane E. Brody, "Women's Heart Risk Linked to Types of Fats, Not Total," Women's Health, *New York Times*, November 20, 1997.

15. Fahey, Ourisson, and Degnan, "Pathogen Detection"; Tang, Zhang, et al., "Potent Activation"; Farnham, Stephenson, and Fahey, "Glucoraphanin Level in Broccoli Seed"; Fahey, Stephenson, Dinkova-Kostova, et al., "Chlorophyll, Chlorophyllin and Related Tetrapyrroles"; Haristoy, Fahey, Scholtus, and Lozniewski, "Evaluation of Antimicrobial Effect."

16. Deena Beasley, "Big U.S. Study Links Breast Cancer to Drinking," ed. Cynthia Osterman, Reuters, April 14, 2008.

17. Ibid.

18. Colwell, "Re-Examining Breast Health."

19. R. Baan, K. Straif, Y. Grosse, et al., "Carcinogenicity of Alcoholic Beverages," *Lancet Oncology* 8, no. 4 (April 2007): 292–93.

20. N. Hamajima, K. Hirose, K. Tajima, et al., "Alcohol, Tobacco and Breast Cancer-Collaborative Reanalysis of Individual Data from 53 Epidemiological Studies, Including 58,515 Women with Breast Cancer and 95,067 Women Without the Disease," *British Journal of Cancer* 87 (2002): 1234–45.

21. Davis and Bradlow, "Can Environmental Estrogens."

22. Michele Morin Doody, John E. Lonstein, Marilyn Stovall, et al., "Breast Cancer Mortality After Diagnostic Radiography: Findings from the U.S. Scoliosis Cohort Study," *Spine* 25, no. 16 (August 15, 2000): 2052–63.

23. www.cancer.org.

24. Mike Stobbe, Associated Press, February 24, 2006.

25. Roni Caryn Rabin, "Benefits of Mammogram Under Debate in Britain, *New York Times*, March 30, 2009.

26. Gina Kolata, "Cancer Risk of Hormones May Linger," *New York Times*, October 24, 2002.

27. Gina Kolata, "Panel Urges Mammograms at 50, Not 40," *New York Times*, November 16, 2009.

28. Gina Kolata, "Mammogram Debate Took Group by Surprise," *New York Times*, November 20, 2009.

29. Samuel S. Epstein, MD, Web site.

30. David B. Thomas, Dao Li Gao, Roberta M. Ray, et al., "Randomized Trial of Breast Self-Examination in Shanghai: Final Results," *Journal of the National Cancer Institute* 94, no. 19 (October 2, 2002): 1445–57.

31. Russell Harris and Linda S. Kinsinger, "Routinely Teaching Breast Self-Examination Is Dead. What Does This Mean?" *Journal of the National Cancer Institute* 94, no. 19 (October 2, 2002): 1420–21.

32. Jane Bennett and Alexandra Pope, *The Pill: Are You Sure It's for You?* (Crows Nest, NSW: Allen and Unwin. 2008), 52–53.

33. Collaborative Group on Hormonal Factors in Breast Cancer, "Breast Cancer and Hormonal Contraceptives: Collaborative Reanalysis of Individual Data on 53,297 Women with Breast Cancer and 100,239 Women Without Breast Cancer from 54 Epidemiological Studies." *The Lancet* 347 (June 1996): 1713–27.

34. Bennett and Pope, *The Pill*.

35. Colwell, "Re-Examining Breast Health."

36. Davis and Bradlow, "Can Environmental Estrogens."

37. *The Lancet* 360 (July 20, 2002): 187–95.

38. Chi-Ling Chen, PhD; Noel S. Weiss, MD; DrPH; Polly Newcomb, PhD; et al., "Hormone Replacement Therapy in Relation to Breast Cancer," *Journal of the American Medical Association* 287 (February 13, 2002): 734–41.

39. Sharon Begley, "The Risks of Estrogen," *Newsweek*, May 29, 2000, 51.

40. Marcia L. Stefanick, PhD; Garnet L. Anderson, PhD; Karen L. Margolis, MD, MPH; et al., "Effects of Conjugated Equine Estrogens on Breast Cancer and Mammography Screening in Postmenopausal Women with Hysterectomy," *Journal of the American Medical Association* 295, no. 14 (April 12, 2006): 1647–57.

41. Gina Kolata, "Studies Challenge Traditional Breast Cancer Treatments," *New York Times*, April 12, 2006.

42. Carolyn J. Crandall, MD, MS; Aaron K. Aragaki, MS; Rowan T. Chlebowski, MD, PhD; et al., "New-Onset Breast Tenderness After Initiation of Estrogen Plus Progestin Therapy and Breast Cancer Risk," *Archives of Internal Medicine* 169, no. 18 (2009): 1684–91.

43. Begley, "The Risks of Estrogen."

44. Denise Grady, "Hormone Therapy Worsens Breast Cancer, Study Finds," *New York Times*, October 20, 2010.

45. Ibid.

46. Tieraona Low Dog, MD; David Riley, MD; and Tony Carter, "Traditional and Alternative Therapies for Breast Cancer," *Alternative Therapies* 7, no. 3 (May–June 2001): 37.

47. Ibid.

48. Brody, "Women's Heart Risk."

49. Fox, "Trans Fats."

50. Elizabeth Neuse, "Soy Story II," *Yoga Journal*, May–June 2002, 40.

51. Jane Sprague Zones, "New Research Links Breast Milk to Cancer Cell Death," *Breast Cancer Action Newsletter* 58 (March–April 2000).

52. *The Lancet* 360 (July 20, 2002): 187–95.

53. Ibid.

54. BBC News, "Breast-feeding 'Cuts Heart Risk,'" May 14, 2004.

55. John B Fagan, PhD, and Robert E Herron, PhD, "Lipophil-Mediated Reduction of Toxicants in Humans: An Evaluation of an Ayurvedic Detoxification Procedure," *Alternative Therapies* 8, no. 5 (September 2002): 40–51.

56. C. M. Friedenreich, G. R. Howe, A. B. Miller, et al., "A Cohort Study of Alcohol Consumption and the Risk of Breast Cancer," *American Journal of Epidemiology* 147 (1993): 512–20.

57. Colwell, "Re-Examining Breast Health."

CHAPTER 14   PERIMENOPAUSE AND MENOPAUSE

1. Jane Bennett and Alexandra Pope, *The Pill: Are You Sure It's for You?* (Crows Nest NSW: Allen and Unwin, 2008), 178.

2. *The John R. Lee, M.D. Medical Letter*, March 2003, 5.

3. Tieraona Low Dog, MD; David Riley, MD; and Tony Carter, "An Integrative Approach to Menopause" *Alternative Therapies* 7, no. 4 (July–August 2001).

4. Ibid.

5. Gina Kolata with Melody Petersen, "Hormone Replacement Study a Shock to the Medical System," *New York Times*, July 10, 2002.

6. Ibid.

7. Natasha Singer, "Medical Papers by Ghostwriters Pushed Therapy," *New York Times*, August 4, 2009.

8. Ibid.

9. Sumit R. Majumdar, MD, MPH; Elizabeth A. Almasi; and Randall S. Stafford, MD, PhD, "Promotion and Prescribing of Hormone Therapy After Report of Harm by the Women's Health Initiative," *Journal of the American Medical Association* 292, no. 16 (October 27, 2004): endnote 1983–88.

10. Kolata, "Hormone Replacement Study."

11. Ibid.

12. Writing Group for the Women's Health Initiative Investigators, "Risks and Benefits of Estrogen Plus Progestin in Healthy Postmenopausal Women: Principal Results from the

Women's Health Initiative Randomized Controlled Trial," *Journal of the American Medical Association* 288, no. 3 (July 17, 2002): 321–33.

13. Ibid.

14. Majumdar, Almasi, and Stafford, "Promotion and Prescribing," endnote.

15. *The John R. Lee, M.D. Medical Letter*, July 2002, 2.

16. Gina Kolata, "Menopause Without Pills: Rethinking Hot Flashes," *New York Times*, November 10, 2002.

17. E. Hing and K. Brett. "Changes in U.S. Prescribing Patterns of Menopausal Hormone Replacement Therapy, 2001–2003," *Obstetrics and Gynecology* 108 (2006): 33–40.

18. Kolata, "Menopause Without Pills."

19. Associated Press, "Hormone-Taking Is Linked to Dementia," May 2003; *Journal of the American Medical Association*, http://jama.ama-assn.org; Women's Health Initiative, http://www.whi.org.

20. Ibid.

21. *Journal of the American Medical Association*, http://jama.ama-assn.org.

22. Gina Kolata, "Cancer Risk of Hormones May Linger," *New York Times*, October 24, 2002.

23. Ibid.

24. Gina Kolata, "Citing Risks, U.S. Will Halt Study of Drugs for Hormones," *New York Times*, July 9, 2002.

25. Ibid.

26. Gina Kolata, "Reversing Trend, Big Drop Is Seen in Breast Cancer," *New York Times*, December 15, 2006.

27. Anthony S. Robbins and Christina A. Clarke, "Regional Changes in Hormone Therapy Use and Breast Cancer Incidence in California from 2001 to 2004," *Journal of Clinical Oncology* 25, no. 23 (August 10, 2007): 3437–39.

28. Rowan T. Chlebowski, MD, PhD; Lewis H. Kuller, MD, DrPH; Ross L. Prentice, PhD; et al. "Breast Cancer after Use of Estrogen plus Progestin in Postmenopausal Women," *New England Journal of Medicine* 360, no. 6 (February 5, 2009): 573–87.

29. BBC News, February 5, 2009, http://news.bbc.co.uk/2/hi/health/7869679.stm.

30. Denise Grady, "Hormone Therapy Worsens Breast Cancer, Study Finds," *New York Times*, October 20, 2010.

31. Gina Kolata, "Menopause Without Pills."

32. Stephen Hulley, MD, MPH and Deborah Grady, MD, MPH, "Postmenopausal Hormone Treatment," *Journal of the American Medical Association* 301, no. 23 (2009): 2493–95.

33. *The John R. Lee, M.D. Medical Letter*, April 2001.

34. H. B. Leonetti, J. N. Anasti, and S. Longo, "Transdermal Progesterone Cream for Vasomotor Symptoms and Postmenopausal Bone Loss," *Obstetrics and Gynecology* 94 (1999): 225–28.

35. Dog, Riley, and Carter, "An Integrative Approach to Menopause."

CHAPTER 15   HEART HEALTH

1. Dr. Dean Ornish presentation at the TED conference, Monterey, California, February 2006.

2. John MacLeod, George Davey Smith, Chris Metcalfe, and Carole Hart, "Interheart," *The Lancet* 365 (January 8, 2005): 118–19.

3. Stephen Hulley, MD, MPH; and Deborah Grady, MD, MPH, "Postmenopausal Hormone Treatment," *Journal of the American Medical Association* 301, no. 23 (2009): 2493–95.

4. Alex Berenson, "End of Drug Trial Is a Big Loss for Pfizer," *New York Times*, December 4, 2006.

5. Jennifer Kahn, "Mending Broken Hearts," *National Geographic*, February 2007, 55.

6. Nieca Goldberg, MD, *Women Are Not Small Men: Life-Saving Strategies for Preventing and Healing Heart Disease in Women* (New York: Ballantine Books, 2002).

7. Denise Grady, "In Heart Disease, the Focus Shifts to Women," *New York Times*, April 18, 2006.

8. Ibid.

9. Ibid.

10. Dr. John Lee has a very informative booklet, *JRL Commonsense Guide to a Healthy Heart*. Available from www.virginiahopkinstestkits.com/product12.html.

11. Hulley and Grady, "Postmenopausal Hormone Treatment."

12. Androniki Naska, PhD; Eleni Oikonomou, BS; Antonia Trichopoulou, MD; et al., "Siesta in Healthy Adults and Coronary Mortality in the General Population," *Archives of Internal Medicine* 167, no. 3 (2007): 296–301.

13. Christine Gorman and Alice Park, "Inflammation Is a Secret Killer: The Surprising Link Between Inflammation and Asthma, Heart Attacks, Cancer, Alzheimer's and Other Diseases," *Time*, February 23, 2004.

14. Daniel Q. Haney, "Inflammation Triggers Heart Attacks," Associated Press, reported in *Wisconsin State Journal*, November 14, 2002.

15. Christiane Northrup, MD, *The Wisdom of Menopause: Creating Physical and Emotional Health and Healing During the Change* (New York: Bantam Books, 2001), 63 and 205.

16. Haney, "Inflammation Triggers Heart Attacks."

17. Jane E. Brody, "Hunt for Heart Disease Tracks a New Suspect," *New York Times*, January 6, 2004.

18. Haney, "Inflammation Triggers Heart Attacks."

19. Ibid.

20. Brody, "Hunt for Heart Disease."

21. www.webmd.com/allerties/news/20070607/pot-chemical-may-curb-inflammation.

22. Roger Highfield, "Smoking Cannabis 'Raises Heart Attack Risk,'" Telegraph.co.uk, June 12, 2001.

23. John R. Lee, MD, with Virginia Hopkins, *What Your Doctor May Not Tell You About Menopause: The Breakthrough Book on Natural Progesterone* (New York: Warner Books, 1996), 189–90.

24. Brad Lemley, "What Does Science Say You Should Eat?" *Discover*, February 2004, 43–47.

25. Lee, "What Your Doctor May Not Tell You."

26. Lemly, "What Does Science Say," 47.

27. Gretchen Reynolds, "Can Touching Your Toes Test Your Arteries?" *New York Times*, December 23, 2009.

28. R. N. Alsever, MD; W. M. Thomas, PhD; C Nevin-Woods, DO; et al., "Reduced Hospitalizations for Acute Myocardial Infarction After Implementation of a Smoke-Free Ordinance—City of Pueblo, Colorado, 2002–2006," *Morbidity and Mortality Weekly Report* 57, no. 51 (2009): 1373–77.

29. Y. Chida and A. Steptoe, "The Association of Anger and Hostility with Future Coronary Heart Disease: A Meta-Analytic Review of Prospective Evidence," *Journal of the American College of Cardiology* 53, no. 11 (March 17, 2009): 936–46.

30. Mimi Guarneri, MD, FACC, *The Heart Speaks: A Cardiologist Reveals the Secret Language of Healing* (New York: Simon & Schuster, 2006), 158.

31. Guarneri, *The Heart Speaks*, 169.

32. Geoffrey Cowley, "Health for Life," *Newsweek*, September 27, 2004.

33. Ilan Wittstein, "Neurohumoral Features of Myocardial Stunning Due to Sudden Emotional Stress," *New England Journal of Medicine* 352 (February 10, 2005): 539–48.

34. Guarneri, *The Heart Speaks*, 162.

35. *The John R. Lee, M.D. Medical Letter*, July 2002, 2.

36. Gina Kolata "Menopause Without Pills: Rethinking Hot Flashes," *New York Times*, November 10, 2002.

37. Ernst Rietzschel and Jennifer Mieres, "Oral Contraceptive Use: More Carotid and Femoral Atheroschlerosis Later in Life," November 6, 2007, news briefing at American Heart Association Scientific Sessions, Orlando, Florida, as reported in *New England Journal of Medicine* (2007): 357.

38. Brody, "Hunt for Heart Disease."

39. Nicholas Bakalar, "For Heart Health, Liquor Is Quicker for Women and Slower for Men," *New York Times*, June 6, 2006.

40. R. Baan, K. Straif, Y. Grosse, et al., "Carcinogenicity of Alcoholic Beverages," *Lancet Oncology* 8, no. 4 (April 2007): 292–93.

41. Joanna Colwell, "Re-Examining Breast Health," *Yoga Journal*, September–October 2001.

42. www.alcoholics-info.com/Statistics_on_Alcoholics.html.

CHAPTER 16   OSTEOPOROSIS

1. Tara Parker-Pope, "How Well Will Your Bones Hold Up?" *New York Times*, May 13, 2008.

2. Miriam E. Nelson, PhD, with Sarah Wernick, PhD, *Strong Women Stay Young* (New York: Bantam Books, 2005).

3. Abdurrahman Altindag, MD; Ozlem Altindag, MD; Mehmet Asoglu, MD; et al., "Major Depression (Stress) a Risk Factor for Osteopenia in Premenopausal Women: Relation of Cortisol Levels and Bone Mineral Density Among Premenopausal Women with Major Depression CME," *International Journal of Clinical Practice* 61, no. 3 (2007): 416–20.

4. *The John R. Lee, M.D. Medical Letter*, March 2003, 6.

5. John R. Lee, MD, with Virginia Hopkins, *What Your Doctor May Not Tell You About Menopause: The Breakthrough Book on Natural Progesterone* (New York: Warner Books. 1996), 155.

6. Tieraona Low Dog, MD; David Riley, MD; and Tony Carter, "An Integrative Approach to Menopause," *Alternative Therapies* 7, no. 4 (July–August 2001).

7. Brad Lemly, "What Does Science Say You Should Eat?" *Discover*, February 2004, 49.

8. John Robbins, *Diet for a New America* (Walpole, NH: Stillpoint Publishing, 1987), 191.

9. Nelson, *Strong Women Stay Young*, 4–10, 50.

10. Ibid., 46.

11. Peter Radetsky, "Got Cancer Killers?" *Discover Magazine*, June 1999, 74.

12. BBC News, "Adults' Antidepressant Bone Risk," January 23, 2007, http://news.bbc.co.uk/go/pr/fr/-/2/hi/health/6286681.st.

13. This article comes from Science Blog, copyright © 2004, www.scienceblog.com/communityhttp://www.scienceblog.com/community; James Blumenthal, "Exercise May Be Just as Effective as Medication for Treating Major Depression," *Archives of Internal Medicine* (October 25, 1999).

14. www.fda.gov/cder/drug/infopage/bisphosphonates/default.htm.

15. Tara Parker-Pope, "Drugs to Build Bones May Weaken Them," *New York Times*, July 15, 2008.

16. Gina Kolata, "Drug for Bones Is Newly Linked to Jaw Disease," *New York Times*, June 2, 2006.

17. Parish P. Sedghizadeh, Kyle Stanley, Matthew Caligiuri, et al., "Oral Bisphosphonate Use and the Prevalence of Osteonecrosis of the Jaw: An Institutional Inquiry," *Journal of the American Dental Association* 140 (2009): 61–66.

18. Natasha Singer, "High Stakes for Merck in Litigation on Fosamax, *New York Times*, September 2, 2009.

19. Nelson, *Strong Women Stay Young*, 50.

20. Lee, *What Your Doctor May Not Tell You About Menopause*, 315–17.

CHAPTER 17   ALZHEIMER'S DISEASE AND DEMENTIA

1. http://naturalmedicinejournal.com/ac_apr10_jennings.shtml.

2. Associated Press, "Hormone-Taking Is Linked to Dementia," May 2003; *Journal of the American Medical Association*, http://jama.ama-assn.org; Women's Health Initiative, http://www.whi.org.

3. S. M. Resnick, PhD; M. A. Espeland, PhD; S. A. Jaramillo, MS; et al., "Postmenopausal Hormone Therapy and Regional Brain Volumes," *Neurology* 72 (2009): 135–42.

4. Janice M. Horowitz, "Brain Strain," *Time*, June 28, 1999.

5. Christine Gorman and Alice Park, "Inflammation Is a Secret Killer: The Surprising Link Between Inflammation and Asthma, Heart Attacks, Cancer, Alzheimer's and Other Diseases," *Time*, February 23, 2004.

6. Norman Doidge, MD, *The Brain That Changes Itself: Stories of Personal Triumph from the Frontiers of Brain Science* (New York: Penguin Books, 2007), 255.

7. www.unsw.edu.au/news/pad/articles/2006/jan/Dementia_brain_reserve.html.

8. Qi Dai, Amy R. Borenstein, Yougui Wu, et al., "Fruit & Vegetable Juices and Alzheimer's Disease: The Kame Project," *American Journal of Medicine* 119 (September 2006): 751–59.

CHAPTER 18   THE IMPORTANCE OF DIET AND
LIFESTYLE: AN OVERVIEW

1. Deepak Chopra, Dean Ornish, Rustum Roy, and Andrew Weil, "'Alternative' Medicine Is Mainstream: The Evidence Is Mounting That Diet and Lifestyle Are the Best Cures for Our Worst Afflictions," Opinion, *Wall Street Journal*, January 9, 2009.

2. Dean Ornish, "Clean Living 'Slows Cell Aging,'" *Lancet Oncology*, reported in BBC News, September 15, 2008.

3. Pam Belluck, "Moose Offer Trail of Clues on Arthritis," *New York Times*, August 16, 2010.

4. Chopra et al., "'Alternative' Medicine Is Mainstream."

5. Belluck, "Moose Offer Trail of Clues on Arthritis."

CHAPTER 19   QUALITY AND QUANTITY OF FOOD

1. Jerry Adler and Jeneen Interlandi, "Caution: Killing Germs May Be Hazardous to Your Health," *Newsweek*, October 20, 2007.

CHAPTER 20   FOOD, MEDICINE, AND POISON

1. Anna Nowak-Wegrzyn, MD; Katherine A. Bloom, MD; Scott. H. Sicherer, MD; et al., "Tolerance to Extensively Heated Milk in Children with Cow's Milk Allergy," *Journal of Allergy and Clinical Immunology* 122, no. 2 (August 2008): 342–47, e2.

2. Anahad O'Connor, "The Claim: Hot Liquids Can Ease Symptoms of a Cold or Flu," *New York Times*, January 26, 2009.

3. From an advertisement from the National Eating Disorders Association.

CHAPTER 21   WHAT TO EAT: GENERAL GUIDELINES

1. Michael Pollan, *In Defense of Food* (New York: Penguin, 2008), 1.

2. Dr. Dean Ornish, presentation at the TED conference, Monterey, CA, February 2006.

3. Martha Rose Shulman, "Rice: The World's Underappreciated Staple," *New York Times*, July 27, 2009.

4. Jorge E. Chavarro, MD, Walter C. Willett, MD, and Patrick J. Skerrett, "Fat, Carbs and the Science of Conception," *Newsweek*, December 10, 2007.

5. Anna Nowak-Wegrzyn, MD; Katherine A. Bloom, MD; Scott. H. Sicherer, MD; et al., "Tolerance to Extensively Heated Milk in Children with Cow's Milk Allergy," *Journal of Allergy and Clinical Immunology* 122, no. 2 (August 2008): 342–47, e2.

6. Turmeric's benefits: A. L. Cheng, C. H. Hsu , J. K. , et al., "Phase I Clinical Trial of Curcumin, a Chemopreventive Agent, in Patients with High-Risk or Pre-Malignant Lesions," *Anticancer Research* 21, no. 4B (2001): 2895–2900; Black pepper multiplies the body's absorption of turmeric two thousandfold: G. Shoba, D. Joy, T. Joseph, et al., "Influence of Piperine on the Pharmacokinetis of Curcumin in Animals and Human Volunteers," *Planta Medica* 64, no.4 (1998): 353–56.

7. J. W. Fahey, P. J. Ourisson, and F. H. Degnan, "Pathogen Detection, Testing, and Control in Fresh Broccoli Sprouts," *Nutrition Journal* 5, no. 1 (April 21, 2006): 13 [e-pub ahead of print]; L. Tang, Y. Zhang, H. E. Jobson, et al., "Potent Activation of Mitochondria-Mediated Apoptosis and Arrest in S and M Phases of Cancer Cells by a Broccoli Sprout Extract," *Molecular Cancer Therapeutics* 5, no. 4 (2006): 935–44; M. W. Farnham, K. K. Stephenson, and J. W. Fahey, "Glucoraphanin Level in Broccoli Seed Is Largely Determined by Genotype," *HortScience* 40(, no. 1 (2005): 50–53; J. W. Fahey, K. K. Stephenson, A. T. Dinkova-Kostova, et al., "Chlorophyll, Chlorophyllin and Related Tetrapyrroles Are Significant Inducers of Mammalian Phase 2 Cytoprotective Genes," *Carcinogenesis* 26 (2005): 1247–55; X. Haristoy, J. W. Fahey, I. Scholtus, and A. Lozniewski, "Evaluation of Antimicrobial Effect of Several Isothiocyanates on *Helicobacter pylori*," *Planta Medica* 71 (2005): 326–30.

8. Tieraona Low Dog, MD; David Riley, MD; and Tony Carter, "Traditional and Alternative Therapies for Breast Cancer," *Alternative Therapies* 7, no. 3 (May–June 2001): 37.

9. Fahey, Ourisson, and Degnan, "Pathogen Detection"; Tang, Zhang, Jobson, et al., "Potent Activation"; Farnham, Stephenson, and Fahey, "Glucoraphanin Level in Broccoli Seed"; Fahey, Stephenson, Dinkova-Kostova, et al., "Chlorophyll, Chlorophyllin and Related Tetrapyrroles"; Haristoy, Fahey, Scholtus, and Lozniewski, "Evaluation of Antimicrobial Effect."

10. Ibid.

11. Ibid.

12. Ibid.

13. Ibid.

14. *American Journal of Medicine* 119 (September 2006): 751–59.

15. BBC News, "Cloudy Apple Juice 'Healthier,'" http://news.bbc.co.uk/go/pr/fr/-/2/hi/health/6262473.stm, published January 15, 2007.

16. Maggie Fox, "Trans Fats Linked to Breast Cancer Risk in Study," ed. Xavier Brand, Reuters, April 14, 2008.

17. Jane E. Brody, "Women's Heart Risk Linked to Types of Fats, Not Total," Women's Health, *New York Times*, November 20, 1997.

18. A. Trichopoulou, P. Lagiou, and J. Am, "Worldwide Patterns of Dietary Lipids Intake and Health Implications," *Clinical Nutrition* 66 (1997): 961S–64S.

19. M. G. Enig, *Know Your Fats: The Complete Primer for Understanding the Nutrition of Fats, Oils and Cholesterol* (Silver Spring, MD: Bethesda Press, 2000), 106.

20. Shane Speer, Carolynn Carreno, "The New Superfoods," *Vegetarian Times*, February 2007.

21. M. V. Kumar, K. Sambaiah, and B. R. Lokesh, "Hypocholesterolemic Effect of Anhydrous Milk Fat Ghee Is Mediated by Increasing the Secretion of Biliary Lipids," *Journal of Nutritional Biochemistry* 11, no. 2 (February 2000): 69–75.

22. Dirk Taubert, MD, PhD, and colleagues at the University of Cologne, Germany, "Dark Chocolate Has Health Benefits Not Seen in Other Varieties," *Journal of the American Medical Association* 290 (August 27, 2003): 1029–30.

CHAPTER 22   MEAT: TO EAT OR NOT TO EAT

1. www.virginiahopkinstestkits.com/prevent_osteoporosis.html.

2. Frances Moore Lappé, *Diet for a Small Planet* (New York: Ballantine Books, 1971), 6–9.

3. George R. Lucas Jr., "Political and Economic Dimensions of Hunger," *Lifeboat Ethics: The Moral Dilemma of World Hunger* (New York: Harper Forum Books, 1976), 9–10.

4. http://desertificationb.tripod.com/id3.html.

5. Michael Pollan, *In Defense of Food* (New York: Penguin Press, 2008).

6. Nina Martin, "Fertility?" *Organic Style*, May–June 2003.

7. John Robbins, *Diet for a New America* (Walpole, NH: Stillpoint Publishing, 1987).

8. John R. Lee, MD, with Virginia Hopkins, *What Your Doctor May Not Tell You About Menopause: The Breakthrough Book on Natural Progesterone* (New York: Warner Books, 1996), 151.

CHAPTER 23   WHAT NOT TO EAT

1. Peter Starck, "Cancer Risk Found in French Fries, Bread," Reuters, April 24, 2002.

2. Henry Fountain, "Garlic for a Healthy Heart? Go Fresh, Study Says," *New York Times*, August 3, 2009.

3. www.bk.com/cms/en/us/cms_out/digital_assets/files/pages/IngredientsAndAllergens.pdf.

4. http://en.wikipedia.org/wiki/Tert-Butylhydroquinone#cite_note-1.

5. http://nutrition.mcdonalds.com/nutritionexchange/ingredientslist.pdf.

6. J. L. Barger, T. Kayo, J. M. Vann, et al., "A Low Dose of Dietary Resveratrol Partially Mimics Caloric Restriction and Retards Aging Parameters in Mice," PLoS ONE 3, no. 6 (2008).

7. Nicholas Wade, "New Hints Seen That Red Wine May Slow Aging," *New York Times*, June 4, 2008.

8. Shane Speer and Carolynn Carreno, "The New Superfoods," *Vegetarian Times*, February 2007.

9. N. Allen, et al., "Moderate Alcohol Intake and Cancer Incidence in Women," *Journal of the National Cancer Institute* 101 (2009): 296–305; Michael Lauer and Paul Sorlie, "Alcohol, Cardiovascular Disease, and Cancer: Treat with Caution," *Journal of the National Cancer Institute* 101 (2009): 282–83.

10. Jane E. Brody, "As Bones Age, Who's at Risk for Fracture?" *New York Times*, December 28, 2009.

11. M. Ezzati, A. Rodgers, A. D. Lopez, et al., "Mortality and Burden of Disease Attributable to Individual Risk Factors," in *Comparative Quantification of Health Risks: Global and Regional Burden of Disease Attributable to Selected Major Risk Factors*, vol. 2, ed. M. Ezzati, A. D. Lopez, A. Rodgers, and C. J. L. Murray (Geneva: World Health Organization, 2004), 2141–66.

12. www.who.int/substance_abuse/facts/alcohol/en/.

13. "Million Women Study Shows Even Moderate Alcohol Consumption Associated with Increased Cancer Risk," *ScienceDaily*, February 26, 2009.

14. K. L. Tucker, K. Morita, N. Qiao, et al., "Colas, but Not Other Carbonated Beverages, Are Associated with Low Bone Mineral Density in Older Women: The Framingham Osteoporosis Study," *American Journal of Clinical Nutrition* 84, no. 4 (2006): 936–42.

15. Michael Pollan, *In Defense of Food* (New York: Penguin, 2008), 118.

CHAPTER 24   THE PROS AND CONS OF SOY

1. Kenneth D. R. Setchell, PhD, "Soy Isoflavones—Benefits and Risks from Nature's Selective Estrogen Receptor Modulators (SERMs)," *Journal of the American College of Nutrition* 20, no. 90005 (2001), 354S–62S. A fantastic article that reviews many of the conflicting soy studies and arrives at a benign conclusion.

2. Ibid.

3. Todd Zwillich, "Studies Can't Prove Soy Formula Risks," FoxNews.com, March 17, 2006.

4. Ibid.

5. Elizabeth Neuse, "Soy Story II," *Yoga Journal*, May–June 2002.

6. "Rao L. Divia, Hebron C. Chang, and Daniel R. Doergea, "Anti-Thyroid Isoflavones from Soybean," National Center for Toxicological Research, Jefferson, AR 72079, available online, December 18, 1997.

7. Tieraona Low Dog, MD; David Riley, MD; and Tony Carter, "An Integrative Approach to Menopause," *Alternative Therapies* 7, no. 4 (July–August 2001).

8. Brad Lemley, "What Does Science Say You Should Eat?" *Discover*, February 2004, 43–44.

9. Sharon Begley, "The Estrogen Complex," *Newsweek*, March 21, 1994, 77.

10. "Three out of four epidemiological studies in Asian populations, who consume more soy than any other group, showed an association between decreased risk of breast cancer and soy intake": Neuse, "Soy Story II," 40.

11. Susan M. Potter, Jo Ann Baum, Hongyu Teng, et al., "Soy Protein and Isoflavones: Their Effects on Blood Lipids and Bone Density in Postmenopausal Women," *American Journal for Clinical Nutrition* 68 (1998): 1375S–79S.

12. P. Albertazzi, F. Pansini, G. Bonaccorsi, et al., "The Effect of Dietary Soy Supplementation on Serum Lipoproteins, Blood Pressure and Menopausal Symptoms in Perimenopausal Women," *Menopause* 6 (1999): 7–13.

13. Lemley, "What Does Science Say."

14. Zwillich, "Studies Can't Prove."

15. Setchell, "Soy Isoflavones."

16. See Setchell's article. Also a study that shows that healthy digestion is essential for absorption of soy: Kenneth D. R. Setchell, Nadine M. Brown, Linda Zimmer-Nechemias, et al., "Evidence for Lack of Absorption of Soy Isoflavone Glycosides in Humans, Supporting the Crucial Role of Intestinal Metabolism for Bioavailability," *American Journal of Clinical Nutrition* 76, no. 2 (August 2002): 447–53.

17. Setchell, "Soy Isoflavones."

18. Ibid.

CHAPTER 25   ESSENTIAL ELEMENTS OF A HEALTHY LIFESTYLE

1. Frank B. Hu, MD, PhD; Tricia Y. Li, MD; Graham A. Colditz, MD, DrPH; et al., "Television Watching and Other Sedentary Behaviors in Relation to Risk of Obesity and Type 2 Diabetes Mellitus in Women," *Journal of the American Medical Association* 289 (2003): 1785–91.

2. Dr. Dean Ornish presentation at the TED conference, Monterey, CA, February 2006.

3. Ibid.

4. C. M. Friedenreich, G. R. Howe, A. B. Miller AB, et al., "A Cohort Study of Alcohol Consumption and the Risk of Breast Cancer," *American Journal of Epidemiology* 147 (1993): 512–20.

5. Ornish presentation.

6. Ibid.

7. 2003–2005 National Ambulatory Medical Care Survey and National Hospital Ambulatory Medical Care Survey data files, available at www.cdc.gov/nchs.

8. Trisha Gura with Linda Sparrowe, "The Graceful Change" *Yoga Journal*, December 2003.

9. Ibid.

10. Joanna Colwell, "Re-Examining Breast Health," *Yoga Journal*, September–October 2001, 100.

11. Gura, "The Graceful Change."

12. Michael R. Irwin, MD; Richard Olmstead, PhD; and Michael N. Oxman, MD, "Augmenting Immune Responses to Varicella Zoster Virus in Older Adults: A Randomized, Controlled Trial of Tai Chi," *Journal of the American Geriatrics Society* 55, no. 4 (2007): 511–17.

13. Norman Doidge, MD, *The Brain That Changes Itself: Stories of Personal Triumph from the Frontiers of Brain Science* (New York: Penguin, 2007), 25.

14. Associated Press, "Walking as Healthy as Running, Study Says," *Providence Journal*, August 26, 1999.

15. Science Blog, 2004, www.scienceblog.com/community; 1999 Duke University Medical Center study: "Exercise May Be Just as Effective as Medication for Treating Major Depression." Duke psychologist James Blumenthal published the results of his team's study in the October 25 issue of *Archives of Internal Medicine*.

16. Associated Press, "Walking as Healthy as Running."

17. www.unm.edu/~lkravitz/Article%20folder/stresscortisol.html.

18. *The John R. Lee, M.D. Medical Letter*, May 2001.

19. A. Rapkin et al., "Prevalence of Self-Reported Poor Sleep in a Healthy Population Age 50–65," *Social Science Medicine* 34, no. 49 (1992): 49.

20. Sharon Lerner, "Good and Bad Marriage: Boon and Bane to Health," *New York Times*, October 22, 2002.

21. Devra Lee Davis and H. Leon Bradlow, "Can Environmental Estrogens Cause Breast Cancer?" *Scientific American*, October 1995, 166.

22. Rick Smith and Bruce Lourie, *Slow Death by Rubber Duck: How The Toxic Chemistry of Everyday Life Affects Our Health* (New York: Alfred A. Knopf, 2009), 27.

23. Polychlorinated biphenyls (PCBs); 2,4 dichlorophenoxyacetic acid (also called 2, 4-D, this is a pesticide used on lawns and an active ingredient in Agent Orange); 2,3 dibromopropyo phosphate (Tris-BP); all the various phthalates, including DEP, DEHP, DINP, DIDP, DNOP, and MMP; certain herbicides; dieldren; DDT (now banned); chlorine; vinyl chloride; pesticides such as endosulfan and atrazine; ozone-destroying CFCs (chlorofluorocarbons); perflourinated compounds (PFCs); perfluoroisobutylene (PFIB); bisphenol-A (BPA); various chlorinated and brominated compounds such as polybrominated biphenyls (PBBs—used as fire retardants and close cousins of PCBs) and polybrominated diphenyl ethers (PBDEs—other common flame retardants); perfluorooctanoic acid (PFOA); perfluorooctane sulphonate (PFOS); dioxins, phthalates; dioxin; triclosan (5-chloro-2, or 2,4-dichlorophenoxy phenol—an ingredient in many "antibacterial" products); POPs (persistent organic pollutants); and many, many others. POPs (persistent organic pollutants) include many halogen (chlorine, bromine, fluorine, or iodine) atoms.

24. Smith and Lourie, *Slow Death by Rubber Duck*, 192.

25. Nina Martin, "Fertility?" *Organic Style*, May–June 2003.

26. Smith and Lourie, *Slow Death by Rubber Duck*, 100.

27. Sharon Begley "The Estrogen Complex," *Newsweek*, March 21. 1994, 76.

28. Oliver A. H. Jones, Mahon L. Maguire, and Julian L. Griffin, "Environmental Pollution and Diabetes: A Neglected Association," *The Lancet* 371 (2008): 287–88; Smith and Lourie, *Slow Death by Rubber Duck*.

29. Jane E. Brody, "Hunt for Heart Disease Tracks a New Suspect," *New York Times*, January 6, 2004.

30. Smith and Lourie, *Slow Death by Rubber Duck*, 22.

31. Ibid., 232.

32. Ibid., 228.

33. Antonia M. Calafat, Xiaoyun Ye, Lee-Yang, et al., "Exposure of the U.S. Population to Bisphenol A and 4-tertiary-octylphenol: 2003–2004," *Environmental Health Perspectives* 116, no. 1 (January 2008): 39–44.

34. Smith and Lourie, *Slow Death by Rubber Duck*, 220.

35. Ibid., 248.

36. BBC News, "Concerns over 'Female Chemicals,'" May 3, 2005.

37. Ibid.

38. S.-M. Ho, W.-Y. Tang, J. Belmonte de Frausto, and G. S. Prins, "Developmental Exposure to Estradiol and Bisphenol A Increases Susceptibility to Prostate Carcinogenesis and Epigenetically Regulates Phosphodiesterase Type 4 Variant 4," *Cancer Research* 66 (2006): 5624–32.

39. Leslie Wayne, "Fight Grows over Labels on Household Cleaners," *New York Times*, September 16, 2009.

40. "California Legislation Seeks to Limit Bisphenol-A and Phthalates in Children's Products," *Monitor* 605 (March 21, 2005), reprinted from Toy Industry Association, Inc., www.toy-tia.org.

41. Environmental News Network staff, "Burn Barrels Fuel Dioxin Levels," CNN News, January 10, 2000.

42. Martin, "Fertility?"

43. Be Safe, "New York City Council Passes Legislation to Reduce Purchase of Products Containing PVC, Lead, Mercury, Toxic Flame Retardants, and Other Toxic Chemicals," news release, December 21, 2005, Besafenet.com.

44. Charles Duhigg, "Debating How Much Weed Killer Is Safe in Your Water Glass," *New York Times*, August 22, 2009.

45. Charles Duhigg, "Clean Water Laws Are Neglected, at a Cost in Human Suffering, *New York Times*, September 12, 2009.

46. Smith and Lourie, *Slow Death By Rubber Duck*, 230.

47. General information in this chapter from Darshak M. Sanghavi, "Factors Linked to a Risk of Early Puberty," *New York Times*, October 18, 2006; Smith and Lourie, *Slow Death by Rubber Duck*.

48. Davis and Bradlow, "Can Environmental Estrogens."

49. Martin, "Fertility?"

50. Johns Hopkins Bloomberg School of Public Health, "Researcher Dispels Myth of Dioxins and Plastic Water Bottles." Interview with Rolf Halden, PhD, PE, assistant professor in the Department of Environmental Health Sciences and the Center for Water and Health at the Johns Hopkins Bloomberg School of Public Health, Johns Hopkins University, 2006.

51. Smith and Lourie, *Slow Death by Rubber Duck*, 247.

52. BBC News, "Chemicals May Damage Male Babies," May 27, 2005.

CHAPTER 26   STRESS MANAGEMENT TECHNIQUES

1. Charaka, *Charaka Samhita: Sutrasthanam* V, ed. and trans. Prof. Priyavrat Sharma (Varanasi, India: Chaukhambha Orientalia: A House of Oriental and Antiquarian Books, 1981), ch. 5, verses 88–89.

2. Kirpal Singh, *The Crown of Life: A Study in Yoga* (Delhi, India: Ruhani Satsang, 1961).

3. L. S. Berk, S. A. Tan, W. F. Fry, et al., "Neurendocrine and Stress Hormone Changes During Mirthful Laughter," *American Journal of the Medical Sciences* (1989).

4. Jennifer Kahn, "Mending Broken Hearts," *National Geographic*, February 2007, 55.

CHAPTER 27   CHANGING LIFESTYLES, CHANGING LIVES

1. Associated Press, "Walking as Healthy as Running, Study Says," *Providence Journal*, August 26, 1999.

2. Eduardo Dias-Ferreira, João C. Sousa, Irene Melo, et al., "Chronic Stress Causes Frontostriatal Reorganization and Affects Decision-Making," *Science* 325, no. 5940 (July 31, 2009): 621–25.

3. Published with permission.

4. http://en.wikipedia.org/wiki/Frank_Buckles.

5. *The John R. Lee, M.D. Medical Letter*, June 2000, 5.

6. Johns Hopkins Bloomberg School of Public Health, "Researcher Dispels Myth of Dioxins and Plastic Water Bottles." Interview with Rolf Halden, PhD, PE, assistant professor in the Department of Environmental Health Sciences and the Center for Water and Health at the Johns Hopkins Bloomberg School of Public Health, Johns Hopkins University, 2006.

7. www.healingdaily.com/detoxification-diet/sugar.htm.

8. Dr. Dean Ornish presentation at the TED conference, Monterey, CA, February 2006.

APPENDIX A   RESOURCES

1. BBC News, "Chemicals May Damage Male Babies," May 27, 2005.

INDEX